T0221143

Parents of Premature Infants:
Their Emotional World

Parents of Premature Infants: Their Emotional World

EDITED BY NORMA TRACEY

Social worker and psychotherapist, Sydney

W

WHURR PUBLISHERS

LONDON AND PHILADELPHIA

British Library Cataloguing in Publication Data
A catalogue record for this book is available from the
British Library.

ISBN: 1 86156 130 X

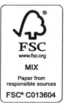

FSC
www.fsc.org

MIX

Paper from
responsible sources

FSC® C013604

Contents

DEDICATION

For Ron Brookes and David Buick

List of Contributors

Bryanne Barnett   Professor of Perinatal and Infant Psychiatry, University of New South Wales.

Peter Blake   Psychotherapist, Sydney.

Deidre Chiu   Social Worker, Sydney.

Jill Ditton   Social Worker, Sydney.

Charles Enfield   Child and Family Psychiatrist and Family Therapist, Sydney.

Sylvia Enfield   Child and Family Psychotherapist, Sydney.

Philip Garner   Psychologist and Psychotherapist, Sydney.

Megan Gosbee   Social Worker, Sydney.

Helen Hardy   Occupational Therapist, Sydney.

Lisianne La Touche   Social Worker, Sydney.

Isla Lonie   Psychiatrist and Psychotherapist, Sydney.

Anne Mayo   Social Worker, Sydney.

Campbell Paul   Associate Professor of Psychiatry, Melbourne.

Louise Poles   Social Worker, Sydney.

Marija Radovic   Clinical Psychologist, Sydney.

Lorraine Rose   Psychologist and Psychotherapist, Sydney.

Frances Salo   Psychoanalyst, Sydney.

Pamela Shein   Social Worker and Psychologist, Sydney.

Terese Sheridan   Family Therapist, Sydney.

Sheila Sim   Head Social Worker, Sydney.

Norma Tracey   Social Worker and Psychotherapist, Sydney.

Lynne Tripet   Social Worker, Sydney.

Beulah Warren   Psychologist and Parent-Infant Therapist, Sydney.

Foreword

The contributions to this book are predicated upon an extraordinary, indeed unique, piece of research. Twelve couples, six of whom experienced a comparatively uneventful pregnancy and birth, and six whose infant arrived more than nine weeks before the due date, were interviewed 18 times each over the first four months of their baby's life. Mothers and fathers were interviewed separately for 50 minutes on each occasion and were encouraged to talk freely about their thoughts and feelings. The interviewer (an analytic psychotherapist) facilitated this reflective process on the part of the parents, while making no comments or interpretations. She placed herself in the role of an attentive bystander, an emotionally available listener. Various publications have emanated from this research, and this present text, although including material from all 12 families, concentrates particularly upon issues relevant to the parents of the premature infants.

As a perinatal and infant psychiatrist, I was struck by some particular aspects as I reviewed the subject matter. First, a traumatic event as severe as the birth of an extremely premature infant clearly invokes major and primitive psychological defensive activity, at least initially, before the parents gradually 'get their act together', a process, incidentally, that does not occur in the same fashion or at the same rate in each partner. Is it possible to recover completely from such a trauma? I think not; a degree of scarring is inevitable. At best, one can hope to work through or resolve the issues sufficiently to move on with life, perhaps with more strength than before; at worst, one would become stuck or ill. So, what facilitates adaptive resolution?

Following on from this, I was impressed that parents – of both sexes – seem readily and naturally to have used the unusual opportunity provided by the research. Elkan (1981) noted 'the urgent desire demonstrated by mothers to recount the birth experience ... whether easy or difficult, seeking recognition and acknowledgement of their emotions, and especially of the uniqueness of their own experience'. She considered that, especially after a traumatic birth, the opportunity to communicate and share her doubts and anxieties might free the mother to attend to her infant. A better understanding of the events might reduce feelings of guilt or anger surrounding possible staff or personal failure.

I then speculated further on the difference that this intervention might have made for the families, both at the time and subsequently. One could, for example, feel horrified that such assistance is not offered to all new parents, especially those with premature infants, but more research is required before any definitive statement can be made in this regard. So far, there is insufficient evidence to support such a conclusion. Only a randomised, controlled clinical trial, on a much larger scale, can tell us whether (a) such interviews affect the development of the infant and the various relationships among the family members in a positive way in the short, medium and longer term, and (b) the qualities of the particular interviewer and the type or number of interviews are significant variables.

Finally, there is the question of other possible interventions. I am constantly reminded when I see expectant or postnatal parents that the commonly used medical phrase 'pregnancy and delivery were uneventful' is bizarre. Pregnancy and delivery are never uneventful for the parents or indeed for any members of the family. They constitute a physical and emotional crisis even when no complications arise. How well do we prepare parents for this? The importance of such preparation when something starts to go wrong has been repeatedly emphasised (e.g. Astbury 1996), and many obstetric units have plans that are then set in motion – but by that point there is often insufficient time. The woman has to be transferred urgently to a different delivery location, and the parents are already in a state of shock, unable to ingest and process what is being offered. To attempt routinely to warn all expectant parents of the possibility of disaster and what a neonatal intensive care unit is like, and invoke anticipatory coping, is not possible within the framework of our current antenatal clinics and classes. It might even prove counterproductive. We do, however, have ample time to ensure that staff are prepared for the arduous tasks that they may have to tackle. We do not do this.

An important aspect of professional training for counselling or psychotherapy concerns strategies to protect the person offering help from being overwhelmed by the process. Staff in obstetric and neonatal intensive care units tend to have to survive as best they can and then support distressed parents. Appropriate training might lessen the strain upon them, increase their job satisfaction and allow them to offer more assistance to both parents and infants.

It is important that we stop avoiding these complex issues, and I am confident that this volume will facilitate progress in an undoubtedly difficult and immensely important field. Norma Tracey's research and the insightful reflections of the various authors upon it are truly inspirational. It is to be hoped that the material offered in this book will encourage all those involved with new parents to reflect first on whether they can offer something more or something different to families, second on whether their own work environment is sufficiently supportive of staff, and third upon the nature of the helping relationship itself.

Bryanne Barnett, MD, FRANZCP
Professor of Perinatal and Infant Psychiatry, University of New South Wales; Area Director, Paediatric Mental Health Service, South Western Sydney Area Health Service, Australia

References

Astbury J (1996) Consumers' Perspective on Preterm Birth. Unpublished consultant's report to the Care Around Preterm Birth Working Party. Cited in Care Around Preterm Birth. A Guide for Parents. NHMRC, February 1997.

Elkan J (1981) Talking about the birth. Journal of Child Psychotherapy 7: 11–15.

Acknowledgements

The writing of the main material for this book began four years ago with the receipt of an Australian Government Grant (RADGAC) and generous assistance from many commercial enterprises, especially Wyeth and Wellcome. It was made possible through an agreement with Professor David Henderson Smart that subjects could be accessed from the Neonatal Intensive Care Unit of the Department of Perinatal Medicine, University of Sydney in King George V Hospital. As the study was immediate rather than retrospective, it required sensitive co-operation between the Ethics Committee (Central Sydney), the chief researcher (Norma Tracey) and the research designer (Henry Luiker).

I wish to thank the enormous number of people who contributed their ideas and support for this project, especially Professor David Henderson Smart, Cristo Wacadlo, Lisa Askie, Marisa Gawley, Kim Suttor and the staff of King George V John Spence Nursery. Professor Bryanne Barnett and Dr Greg Rough were the two outstanding people who gave support to the project from beginning to end. Special thanks need to be given to the research designer Henry Luiker, without whom the project would not have begun. Thanks are also due to Angela Todd for analysing the data.

Professor Julian Katz and the late Dr Alan Bull assisted many of the chapter authors in developing their professionality, and for that they are gratefully acknowledged here.

Thanks go to Routledge for permission to reproduce in Chapters 5 and 10 amended versions of the articles 'Narrative of a mother with a premature baby' and 'Narrative of a father with a premature baby', which first appeared in the *Journal of Child Psychotherapy*, volume 22, number 2, pages 168–94, and volume 21, number 1, pages 43–64, respectively.

Lorraine Rose contributed to the formation of this book in many ways, reading, commenting and advising on chapters. Beulah Warren was supportive throughout. Caroline Andrews helped by designing the rating scales and Liz Jackman transcribed all the interviews. Louise Kobler gave assistance with making the text understandable. Sally Melhuish was the editor-in-chief, and it is her working of the manuscript that has made publication possible. Colin Whurr, the publisher, was untiringly supportive and encouraging from beginning to end.

PART 1
BACKGROUND — A MAP

Chapter 1
Background — a map of this book

NORMA TRACEY

> This book is about the inner emotional world of the mother and father in the first 12 weeks of the life of their premature baby.

The interviews that form the basis of this book are part of research that took place at an inner city hospital neonatal intensive care unit (NICU). In a NICU, the premature infant, instead of being in the mother's womb, is in a plastic 'box', being cared for by others in strange space-age-like equipment, dependent for his or her life on the doctors and ward team rather than on the mother. Our research question was, 'For the parents of a premature baby, what normal vulnerable psychic processes are disturbed, disrupted or fractured at this time?'. Our book is a way of seeking answers to this question. As I was doing these interviews with the parents, I began thinking about them as taking place in an inner world space somewhere between life and death. As I, the interviewer, was affected by emotions I had never before accessed, I wondered what was happening to these parents.

The Research Project

To answer the research question, we designed a project comprising 216 interviews with 24 mothers and fathers of newborn babies (12 couples). Of these 12 couples, six had babies between 640 g and 1200 g and/or under 32 weeks' gestation, and six were the parents of full-term babies. The parents of the full-term babies were interviewed to provide a contrast with the parents of the premature babies, but they were not considered to be a control group. The first four interviews with each parent were conducted weekly and commenced within a week of the baby's birth. These were followed by four interviews conducted fortnightly, a final

3

interview taking place one month later. This amounted to 18 hours of audiotaped interviewing with each family – nine hours with the mother and nine hours with the father – over a period of four months.

These interviews sought an in-depth explanation and understanding of the inner psychic world of emotions, thoughts and fantasies of the parents. The interviews were explained to each subject in the following way:

> These interviews are a space to think and to talk about how you are feeling. They are designed for us to understand closely and intimately the emotions you are experiencing during this time about yourself, your partner and your baby. There are no questions; you may just speak as you wish.

The interviewer was empathic, as all the subjects were severely affected by trauma, but remarks were limited to clarification of the information, with no interpretations. The interviewer was purposely not briefed medically and knew only that the mothers were all first-time parents, that all had partners and that the couple's baby was expected to have a good outcome.

As the recipient of these parents' raw, unconscious and often unprocessed emotions, this was a unique experience. I sought to share this experience through the audiotapes and transcribed interviews with chosen professionals in the field of parent–infant relations. Each author, coming from a slightly different theoretical background, was asked to listen to chosen material, read the transcript and write a chapter on their own thoughts and conclusions. Some wrote in a group, some individually, others with a colleague. Some chose to do one interview in depth; some compared the nine interviews. Others (such as Philip Garner and Sheila Sim) listened to and studied the 108 interviews with mothers with premature and full-term babies, using a rating scale that might show up differences between the two. Lorraine Rose listened to and studied all the tapes of the full-term mothers and fathers. This book is the result of their work.

To give the book a total perspective, we have included a chapter on the premature baby, asking what might be happening for the baby at this time and how we could help the parents to bond with and be active in the care of their baby. We have also included chapters on what was happening to the staff and how they could be helped to cope in this vulnerable life-and-death environment. It became central to our task to consider how they could create a space on the ward where the mother–baby unit was able to thrive.

Map of the book

The book is divided into sections for easy access. In the first section – 'Beginning the Journey: the Mothers' – Lorraine Rose shares her own thinking of what might be happening for the mothers of full-term babies, using some of their revealing interviews as a basis. In Chapters 3 and 4, I use a dynamic model to give a theoretical base for a full-term pregnancy and birth, and then contrast these with the distortions caused by prematurity. Chapter 5 is one of two chapters written by a special parent–baby interest group made up of different professionals with different theoretical approaches. This group met fortnightly for 18 months, listening to each of the nine interviews of one mother and one father. They wanted to understand the significance of this material (included here from the *Journal of Child Psychotherapy*, with kind permission of Routledge, London). Beulah Warren's Chapter 6 uses a 'self-regulation' perspective to explore one mother's perceptions of her premature baby and how these changed over the first three months of his life as he began to thrive and develop. Frances Salo (Chapter 7), using a psychoanalytic approach, writes on the internal mother of the mother, asking what happens to a new mother when her own mother has died.

In the next section, 'The Fathers', Lorraine Rose (Chapter 8) begins with her study of the fathers of full-term babies. In Chapter 9, Peter Blake, taking one interview from a psychodynamic perspective, gives a brief account of one father's reactions to the arrival of his premature baby and what is awakened from his past. The parent–baby group again presents an in-depth study of a father with a premature baby, from birth to four months of age (Chapter 10). We know of no literature about the father that has been presented in such detail.

Charles Enfield (Chapter 11) begins the next section on 'The Family' by concentrating on the family system and intergenerational aspects as he studies one couple over the three month period. Isla Lonie (Chapter 12) writes about a young migrant couple and how the condition of migration and cultural difference colours their experience of the birth and first few months with their premature baby. In the last chapter in this section, Bryanne Barnett and Marija Radojevic use attachment theory as a basis for discussing the experience of a mother with her partner.

The first three sections of the book lean heavily on the narrative of the parents, which, with their permission, is included in as much detail as space in the book allows. These narratives are revealingly sensitive and poignant, speaking louder than any theory.

The next section, comprising Helen Hardy's singular chapter on the premature baby (Chapter 14), asks, 'What might it be like for the baby?'. She gives a unique view of how parents may care for their babies on the ward and how the staff can be involved in linking the parents with their babies.

This leads to the next section, where the area of focus becomes 'The Ward'. Bryanne Barnett (Chapter 15) begins by asking, 'Whose baby is it?'.

Campbell Paul (Chapter 16), from his experience as a psychiatric consultant, writes about how staff of an NICU are affected by the work they do
and how this affects their relationship with the parents and the baby. The
chapter following this was 'workshopped' by a group comprising professionals (mostly social workers) from each of the major NICU centres in
Sydney, Australia. They discuss the way in which the problems they experience mirror what the parents on the ward are suffering. This section
concludes with a chapter by Sheila Sim, a social worker in neonatal intensive care for many years. After listening to 108 interviews of the mothers of
both premature and full-term babies, she explores how parents experience the environment of neonatal intensive care from a 'humanist'
perspective.

We end the book with two chapters on the nature of the parents'
trauma. When Philip Garner (who rated 106 mothers' interviews) began to
write the more formal part of the research, I had no idea that there would
evolve a chapter in which his experience mirrors the suffering of these
parents. My final chapter (Chapter 20), distilled over many months,
formulates a theory of trauma. Our concluding remarks address the
question, 'What do these parents need, and how can we help them?'

Why this book has been written

The authors of these chapters want to take the reader via several theoretical approaches into the hearts and minds of these parents. The crucial
four months of early life for mother, father and baby are focused on from
many perspectives. We make no apologies for repetitions: indeed, we
think it adds to the quality of the work. For example, and to our own
surprise, the question of 'Whose baby is it?' came up in chapter after
chapter, but each author gave his or her own view of what the answer to
this might be. Another question that emerged in many chapters is 'Where
is the baby?' The answers 'Born?', 'Not yet born?' and 'In the mind of the
mother?' confused us throughout.

This book is about a different and important kind of 'knowing' that is
beyond mental processes. It invites the readers' involvement and the experience of an emotional empathy that will give added meaning to their interaction with mothers, fathers and babies. We want to open doors and make
links rather than focus on answers. The book has been written so that each
chapter can be absorbed as an entity even though it is part of the whole. We
are hoping that the minute variations and several different perspectives that
gather in the mind of the reader will allow for a substantive whole eventually
to be born, revealing the horror and trauma of this period – for the parents,
the premature baby and the staff who work with them.

We hope that the chapters about the ward will give staff a tolerance of their own feelings aroused by working in this vulnerable life-and-death situation. Our main thrust is that it is not enough to save a baby's life if the baby's parents are so traumatised that they have lost the basic links with their baby and their trust in themselves as parents. While it is the authors' hope that a deeper understanding of what these parents are going through will lead more staff such as therapists, social workers and psychologists to be focused on the parents' needs, it is the whole ward team who, with insight, can create a safe and meaningful space for the parents in their unit. Parents need to be seen as an integral part of their baby's care. What they are suffering needs to be acknowledged.

Beyond this, the authors hope that the staff will receive the support they need to continue to work successfully in this extraordinary environment. If only the ward had known how Debbie felt, she would have been told of her baby's transfusion prior to it being given; the nurse would not have taken over the bathing of the baby from Jack and robbed him of his first anticipated contact; Joanne might not have felt alienated on the ward, like 'a shag on a rock'. It would have helped the staff to know that Rita had resisted taking her baby home not because she was rejecting her baby, but because she was terrified that she would repeat her failure to 'hold' the baby. They might have supported her living in with the baby a lot longer than 24 hours even though they were desperate for the space. Someone might have let Susan talk about her mother's suicide five years previously and seen how, with her own baby's birth and her now becoming a mother, the trauma had all been reawakened. It would have helped the staff to understand Michelle's panic if they had known that her brother had taken his own life with drugs only two years before, aged 32: they would have made sense of Michelle's terror that her newborn male baby was going to die, regardless of who told her otherwise. The need for the space for these parents to talk, a person to hear them and a place on the ward to just 'be' parents to their babies repeatedly stands out in every narration. We make no apology for the repetition since the cries of pain are so remarkably similar.

Who is this book is for?

We have written this book for the entire staff of neonatal intensive care and associated teaching units. This includes medical staff – both junior and senior – nursing staff at all levels, including nurse educators, occupational therapists, social workers, physiotherapists, psychologists, consultant psychiatrists and psychotherapists. While physical science has made massive advances that permit survival at a high-quality level for many of these babies, it is extremely important to understand the effects of such a trauma on the inner world of the parents, on their baby and on the staff who work in these wards. These chapters are an opportunity to explore how some of the highest technical achievements in the field of medicine affect the most primitive area of human existence. Consider the situation – a baby suspended somewhere between the womb and birth, dependent on space-age machines, scientific and medical care; and the traumatised parents, hanging between life and death for their baby, sometimes even with a fear of death for the mother herself.

For many, this book will be a validation of what they have emotionally 'sensed' and unconsciously 'known' but not easily articulated in their consciousness. For others, it will open doors that they would rather leave closed as it demands not only expert care in the medical and scientific field, but care in an emotional sense as well. This emotional care is of great importance if parents and babies are to survive the psychological trauma of such terrible beginnings.

PART 2
BEGINNING THE JOURNEY: THE MOTHERS

Chapter 2
Mothers of full-term infants

LORRAINE ROSE

This chapter will study the development of the relationship between the mother and baby, looking at those mothers who had a full-term pregnancy. The sample comprised six mothers and babies. Each parent had nine 50-minute unstructured interviews with Norma Tracey over a four month period. Where possible, I will let these families tell their own stories, which they generously shared on audiotape with the interviewer. No attempt is made to compare and contrast the mothers of full-term babies with those of premature babies. It is left to readers to draw their own conclusions.

Background information

There was enormous diversity among the parents studied, from not being married and not planning to have a baby but becoming pregnant and living most of the pregnancy with the family of origin, to being married and trying to become pregnant for seven years. Apart from the couple who had been trying for seven years to become pregnant, most of the other families had not especially planned the birth.

Internal and external circumstances also varied for the mothers. One was concerned with her eating disorder and her self-esteem, while another mother was grieving the loss of her young nephew who had died a week earlier and whose funeral was held while she was giving birth.

The birth

Looking at this sample of mothers, there seems to have been little in the way of 'natural birth'. Half of the group had a caesarean birth and the other half assistance, mainly in the form of an epidural. In fact, from a medical point of view, there was little that was 'normal'. Those who had a caesarean birth did so for medical reasons, for example pre-eclampsia, pregnancy-onset diabetes, or fibroids coupled with only two vessels in the umbilical cord rather than three, creating the potential for an abnormality in the baby. Of those who went into labour, one suffered damage to her urethra accompanied by a loss of control of the bladder and another was induced, while a third had stitches. A certain amount of trauma was experienced by all the mothers as a result of the birth.

As I listened to the mothers' accounts of the births, I could feel their sense of urgency and need to recount every detail of the experience. This was in part a response to the larger-than-life event that they had experienced, and they needed to share their excitement and heightened state with others, having successfully survived their ordeal. It had also provoked life-and-death anxieties about what would happen to them and the baby during the labour and birth. These fears were accessible to them and able to be shared, indicating that the level of trauma had not been so overwhelming that they were forced to split off and cut off from their experiences.

The following two accounts give some idea of what these mothers experienced. While I have considerably reduced the length of the verbatim material, I wish to convey something of the sense of what had to be endured, what these mothers had to see through, no matter what they were feeling at any one time:

I was quite surprised because I had to be induced. I was expecting to give birth later on – I was a bit worried because I thought there might be complications that might harm the baby. When I went into the hospital that night, I was three centimetres dilated and they gave me some gel, and soon after I started to feel the contractions. I wasn't aware of them being contractions, because they were coming one after the other, and I didn't realise. I also had a bad belly ache and the pains got worse. It was about 5 o'clock in the morning when I rang my husband to say come into the hospital. He came in and he was very supportive. We went into the labour room and he was there helping me out, and the pains got worse. I didn't think much about the baby.

I blanked out in a way. I was busy concentrating on the breathing techniques. They offered me the gas but that just made me feel nauseous. I was in labour about thirteen hours, and after that I had an epidural because it was getting too much for me – I hadn't slept and I was feeling very very tired. I felt more relaxed then. Once the epidural wore off, I pushed and brought the baby out and I was quite surprised because that was the best part of it. I was working for the baby now; it wasn't just feeling the contractions and the pain. Of course, my husband was there and he was spurring me on and encouraging me. The baby's head came out and the whole body came out. They said, 'It's a baby boy'. After they said, 'It's a boy', we were very happy and the baby was taken out to get weighed. It was a big relief when the baby came out. I felt ... it's hard to describe. I didn't get to hold him straight after the birth because I think they had to give him something to help him breathe; he was a bit sort of purply coloured, but soon after they cleaned him up I got to hold the little baby in my arms, which was a really special thing. It's really incredible, you've got this little baby in your arms and you forget about all those hours of pain!

The second abridged account illustrates that the mother is in a highly charged and volatile situation in which anything can happen at any time. This means that it is hard to process everything that is happening to her, making it difficult for her to be available to meet the baby:

There was a bit of meconium but it was quite thick, which meant that they couldn't keep us at the birth centre. We went upstairs and they plugged us into the machine and put straps around me. I'm sure those straps made the contractions feel worse because they were pressing in the wrong area. It was painful and the tears were flowing. It was just the whole situation I think, spreadeagled in front of everyone, with no control over what's happening, and the pains were getting really bad. Whenever I was having a contraction, the baby wasn't responding quite well enough, so they put one of those things on his head. I don't know what it is called.

Then a new registrar came in and assessed the situation quite quickly and said, 'We are going to do a caesarean'. So all the tears started flowing again. I knew it was the best thing and they were all trying to explain it to me. It was just the fact that everything had changed, and the fact that I knew I would be awake for an operation scared me. They gave me an epidural, and I was shaking as I was going down. Once there, my husband put on a gown, and there's all this pushing and pulling. Finally, half of it arrives and they're saying, 'Here he is'. I said, 'Is it a boy or a girl?', and they said that they couldn't tell yet. Finally, they told me it was a boy. They had to race him straight off because he'd swallowed some of the gunk, so they suctioned him out. Finally, they brought him back to me and it was still not real ... it had all been so quick and everything. I really thought I was having a girl, and when they said it was a boy, I thought that can't be right. But it doesn't make any difference. They laid him by my head so I couldn't focus on him. I don't know whether it was the drugs or whether he was just too close. I could see this little thing lying there, but I could barely move to do any more.

As I heard what each of the women had to say, I felt a sense of relief that the interviewer was there to receive these women's stories. These experiences needed to be thought about and shared with someone else who could understand how profound they were for them. It brought to mind for me the notion of 'women's business' around the birth and the natural desire for mothers to get together and recount and exchange their birth experiences. The physiological birth is the first working together that the mother and baby engage in, in order to achieve the transition from pregnancy, and it is the first separation and rupture that the mother and baby have to face. Their working together at this time sets a pattern and a tone for their relationship in the future.

The experience of hearing these mothers raised concerns in me about the brevity of the stay in hospital, when mothers do not always get an opportunity to process the birth with others. Without the opportunity to ventilate their experience, the mothers are not freed to get on to the next step of the process, that is, to meet their new baby. Unprocessed, the birth can get in the way of that meeting being a full one at the emotional level.

The world is irrevocably changed for a woman as she becomes a mother, as it is for the baby, and this shift and transformation have to be traversed at deep psychological levels. The mother now has to find a place in her mind to hold the welfare of her newborn baby, who will similarly have to find out whether he/she has been born into an environment that will meet their needs for safety and care. It will be through the mother's thoughts and preoccupation that the birth of the personality of her baby will be able to take place. The mother, however, requires others to tend to her interests so that she is enabled to engage in this process with her new baby. Nourished by this support, mother and baby can move on to begin to share the mutual task of getting to know each other.

Mother and baby meet

The newness of being a mother was very evident from the first interview after the birth. All the women were shell-shocked and experiencing a sense of dislocation, but they were at the same time aware of the enormity of the changes in their life. It was obvious that the development of the connection with their baby was a process rather than just an instant transformation, and they needed time to adjust to the new physical and emotional demands of becoming a mother.

One mother movingly shares her process with us in this way:

I think about being a mother – I don't actually feel like a mother. I think it's still very weird; it's coming to the reality of it all. I felt very happy ... it's a joy to have the baby around and you see little things about him – it just makes you feel so happy, and so happy to be part of that. To think that you're responsible for this little life, it's really incredible, it's just a little miracle. And I'm definitely glad we've had him ... I think we will be very happy.

Another mother expressed the changes to herself and to her life in another way:

I get teary – it seems to be like every second day when I'm just a bit teary and everything ... it is so sort of new to me ... I'm not usually a teary person at all. And I was thinking, ooh what is it, and you know, is it because I'm not coping, and I'm thinking I'm doing all the right things; it was just a completely new experience – the whole thing – and you start thinking, I'm attached to this thing forever!

It was possible very early on to observe those mothers who had room in their mind for their new infant and hence were almost immediately available to meet their new offspring. Others were preoccupied to varying degrees with their past, especially their past relationships with their own parents, in particular their mothers. The degree to which these issues were unresolved determined the capacity in the mother to make available a space in her mind for the new individual born into the couple.

While most of the mothers in the sample were engaged with the process of grappling with the enormity of the changes to their lives as a result of the birth of their babies, another mother was preoccupied with her unresolved past:

It is really quite overwhelming. A lot of the time, I find myself just crying at the thought that ... she's here and I love her so much and fear – fear that I might lose her ... [crying]. It's funny because it took a few days to feel anything much, especially after having had a caesarean, and I had a terrible time with the drugs afterwards, and pethidine. I was having nightmares as well from the blood pressure drugs ... it took a couple of days to bond with her, to start feeling anything much. I'd lie there feeling very afraid of her, thinking I can't look after her – I can't even look after myself [crying].

I suppose I am afraid of being sick too. My mother was sick when I was little. She died of cancer when I was five ... it hit me what my mother must have felt, it had never struck me before just how traumatic that must have been for her not just to face death herself but to know her babies weren't going to be looked after.

This very poignant story shows graphically how unresolved past issues surface at the crucial time of birth. It is inevitable that some return to our own childhoods will be activated, but if there are many unresolved issues left unprocessed, they can get in the way of the mothers forming a connection with their newborn. Another mother spent much of her initial interview discussing her family, her parents and her sisters, who were spread all around the world, and it was obvious that she needed to connect up to her family, even though a certain amount of ambivalence surrounded her relationship with her mother. It does seem that the mother–daughter relationship in the previous generation is a significant factor in the new mother's adjustment to her role as mother.

Listening to these new mothers evoked strong feelings of protectiveness in me, and I became poignantly aware of their heightened sensitivity and openness, as well as their different way of being in the world. I was painfully aware of their need for a protective, safe environment in which they could incorporate their 'hypersensitive' self and be allowed the time and space to do this without having prematurely to close down on this new emotional state.

Unfortunately, this was not always possible, and when there were intrusions from the external world, they had a major impact. The mother who had to face the death of her nephew was unable to breastfeed because of the difficulties arising from her grief surrounding her nephew. Another mother had difficulty with a drug-addicted, highly agitated woman who shared her hospital room. This mother was quite rightly disturbed by these circumstances and needed someone who would intervene to protect her and her baby from such an intrusion. Such circumstances demonstrate an important role of the father in protecting, where possible, the mother–baby dyad in the early days of the relationship.

A major source of support did, in fact, come from the partners. On the whole, they were able to be available to their wives while they were grappling with their own changed conception of themselves, and this support was greatly appreciated.

As one mother said, 'My husband was just so supportive; I guess it's really important that both parties communicate a lot, and that they want to give to each other.'

The mothers' ability to incorporate the fathers varied, some being more active than others in incorporating the father into the new family:

> James is really rapt. I didn't think he'd be as rapt as I was, but he's really good. Especially, I think because the baby looks like him. James has been very good with him. He's been a good dad so far, hasn't he? [pause, baby sounds] I think I feel more now for James ... it feels different because I loved him before the baby, but it just seems to have gotten more after the baby.

Others felt less unified in their task:

> I think our decision to have a baby, at this stage, was probably more mine than his ... something I definitely wanted ... maybe I felt unfulfilled, I don't know.

While the overall sense of these mothers was that they were well supported, the mother who was struggling to become a mother felt somewhat accused by her husband's less ambiguous feelings:

> [He] was over the moon and besotted about her straight away, so he was obviously doing all the right sort of emotional things. I didn't really feel anything much.

The support of family and friends was also an important variable that served either to facilitate the developing relationship between the mother and the baby or to leave the mother feeling less resourceful in her capacity to meet the needs of her newborn. The lack of current parental support, no matter what the past, was keenly felt. Conversely, those who were well supported by family or friends were deeply appreciative of their current support.

It can be seen in the first interview that while all the mothers, in their own way, suffered some degree of trauma from the process of birth and the medical interventions that were required, they were largely in touch with their thoughts and feelings about what had happened to them and were able to freely communicate their experiences. Most were able to respond very quickly to the new arrival on the scene and to experience the joy of the birth of their baby alongside the physical and emotional pain that they experienced. As seen so clearly from the texts, the past histories of the mothers had a profound influence on their capacity to become mothers, while current levels of support from family and husband were critical factors in facilitating these mothers' transformation into their new role. Depending on the degree of support that they had received in the past and in the current situation, they were better able to begin to think about the new baby who had arrived. If those around them had a space for them and showed concern for their concerns, and this had also been available in the past, these mothers were better able to provide a space for their babies in their mind.

4–6 weeks

At this stage, the mothers were well immersed in both the joys and the difficulties of motherhood. Most were working hard at their task and doing what they could to meet the challenges and needs of their baby. Some issues were still needing to be worked out between mother, father and baby, these being accompanied by some uncertainty on the part of the mothers. Most were still grappling with the idea of themselves as mothers and were concerned with their competency, as they endeavoured to work out how they wanted to be with and manage their babies against all the differing pieces of advice they were receiving from professionals, parents, in-laws and friends. Most were engaged in a preoccupation with their baby and were struggling with what was best for them both.

The baby, on the other hand, initially experiences itself as a stream of sensations and only gradually comes into the relationship with the parents. In the face of many new stimuli, the baby will begin to attempt to structure his/her world by dividing experiences into 'soft' ones and 'hard' ones. 'Soft' experiences will be the warm, holding, feeding ones, when the infant feels 'held' both psychologically and emotionally. 'Hard' experiences may arise from having to be unwrapped and have a nappy change, needing to be bathed, being put down to sleep or experiencing discomfort and pain. 'Soft' experiences enable the baby to feel at 'one' with the mother, and the 'hard' experiences confront it with the fact that it is now apart and a separate being from its mother. Both aspects are important if the baby is to develop.

It is the mother who, by her preoccupation and attentive, reflective care, gradually enables the baby to feel secure and held, experiencing the world but not being overwhelmed by it. The mother, through her maternal reverie, develops a mental skin around this stream of sensations that is her baby. When experiences, both pleasurable and unpleasurable, escalate, someone needs to be there to help the baby to deal with its intolerable level of stimulation or anxiety. By knowing about the baby's feelings, the mother helps the baby to make these feelings more bearable and less overwhelming.

Some mothers can react negatively to the baby seeking to have its needs met, and especially if their own needs have not been responded to, or have been only inadequately addressed, they may see the baby only as taking from them at their expense. On the other hand, the mother may be disappointed that the new baby cannot give her what she has missed out on and is still waiting for.

While the mothers in these interviews had doubts and anxieties, it was also evident that the joys of having a baby certainly compensated for the difficulties that they were experiencing. At this point, I would like to introduce the mothers and babies in turn so that it is possible to get a sense of where each of the six mothers was at this point in the process:

> I think everything's still going fine ... Lack of sleep is a big problem ... it's just trial and error ... you can't really plan what you are going to do in a day. We're having some trouble at night, just sometimes, because when he does start playing up he plays up for a long time. I made an appointment to go to Possum Cottage [a mother–infant centre]. I've got this sense that I'm failing and I don't want to fail. The protective instinct is there, but not knowing how to handle things is there too.
>
> He didn't breastfeed well ... so I took him off the breast and put him straight on to the formula. He seems to be going well now. Like with any relationship or anything that's new, you have your ups and downs, but it's still lovely to have him and we wouldn't give him back even though he does keep you up and cries or is in pain or whatever.

This mother is clearly feeling her way with her baby and trying to negotiate her way of being with her baby boy. Despite her difficulties, she is happy to be engaged in the emerging relationship with her son and is perhaps in need of some reassurance that she is doing well and that being unsure and finding her way is natural at this point.

Our next mother expressed it thus:

We've had a bit of a rough week. We went up to the clinic because of our regular visit to get him weighed. I said that he hasn't been sleeping during the day at all, he just wants to drink and feed ... although at night he was sleeping beautifully so we had no problems there. Anyway, the clinic Sister booked us into a care place. They tried their control crying techniques. We came home with all the right things to do ... we couldn't do it ... as soon as we put him in his bassinet he'd cry, and we'd try and wrap him up and he'd start bawling. Now when he goes to sleep he jerks and thrashes around. He used to sleep very soundly, but now he is waking and I keep thinking he's having a nightmare about being wrapped in those blankets. They say it's all follow your instincts, but being a new mother you worry. I wanted to get him into some sort of routine because we have to leave him with people when I go back to work. I am breastfeeding but I have to get him used to the bottle. I'm all right until everyone starts telling me you've got to do this, you've got to do that, and then all common sense just falls out the window.

This mother is struggling with her instincts and attempting to discriminate what would be helpful for her baby. The intervention of controlled crying seems to have interfered with a reasonably workable relationship between herself and her baby. It also seems that the need to return to work places pressure on this mother to establish routines that may be premature for both herself and her baby. Mother and baby did seem to be able to establish a good rapport, but external pressures were limiting their ability to keep responding flexibly to the changing needs of the developing baby and their developing relationship.

Our next mother is also grappling with her doubts and the differing advice she is getting, but she is gradually deciding how she wants to be with her baby:

I've had a pretty good week. The baby's settling down a bit more which is good. I think it's because of the formula milk more than anything. I feel awkward and a bit nervous sometimes about leaving the baby with my parents or with someone else. I guess I'm very protective in that way.

I haven't managed to sleep during the day because the baby still vomits, and when he vomits it goes up his nose; it's really bad so I usually watch out for him. Other than that, I am feeling fine. I haven't been feeling depressed at all. Actually, as time goes on, I'm feeling more confident about the baby. I feel like I know the baby a lot better now as well. I've stopped breastfeeding altogether now and I'm just bottle feeding. I am feeling happy and confident about the decision to put him on to the bottle, but I felt a bit bad about it at first.

I think he's absolutely gorgeous really. Sometimes I think how sweet he is and how gorgeous he is, just while I'm changing him. And I just love giving him a bath because he just shows so much expression on his face. It's really weird, you get so many different people giving you advice. And it's very different advice. One person says this, and another person says that, and it's just almost opposing, so it's just hard to know.

I'm hoping to go back to work in May [a couple of months].

While this mother is also returning to work, she still has some time to 'go with' the relationship with her baby and feel her way with it. There is still, for the time being, the sense of time to engage in the relationship and the sense of pleasure in the everyday activities and routine of having a baby, even though he has been weaned perhaps in preparation for her going back to work.

Our next mother is very involved with her baby girl, who seems able to ask for what she needs from her mother:

She's going through a growth spurt ... she only sleeps for about ten minutes and she wants to be up again. She seems to be genuinely hungry and she spits the bottle out when she doesn't want it. She has a large feed prior to going to bed at night time, and then she'll sleep for about five hours, and then she's back on the four-hourly feeds. During the day, she's on two- or three-hourly feeds.

She's really gooing and gaahing and heaps of smiles now, especially when I take her nappy off; she loves to have her nappy taken off. It's lovely in the morning because she wakes up about 6 o'clock, sun shining on her face, so her dad brings her in to bed and she has this lovely time, about three-quarters of an hour, smiling and it's really nice. This is her time with dad.

It's still hard to believe that I've got my own little girl ... it's all worth it.

While this mother had many financial worries at this time and was in the thick of renovations of the house, she is clearly enjoying her contact with her baby and is very inclusive of the baby in her conversation. She clearly sees her baby as a little personality in her own right, and while the baby is making quite a lot of appropriate demands on her mother, there is a sense that the mother has a great deal of nurturing to offer and that she is well able to respond to the dependency needs of her baby.

The next mother is dealing with difficult circumstances – the absence of her partner:

Well, I've had a very busy morning. My husband's away this week. I think the nights are the worst, especially the beginning of the night. I'm just so tired, and there's nobody to get up to him if he starts really crying, so I think the poor little love's been left a lot longer than he's used to. Like this morning, I was just so tired, I couldn't keep my eyes open and I was having a feed about 7 am. I'd already been up twice in the night and I was just so exhausted. I just thought I'll just put him back and I realised afterwards that he'd actually been crying, sort of grizzling; it must have been over an hour, and I really didn't hear it. I actually wonder how single parents ever cope; I just can't imagine how they do. I think I'd go absolutely bananas if it was just me. I think he would be left an awful lot

of the time, just to get on with it, or else I think I'd be worried about what I'd do
to the poor little love. I find it quite difficult to know how much attention they
need at this stage, and whether I'm giving him enough or not.

I probably have missed my husband ... but I've been very busy so I haven't
been sitting pining for him or anything like that. But I really have missed his
company and certainly missed his help with the baby. I wrote a letter to my
Dad, and I actually found myself feeling very sad about him not seeing his
grandson at this stage ... being a proud Mum and thinking he's so yummy.

With the absence of both her family and her husband, this mother is struggling to be available to her baby boy. In the absence of thought and attention for herself, she is less able to hold things together, and the baby is
dropping out of her mind. Additionally, in order to cope with the
emotional feelings of loss surrounding her partner, this mother is keeping
herself busy and is hence less able to be emotionally available to her baby's
different states of mind and the baby's need for closeness, both emotionally and physically. Her comments on the difficulty of being a single
mother highlight the problems of lack of support and need for nurturing
of the mother.

Finally, some comments from the mother who suffered the early loss of
her own mother and has struggled to come to grips with her new role:

This week was easier. Everything feels like it's more bearable. I'm sure that's
being off the tablets. Not breastfeeding means I'm feeling like my body's
starting to be my own again. I'm much happier with the routine of making up
bottles, sterilising bottles, doing that sort of thing. It's something that is away
from me, it's not encroaching on myself and my body the way it was.

Most of the time, I don't think about the misery and the low things, the
things that make me cry, whereas even a week ago I was dwelling on that sort of
thing quite a lot. Although I think if the baby weren't settled and if I didn't have
the kind of help and support I've got from my partner, I think I'd still be in that
pit of despair a lot more. I am actually starting to get a little bit bored with just
being at home. I am starting to feel more useful beyond just being a mother and
looking after a baby. She's a good baby. It'll be good to go back to work. I
suppose I won't be leaving her, because I'll be leaving her with her dad
sometimes and I'll be taking her to day care on campus with me. I am itching to
get back to work you know, not the day-to-day slog of teaching but to my study
leave, the books and the conferences and things I want to write.

This mother finds it easier to create some distance in her relationship with
her baby and has begun partly to disengage both mentally and emotionally
from her baby. This may also be a protective measure against the anger she
must carry because of her own difficult experiences. Because of this lack of
involvement, the relationship is not as fulfilling and she correspondingly
looks for stimulation from her place of work. The baby has adapted to her

mother's needs and is not making too many demands on her mother, who is grappling with her own issues of not being mothered herself.

Listening to these mothers, you cannot help but admire their attempts to come to grips with the difficult and demanding role of becoming a mother. While developing bonds with their baby, the hard task of being a mother was being met with much courage and fortitude, which commanded my respect for their efforts. I felt very keenly that these mothers needed support just to stay in the struggle and see it through. Realistically, this period can only be one of uncertainty and discovery on both sides for mother and baby. These mothers needed support, holding and encouragement, rather than solutions imposed on them, to help them to stay in touch with their task.

It was also painful to feel that the gently developing relationship with the baby was often being dictated by the external demands of making a living rather than by the needs of the mother and baby, and painful to see the impact of this on the tenuous links that were being forged. Most mothers weaned at this early time and spoke with a mixture of relief and bravado of the early weaning of their babies. I experienced a sense of great sadness that there did not seem to be enough time for the full relationship to blossom, and that there was thus a lack of satisfaction and some pulling back from the intensity of the engagement with the new little being in their life.

10–12 weeks

By now, the baby well and truly recognises who its parents are and will smile in response to consistent care. All are usually getting to know each other a little better, and this mutual recognition is acknowledged on all sides. While everyone is still finding their way, a little more organisation and routine are usually possible. Babies love the rhythm of a routine that helps them to locate who they are – not a routine that is rigidly applied but one that takes them into account and is given shape by their needs, while at the same time having predictability and reliability. This helps their surroundings to be a little more manageable for them as they struggle to sort out how this new world works. The early distinction between 'soft' and 'hard' experiences is now more differentiated into 'good' and 'bad' experiences. What is built up in the baby's mind is an idea of 'a mother who soothes me' or, conversely, 'a mother who leaves me to be a separate little person'. To bring the baby gently into reality, we have to be both the good provider and the one who takes it away; both mothers are essential to development. Both mother and baby work together to find the real world and their real relationship as opposed to an idealised one. Important here is the notion of 'good enough mothering', a term coined by Winnicott (1960).

Most of the mothers in this study were bonding with their growing babies, who were no longer newborns, and enjoying the process of their development. By now, they were noticing more complex states of mind in their babies and were able to begin to decipher expressions on their babies' faces and to note aspects of their personalities, for example whether their baby was 'alert', 'fun' or 'thoughtful'.

The mothers had begun to resolve ambivalent attitudes towards having a baby and seemed to have decided that, while it had been difficult, it had been more than worthwhile:

> I think at the beginning I didn't really know how I would feel about mother-hood and babyhood, but I would say to anyone that I would recommend it, even the bits that I thought would be really dreadful haven't been that bad. I've just enjoyed it, and I would recommend it to anyone.

At this stage, the mother's feelings are highly volatile as the relationship with the baby grows in intensity. For both sides of the relationship, every-thing can be all wonderful or all terrible in quick succession as the roller coaster of being 'in love' is experienced.

One mother, in speaking so clearly of this experience, is representative of a mother's feelings at this time:

> You notice your life a lot more when you have a baby. It has meaning to it – you feel depressed, you feel happy, you feel wonderful when they smile, you have so many more emotions that you are aware of, more than you did before. It's hard to believe that a child does that. You are so aware of everything that goes on around you and you are so protective. I never thought that I would be so protective, and I never thought I would feel so much for a child, even though I still feel really tired and really weak for some reason and it's a real effort to get up to him.
>
> When he smiles his whole face lights up and it makes everything worth it; the tiredness, the late nights, the feeding and the grumpiness, it makes it all worth-while. You have your down times too, when he cries and you can't settle him and you think, what did I do this for? Your moods do swing, they swing a lot.

Separation and individuation issues naturally arise at this point for many mothers and centre around whether and when to return to work. It seemed that the issue of separation hovered over most of these mothers from the beginning of their relationship with their babies since most were considering returning to work at some point:

> I love going to work and having time from him, but I really miss him. By the time I'm coming home, I just can't wait to see him. And leaving him in the morning – in the morning we have him in the bed with us. Because I am too

lazy, I just feed him in bed and we drift off to sleep together, and he just giggles and smiles the whole time, and it's so hard to leave him when he's just laughing at you and smiling at you. He's so gorgeous.

This is a very clear expression of the difficulties that this mother faces in leaving her baby, and I felt deeply for her in her dilemma. Later, she discusses in her interview all the toys that her baby now has to play with and her considerable outlay on activities for him to enjoy, as if to occupy him in her absence. While the baby is often left with the father or with someone felt to be very warm and caring of him, some psychological issues around separation remain. Here the baby is being breastfed after his mother gets home from work in the afternoon:

I'm just beginning to worry though, because whenever I feed him then put him to bed he's already asleep. I can't get him to go to sleep by himself yet, and I keep thinking he's got to be able to do that soon. I can't keep feeding him for the rest of his life like this. I don't know how to stop it because I've tried, and every time I try he cries and cries and cries.

This mother is not wishing to cause her baby pain by separating from him and returning to work, but there is a sense of attempting to avoid the consequences of separating, which may mean that the baby is not as happy about her being away at work, even though he is generally coping with the separation. It will be important for this mother to manage the ambivalent feelings of the baby, who will quite naturally be both happy and unhappy with his mother as a result of her absences, and that she bear her ambivalent and guilty feelings towards him.

Another mother who obviously enjoys her little girl, the ambivalence clearly being resolved on the side of the positive, is able to articulate the mixed feelings that both mothers and babies feel at this time:

She's very happy, believe it or not. She's a very happy little girl; she doesn't cry an awful lot. Grizzles when she's hungry, but she's not someone who spends her time screaming – she's just a happy gorgeous little girl.

Later, she is able to say:

I feel dread if she doesn't wake up at 11.30 though, because then it's usually 3.30 or 4.00 in the morning before she wakes up.

The growing sense of self in the baby can provoke, on the other hand, fears about separating and whether one will still be loved if separate development is allowed. There also can be the worry that growing up and separating might be a dangerous rather than a good development:

He's really wonderful, and he's an extension of Donald and I ... I've been enjoying Christopher so much, and I'm so glad I haven't returned to work because I think I'd just feel I'd be missing out on those precious hours of being with him. He's growing and he's changing all the time. Growing up, I felt very distant from my parents. I think I am very insecure and very fearful of losing things. You get the feeling that once you have something and you're really happy with it, it will go, or if you really want something you can never get it, or if some things are really good it just doesn't last for long.

Other issues that arose included the mothers' self-image with regard to their body, which either they decided did not matter or felt it was important to 'do something about'. All the mothers commented on the amount of time it took to look after a baby and noted the lack of time they now had for themselves and their relationship with the baby. While many were still grappling with the issue of having another human being in their lives, most were talking about having another child, which perhaps also reflected their preoccupation with coming to grips with the new family that had just been formed. Perhaps being successful with this baby made them confident of the next. On the other hand, I experienced a sense of the process of the birth and the early months with their baby as being very rapid, passing too quickly and being partly missed out on. If this is so, some of the desire for another child might have been a longing for the time and space to have a fuller experience of motherhood. Being a parent was, however, something they all welcomed and were pleased to embrace.

Conclusion

The six mothers and babies who formed the basis of this discussion came from very diverse situations. All had experienced some difficulty of a medical nature at the birth of their baby. Despite these difficulties, the emotional impact of their experience could be discussed readily and easily with the interviewer, which facilitated their moving into the next phase of getting to know their newborn.

The factors that assisted the mothers in their task of relating to their baby included their own mothering experience with their mother when they were young, and the support that they received from the father of the baby and from family and friends. All the mothers experienced a great deal of uncertainty as they negotiated their transition to motherhood and were sensitive to advice from others, needing considerable support and validation of their handling of the situation as they struggled to gain their own confidence in dealing with their baby.

It was also clear that the maternal preoccupation of the mothers was very fragile and that external and internal events could easily fracture the new relationship, which needed a great deal of protection in the early months. Most mothers also chose to wean their babies gradually from breastfeeding in the first six weeks. While most of the mothers took some time off to be with their babies, the question of returning to work preoccupied them and seemed to have the impact of 'rushing' the relationship. As the relationship between the mothers and their babies grew, the mothers began to connect more to their babies and experienced a wide range of emotional states in line with their baby's growing emotional complexity. If bonded, the mothers and their babies faced the issue of separation, which required great understanding on the part of both mother and baby.

As their babies grew, the mothers began to feel the need to reclaim their bodies as their own, which was often expressed in terms of regaining the body size they had had prior to having a baby. This also seemed to be connected to reclaiming their relationship with their partner. All of the mothers felt strongly about the loss of time for themselves and for this relationship since the birth of the baby. While experiencing these difficulties of integrating a new little person into their couple and making the transition to being a family, all the mothers contemplated a further addition to their family. The overriding feeling from all the mothers involved in these interviews was that, despite the ups and downs, becoming a parent was well worth while.

References

Winnicott DW (1960) Ego distortion in terms of true and false self. In The Maturational Process and the Facilitating Environment. London: Hogarth Press/Institute of Psychoanalysis.

Chapter 3
Prematurity and the dynamics of pregnancy

NORMA TRACEY

When a woman is pregnant, she is also pregnant with herself as a mother, just as a man is pregnant with himself as a father. In this chapter, I think about how the important processes of this time are fractured by the premature interruption of a pregnancy and having a newborn infant at risk of death in neonatal intensive care. To understand what happens to the mother and father of the premature infant, we need to understand some of the normal changes during pregnancy and birth, and the relevance of the sensitive period called primary maternal preoccupation, which begins prior to birth and continues for the first six or more weeks after birth.

In this chapter, I use two primary concepts – inner world phantasy and dynamic theory – to develop a way of thinking about the processes taking place in a woman's psyche during pregnancy. The inner-world opposites that a mother- and father-to-be have to negotiate in pregnancy take them emotionally into the world of parenthood. They concern their own self-image and their internal representation of their infant. Their resolution has far-reaching consequences for the mother–father–infant interaction in the future. My thoughts in this chapter are about how much a premature birth distorts and disrupts these dynamics.

What happens in a normal pregnancy? There is chaos in surrendering the old internal order as the new order redefines the parent's identity as mother or father. We know now that the transitional crisis of pregnancy and childbirth involves profound endocrine, somatic and psychological changes. Several authorities have recognised pregnancy as a normal transitional crisis. Deutsch (1945), Benedek (1952), Bibring (1959), Kaplan and Mason (1960), Bibring et al (1961) and Pines (1982) have stressed the profoundly sensitive emotional equilibrium of the pregnant woman and her vulnerability to psychological disturbances. The documented emotions of pregnant women include anxiety, worry, mood lability, insomnia, impaired cognitive functioning, emotional conflicts, severe disturbances of thought and behaviour, premonitions, magical thinking, paranoid and depressive reactions, regressive shifts with the emergence of early attitudes and conflicts, and increased dependency needs.

For the father, it is also a time of crisis. He needs to cope with the responsibility of a changing wife, preoccupied and emotionally labile. In addition, he must cope with his emerging identity as a father, his identity in relation to his baby, and his past experiences of rivalry and identity in terms of his own father. As well as this, there is the awakening of his former relationship with 'his' own mother as he comes to terms with the 'mother' in his wife and his own envy, fear of replacement and fear of not being able to produce 'good' babies with her. Emotions to do with his own potency, his fathering of his own infant and who his infant will be to him are unconscious and conscious during pregnancy and birth, as we will see from the ensuing chapters.

The dynamics of the inner world during pregnancy

The opposites that a mother- and father-to-be negotiate I have called the inner world dynamics of pregnancy. In order to have a shared language base, I will begin by defining what is meant in this chapter by 'a dynamic' and by 'inner world'. The *Oxford Dictionary* (1987) defines dynamic theory as 'a theory that phenomena of matter and mind are caused by action of opposing forces'. Ogden (1985) writes that 'a dynamic is a process in which two opposing concepts each create, inform, preserve and negate the other, each standing in a dynamic ever changing relationship with the other'. He also quotes Hegel (1807) and Kojever (1947), who both wrote of the dialectical process moving towards integration, 'but integration is never complete; each integration creates a new dialectical opposition and a new dynamic tension'.

This is a useful way of conceptualising what occurs in pregnancy.

Since these dynamics take place in the inner world of the mother and father, the concept of inner world objects is central to all our thinking in this book. We think about the inner world as a space in our mind where our previous relationships are ever present, active and alive.

Freud (1909) initially gave us the concept that within the child's mind are images of intimate relationships with key people such as parents and siblings. Freud postulated that these emotions from previously experienced relationships affect all future relationships. Klein (1928) saw these relationships not only as the past relived, but also as the present, always immediately actively generating a continuing life of their own. Frances Salo, one of the contributors to this volume, says:

For infants, bodily experiences such as hunger or satisfaction seem very intensely felt, and it seems as if, in a similar intense bodily way, infants initially feel that they have important aspects of their important attachment figures inside them, such as a good mother when they feel satisfied, and a bad mother when they feel frustrated and hungry.

Winnicott (1952) explained that, in the earliest stages, the infant and mother are not psychically separate: they are 'part' of each other. As they separate out, the infant, as well as having a real and present mother, also has a living image or imago of a mother inside him. Similarly, the mother has an internal image of her infant and indeed of her own mother. Bion (1977) added that being able to 'think through' the emotions in our experiences is what allows the experience to be symbolised and made into a model. This processing of inner world dynamics, so richly present when a woman is pregnant, is what this chapter concerns.

I will now go on to discuss some of these dynamics.

Preconceptive ambivalence and the dynamic of wanting and not wanting a pregnancy

Before conceiving their own infant, parents-to-be face a vast array of confusing and conflicting emotions. The ambivalence of both wanting and not wanting an infant is present for every parent. This ambivalence is born out of childhood fantasies and experiences, internal representations of their parents, and their partner's experiences and fantasies, as well as their present social and emotional *milieu*. Unconscious fantasising about sexuality, parenting, pregnancy and birth happens from earliest childhood. Children fantasise about having babies – 'Can I have one?', 'With whom?', 'How?', 'When?' – and this will occupy their minds and play through dolls, cars and other toys or symbols from a very early age (Kerstenberg 1956). Feder (1980) writes that 'The mutually attracted heterosexual couple awaken and stimulate in each other a series of interpersonal, ambivalent and contrary conflicts, usually unconscious' and adds that there is 'evidence of procreative joy' as opposed to 'procreative panic'.

For the mother and father of a premature infant in intensive care, it seems as though a premature infant is the fulfilment of their worst fantasies. The parents may have a primitive fear that they have 'caused' the prematurity and the infant's illness. The parents may fear that their own negative fantasies to do with not wanting their infant have overcome the positive ones. This is more so when there have been previous miscarriages. These miscarriages become bound up and confused with the prematurity and further confused with whether the infant was or was not wanted. There is also increased guilt for these normal feelings. The balance is lost:

> I hadn't felt as if I wanted a baby this time. I'd had a previous miscarriage which made being pregnant feel like I was just getting ready for another miscarriage. When he was born so premature, it was like this was true, like I had had another miscarriage. I felt so bad about not wanting to be pregnant in the first place.
>
> I wasn't meant to get pregnant, but I did and then at 12 weeks I had a bleed and I just thought I had lost it again. I'd been on bed rest and pottering around ... I shouldn't have got pregnant I kept thinking. I don't know that I could ever put myself and my husband through something like this again.

Prematurity interrupts and disturbs the dynamic between fusion and separation in pregnancy

The early part of the first stage of pregnancy may be likened to an autistic phase – 'a state of alert inactivity during which the woman, like the newborn, is involved in minimising her disorientation and achieving a state of well being, without much recognition of its source' (Raphael-Leff 1982). Others define a state of fusion so strong that the mother often denies to herself that she is pregnant. The next stage, in which there is movement, is similar to hatching, involving a gradual individuation, the fetus becoming separate. At this stage, the pregnant woman feels a movement of something foreign to her. The final stage culminates in the actual physical separation of birthing. After birth, the idea of two people in one skin is very strong. The mother holds the infant psychically in the 'womb of her mind'. In prematurity, there is a rupturing of the individuation processes and a disruption of the fantasy of fusion or symbiosis. The defence against the massive intrusion is invariably a feeling of the baby not being hers. Many mothers speak of a feeling of alienation: 'I still feel as if he is someone else's baby and I am visiting him'.

Prematurity disturbs the dynamic between the dream, the dread and the reality

There are three separate paths existing throughout life that are repeated at every developmental phase: the dream, the dread and the reality. There is a dream of what parents want their baby to be, and there is the opposite, which is the terror of what he or she might be. Is he/she going to be the fulfilment of their love? Is he/she going to be the declaration of their right to impulsiveness in their sexuality? Is he/she their sin, their punishment? Is he/she the embodiment of their evil or their virtue?

From the fetus, the infant carries some parental myth of his or her destiny. Such mythological expectations are seriously affected by prematurity. Dread is so close to reality. We believe that the harsh imposition of reality brought on by a premature birth fractures and disturbs these myths. In prematurity, the dread of a dead, sick or damaged infant is the harsh imposition of reality. It cuts across the 'dreaming'. Here are some of the mothers' comments after the birth:

> I nearly died, she nearly died. It is just dawning on me. It was like all my worst fears came true.

> I thought I will never see that baby like any other baby, he will come dead or something. So every time I go in the nursery and see him I cry and cry. I dream of him coming home and screaming the house down. Then I will be happy.

The dynamic between being and reacting is disturbed by prematurity

Being and reacting are opposites: in reacting, being is lost. Winnicott (1949) and Bion (1962) both speak of 'a state of being' for the infant in the womb, a place where no action or response is needed, where everything is provided. For the mother too, pregnancy is a passive state of being. With the propulsion of birth, both mother and infant are forced to react and lose being, only to regain it again after birth. If there is trauma, the psychic pain is too severe, and the state of safe 'being together' is lost. Each of the mothers with a premature baby seemed to suffer the loss of equilibrium a great deal more and for longer than did the mothers of the full-term infants. One mother said:

> I have been moody all the time and I cry all the time. He [her partner] can't understand why I am crying all the time and it upsets him, and that makes me worse because I see him getting upset.

The dynamic between fullness and emptiness, the normal narcissism, of pregnancy is disturbed by prematurity

A baby's kick or movement reassures a pregnant woman that she is full of life. Some pregnant women speak of a sense of superiority and elation. Lemoine-Luccioni (1987) speaks of the woman's fullness as being full of 'penis? breast? baby? ... full of grace, blessed among women and blessed in the fruit of her womb'. The time after birth is a normal psychically depressed time. It is mourning the loss of the fullness. If the baby is healthy and feeding, it rivals the narcissistic loss of the fullness, and the reality of a thriving infant hopefully repays the mother adequately. She settles for her baby being outside her womb and experiences the intense sensitivity that goes with being vulnerable and separate (Lemoine-Luccioni 1987).

If the infant is premature and in an intensive care nursery, however, the mother's emotions become confused and unresolved. The healthy surrender of fullness is not replaced with a healthy living baby but with a very small, immature infant, with whom the mother has limited contact and fears to attach. There is real tragedy if the baby dies. There is a total narcissistic loss.

> I've got one photo of Jacky and that was taken 15 minutes after he was born, and I look at it all the time while I am expressing with the machine. He doesn't even look like that any more [crying].

> I touched her little hand and her little foot and, um, very tentatively of course. The next time I went to see her she went from lobster red into sort of suntan Bahamas glow, and then she had the little lights and the blindfoldy things. And she's been doing well and I've lost, ah well, I probably feel that I've lost a bit of the bonding process by not being conscious for this operation [the birth] and then not being able to hold her. I'm still thinking about when I have a baby. Then I think, 'hey! I've had one'.

It appears here that these mothers do not get a healthy baby to make up for the emptiness and replace the fullness. What they have is only a tenuous hold on a vulnerable infant, one whom they are not really sure they even have or will continue to have.

Primary maternal preoccupation: the dynamic between primary maternal protection and primary maternal persecution is disturbed by prematurity

In the inner world of archaic internal objects, opposites are ever present. There is the imago of a mother who will protect from all harm, be omnipotent in shielding the infant and be powerful in protecting the mother–infant duo. Also present is the fantasy of an evil mother who will rob the womb or kill the baby. There is a lack of control over what is growing inside her – it could be a Christ child or monster, living or dying, healthy or ill. Both idealising and negative forces may be projected onto her real mother, mother-in-law or husband. Neither is the fetus safe from projections. It may be seen in turn as the saviour of the family or as a foreign intruder ready to tear the mother's womb apart and endanger her life. These opposites of primary maternal persecution and primary maternal protection are dealt with by the mother in a stage towards the end of the pregnancy and immediately after birth known as primary maternal preoccupation. It is our understanding that the father also experiences this preoccupation, which, for him, includes the mother and the infant.

An infant born prematurely heightens the mother's fear of negative and persecutory forces, as though they are more powerful than her benign positive ones. The loss of the full-term healthy infant may well awaken a terror of what the 'bad' internal mother is capable of doing. This is sometimes projected onto the staff, with the feeling that they have stolen her baby. At other times, the 'bad' is projected back onto herself, with feelings that she deserves to have her baby taken since her womb was not 'good enough' to hold her infant to full term:

> I feel like I didn't make it. Like I let him down somehow. It makes me feel what I think they call postnatal depression. It's all been awful!

The dynamic between knowing and unknowing is disturbed by prematurity

A pregnant woman faces a very long period of unknowing. In the inexorable process of development, over which she has no influence, she must tolerate changes that are beyond her control. When her baby is born, she begins a dynamic process between knowing and not knowing her baby, a process that both parents will go through throughout their child's life. With prematurity, the unknowing takes over and fear freezes the capacity to dare to not know. Because of a lack of handling, mothers cannot even physically 'feel' that they are getting to know their baby, and dare not know the baby as theirs in an emotional sense until they are assured that the infant will live and is at home with them:

> I don't know that I had any maternal instinct before and I am short on it now for sure.

The dynamic between autonomy and deep dependency in pregnancy

There is a special autonomous space in which the mother and infant reside, the mature father being the protector of this space. An embryo is in an amniotic sac – in a mother's womb. Although the baby is in the mother, the baby has their own internal space. At birth, the infant is 'in the womb of the mother's mind' (Tustin 1981), because she thinks about and for that infant, who cannot think for itself. It is the mother's capacity to reflect on the infant's needs that keeps the infant in a psychic, safe holding place. By holding the infant in her mind, the mother protects them with her own psychic skin until the infant has a skin of their own.

Any intrusion on this is threatening. It destroys the infant's safe place in the mother's mind. An intrusion into this vulnerable womb/mind can cause psychic distress or psychic death, just as an intrusion on the fetus can cause distress or death. This can be seen most vividly in a premature infant hospital ward – the place is public, the holder is a humidicrib, and the feeder is a tube. The care-taker is not the mother but a ward team.

The dynamic between chaos and order is affected by prematurity

This dynamic is central to understanding the full extent of the trauma for the mother of a premature infant. The three main stages in a woman's life during which she experiences deep emotional and physical changes are the onset of puberty, pregnancy and menopause. In each of these, there is a maturational crisis marked by chaos. This chaos is a result of the surrender of the old order as it gives way to the new. From this chaos comes the push towards 'getting things right' in the new phase. Pines (1972) wrote thus of the third trimester of pregnancy:

> This stage is marked by bodily discomfort and fatigue. There is a need for mothering. There are characteristic mood swings from pleasure at the imminent possibility of her baby's reality to unconscious anxiety that either she or the baby may die at birth. However strongly the outside world reassures her, the anxieties persist and there can be revivals of old guilts about whether she can produce anything good or not.

The preoccupation of this final trimester is so great and so intense that were it not for the baby, the mother would be considered insane (Winnicott 1956). Those at risk, even if they are emotionally well, are the mothers and fathers of premature infants in neonatal intensive care units (NICUs). The preoccupation may become heightened and extended, or it may be blocked out altogether. The mother of the premature infant in NICU does not know who she is or at what stage she is – whether she is pregnant, has given birth, is a mother, is not a mother; the confusion is terrible. This is often made worse because she may well have been unconscious during the birth and therefore not have 'had' the birth. For the mother of a healthy full-term infant, the inward-turning in late pregnancy and the first weeks of her infant's life has the quality of a depressive state that is quite different from that of postnatal depression. With the mothers of infants in NICU, the depression becomes much more severe and entrenched, and cannot be processed for sometimes months or years after the infant has recovered. The foundation between mother/father and infant is severely intruded on. Here is a typical quote:

> I had been in hospital for two weeks with high blood pressure. So I had the caesarian ... I wasn't getting any sleep and my blood pressure was really high.

So that was quite stressful and my blood pressure didn't come down after the birth like they said it probably would. So they cut my tablets down and then I just wasn't getting any sleep, I was so I was worried about myself and worried about the baby. It's a terrible time. It was more not being in control of your feelings, and I think it was just made worse because I wasn't that well. I was worried about my blood pressure and they kept saying it should come down and it didn't, and then, yeah I don't know, the postnatal depression, you can't describe it. It's just you're just in tears all the time for no reason.

In pregnancy, a woman is born again as a mother. One of the most satisfying emotions of pregnancy is the identification with an omnipotent, fertile, life-giving mother. She experiences herself as maturing to become a mother in her own right. She is now a physiologically mature woman, impregnated by her sexual partner and powerful enough to create life within herself and to hold it (Pines 1978). If she cannot hold her baby and her womb is, in her mind, 'not good enough' (a mother's words), her image of herself is fractured. Pines adds that, for the pregnant woman, there may be rivalrous feelings towards her mother and a desire at the same time to be like her. There might be gratitude that she is able to be a mother and a fear of this being taken from her. As Pines (1978) writes:

> These are not always either-or, such paradoxes and ambivalence can occur in a short space of time, or even coexist during pregnancy. It is not the absence of, but the mediation of these dialectics that allows a woman to become a mother.

How difficult that resolution is with prematurity.

Conclusion

It is the 'spaced out' initial shock of the trauma of the prematurity and the fracturing of the mother image and father image that stands out most when a pregnancy is prematurely ruptured. This chapter highlights how normal it is for a pregnant woman to feel cheated of her full pregnancy and birth, and the closeness of her infant to her after birth, by prematurity. There is a painful sense of loss in separating from her baby before they are psychologically and physically ready. For me, it was not their emotions or words but the absence of any appropriate affect that made their suffering so obvious.

References

Benedek T (1952) Psychosexual Functions in Women. New York: Ronald Press.
Bibring GL (1959) Some considerations of the psychological processes in pregnancy. In Eissler RS, Freud A, Hartmann H et al (Eds) The Psychoanalytical Study of the Child, Volume 14. New York: International Universities Press.

Bibring GL, Dwyer TF, Huntington DS, Valenstein AF (1961) A study of the psychological processes in pregnancy and of the earliest mother–child relationship. I: Some propositions and comments. II: Methodological considerations. In Eissler RS, Freud A, Hartmann H et al (Eds) Psychoanalytic Study of the Child, Volume 16. New York: International Universities Press.

Bion WR (1977) Learning from Experience. London: Heinemann.

Deutsch H (1945) The Psychology of Women, Volume 2. New York: Grune & Stratton.

Feder L (1980) Preconceptive ambivalence and external reality. International Journal of Psychoanalysis 61: 161–78.

Freud S (1909) Some general remarks on hysterical attacks. CP II, 100. SE IX: The Standard Edition of the Complete Psychological Works of Sigmund Freud (1980). London: Hogarth Press/Institute of Psychoanalysis.

Kaplan DM, Mason EA (1960) Maternal reaction to premature birth viewed as an acute emotional disorder. American Journal of Orthopsychiatry 30: 539–52.

Kerstenberg JS (1956) On the development of maternal feelings in early childhood. Observations and reflections. In Eissler RS, Freud A, Hartmann H et al (Eds) Psychoanalytic Study of the Child, Volume 11. New York: International Universities Press.

Lemoine-Luccioni E (1987) The Dividing of Woman or Woman's Lot. London: Free Association Books.

Ogden TH (1985) On potential space. International Journal of Psychoanalysis 66: 130–1.

Pines D (1972) Pregnancy and motherhood. Interaction between fantasy and reality. British Journal of Medical Psychology 45: 333–43

Pines D (1978) On becoming a parent. Journal of Child Psychotherapy 4(4): 19–31.

Pines D (1982) The relevance of early psychic development to pregnancy and abortion. International Journal of Psychoanalysis 63: 311–19.

Raphael-Leff J (1982) Psychotherapeutic needs of mothers to be. Journal of Child Psychotherapy 8: 3–13.

Tustin F (1981) Psychological birth and psychological catastrophe. In Grotstein JS (Ed.) Dare I Disturb the Universe (1983 edition). London: Caesura Press.

Winnicott DW (1952) Anxiety Associated with Insecurity. Through Paediatrics to Psychoanalysis. London: Hogarth Press/Institute of Psychoanalysis.

Winnicott DW (1956) Primary maternal preoccupation. In Through Paediatrics to Psychoanalysis (1958 edition). London: Hogarth Press/Institute of Psychoanalysis.

Chapter 4
Prematurity and the dynamics of birth

Norma Tracey

In this chapter, I will consider the mother of the premature infant during the actual birth process and the period after birth, when her infant is cared for on a neonatal intensive care ward. Both Winnicott (1949) and Tustin (1983) have written that birth too sudden and too soon can produce an extreme sense of paranoia in the infant. I propose that this paranoid 'psychotic-like' state is also produced in the mother. A pattern of unexpected interference with basic 'being' is imposed on infant and mother, and the autonomy of the mother–infant unit is ruptured.

Labour and delivery

A normal full-term labour and delivery constitute an acute crisis for a new mother and father and their infant. Mahler (1958), speaking of the mother as well as the infant, says:

> The process of human birth actually does combine some of these opposites of life and death. It probably does involve something of a blackout, an apparent almost complete interruption in the life of the organism but one through which a new arrangement of organismic energy is affected.

Bibring (1959) and Bibring et al (1961) say that, for the mother, there is initially both acute physiological and psychological disequilibrium, and it may take months for the latter to subside and for the mother's personality to reintegrate to include her new role as a mother. Benedek (1952, 1959) writes that the likelihood of a favourable resolution of the maturational crisis of motherhood is increased when the pregnancy has induced feelings of enjoyment and enhances the woman's sense of well-being, and this enjoyment will also affect the extent to which the mother experiences love and acceptance of her baby after delivery.

Prematurity places a great strain on the resolution of this process. Stern (1995) writes that the new mother, and to some extent the father, passes into a unique stage of life with a new set of tendencies, sensibilities, fantasies, fears and wishes. He calls this new organisation of mental life 'the motherhood constellation'. Our proposition in this chapter is that the motherhood constellation is seriously distorted by prematurity.

Here are some of the mothers' reports of the trauma of birth.

One mother, speaking of the central line said:

> He tried and tried on both arms, and he couldn't get it in. Because of the pneumonia I couldn't lay down. He ended up putting it in my chest with a local anaesthetic. I kept saying to the Sister, 'Oh please! Is it over yet?' I was terrified he was going to lie me down because I knew once I was laid down I couldn't breathe and I was dead.

> I had this really bad headache and I couldn't go to sleep. So next day I went to the hospital and my blood pressure was up. They transferred me straight away and they told me, 'We are going to deliver you straight away.' I thought, 'He's gonna come dead or something' [bursts into tears]. Like when I saw him I couldn't believe it, because I was only 30 weeks pregnant, and I cried, because I was relieved he was alive because the doctors said, 'We will give you an epidural so you can see him because he'll probably come you know, dead'. I didn't expect it, the birth, I didn't expect it – I just had this headache.

This was repeated six times during this interview and again in subsequent ones, as was the whole story of the birth as this mother struggled to come to terms with it.

> The next day they came and they told me, 'We are going to deliver you in the evening'. No one was there, only me. I was the only one that knew. I got such a shock, I called my husband. The whole family got a shock, everybody got a shock, I mean how could it happen so fast!

The mother experiences a painful sense of loss in separating from her baby before they are psychologically and physically ready. It also places an immense strain on the father in a way that no full-term birth is likely to do. Because of the cost of the birth on the mother, the father is often the primary initial bonder with the infant. There is, for the parents, a sense of things being out of their control. The mother feels hurled into motherhood before either she or baby are ready. In some ways, she is also deprived of motherhood – here is a very small baby with a tenuous hold on life and she, as his mother, is unable to carry, directly feed or protect him. She depends on other people and machines for his life. She may feel guilty for not holding him to full term but also angry and disappointed at the intrusion of the whole medical ward into the privacy of their life together.

Caesarean section

Many of the infants in neonatal intensive care units are not only premature, but also born by caesarean section. Trowell (1982) reported that
mothers who had given birth by caesarean section expressed more anxiety
and apprehension about parenthood and its responsibilities. One month
after the birth, they felt more depression, more resentment of the fathers
and more anxiety concerning somatic symptoms. One year after the birth,
these mothers generally complained more about their child than did
mothers from the control group, and thought that they had experienced
more problems with their child and themselves during the year. Their
labours were longer and they had more medication before and after
delivery, as well as being unconscious at the time of delivery. It is interesting to note that these were mothers of full-term infants. We suggest that
it is worse for the mother of the premature infant, for she does not even
have an infant with her to demonstrate the worthwhile nature of what she
has gone through.

The birth

Lewis (1976) saw the happiness of a successful birth as the celebration of a
'victory of life over death'. I suggest that such a victory is not experienced
by the mother whose infant is rushed to intensive care. Since the baby is
still at serious risk of death, there is as yet no victory. Even with survival,
the mother is unsure whether victory is hers or whether she is a failure,
and the staff, having saved the baby's life, are the 'victors'.

For many mothers, with the birth comes a kind of ecstasy. Meltzer
(1987) writes of truth, beauty, awe, wonder and joy as being present for
both mother and infant. These emotions are, of course, not present for all
mothers, but they seem to be more absent for the mother of the premature infant, and she may feel 'robbed' of all of this and in a way 'robbed' of
her infant too:

> Everyone asks me, 'How does it feel to be a mother?' I don't know. I don't have
> a baby with me. I don't even know if I have had a baby. I've got this beautiful
> baby's room all ready, but there isn't a baby in it.

I wondered whether this mother was really meaning the room in her
womb or, more ominously, the room in her mind for the baby.

The mother of the healthy full-term baby initially falls in love with not
only the infant *per se*, but also the potential of what they are to become
(Meltzer 1987). If this potential is intruded on by illness or the danger of
death, the mother is devastated. Meltzer adds that the general qualities of
a baby – the proportions, helplessness, vulnerability, delicacy of texture

and colouring and family resemblance – have a universal impact, but most important is the absence of blemish or damage. The mother of the premature infant often does not find her baby beautiful, and she rarely describes her experience of motherhood as satisfying, feeling terror in place of wonderment:

> I was like a Dracula or something all swollen up, like I really was a monster, and they had to take my baby away from me. I knew he was on the next floor, but with the drip in I couldn't move. I was crying all the time and I didn't know if it was for him or for me. I thought if I look like a monster, what does the baby look like? Why can't I get to see him? Is he a monster?

In the next interview, this subject spent the whole time in black silence. She was not only enraged, but also stunned. I could only think how different she was from the full-term mother I had seen that same week who could not stop talking with the excitement of it all, laughing as she said to me, 'Do you think everyone else knows this is the most beautiful baby in the world, or am I the only one that knows?'.

The mother's relationship with her infant is distorted by prematurity

The task that a young woman has in motherhood is to integrate reality with unconscious fantasy, hopes and daydreams. After birth, there is a long period of adjustment for any mother and her infant. The actual physical separation leaves the mother, whose body has sheltered her baby for nine months, with a feeling of emptiness. She reconciles herself with being separate and alone again. She moves between emotional fusion with her baby, as if they were still one unit, and learning to recognise him as a separate individual and part of the outside world. Such a paradoxical and complicated process may take days, weeks or months to complete.

One of the main supports for the mother at this crucial time is that her baby is well. The vital elements of bodily contact and smell, which are a normal part of every intimate relationship, are essential to the new mother's bonding with her real baby. This physical contact is denied to her when her baby is in a humidicrib. Even when she is able to nurse her baby, she is put off by the equipment attached to the baby's body and the public place in which she is expected to be intimate and private with her baby. Those parents of premature infants who had the best outcomes in previous studies were those who maintained contact with their infants while on the ward. They felt more empowered and more involved in the recovery of their baby.

I think I missed out on a lot not having her put on my tummy after birth and straight to the breast, but I really feel close to her now. I have nursed her twice, and changed her nappy once. There is something magic about touching such a little thing like that, like putting your hand into the womb and touching the baby inside there.

It's a totally medical environment down there. Mixture of everything as far as procedures go – throbbing machines and lots of graphs and all that sort of thing. I got a Texta and I said, 'Can I write her name down?' and they said, 'Yes', and it helped. Once I wrote her name, I felt I wasn't scared to touch her.

There are times when I forget that I am a mother. I mean, how does a mother know she is a mother? Because she has a baby around her. I had a sort of period yesterday and I thought period means ovulation, ovulation means fertility. Then I thought, how come I'm thinking of having a baby and being fertile? I've got a baby, but you see I haven't got a baby.

The actuality of a birth brings reality to the parents. Their dreams are easily modified and accepted when the real baby is close to what they dreamt of, but when the discrepancy is too great, as can sometimes be the case in prematurity, it is as if the dream is shattered. Menzies-Lyth (1976) writes that:

> for the mother of a full-term healthy infant there is the pleasure of anticipation and the fulfilment of long desired wishes, and a pride in such an overwhelming adult achievement, which must now be measured against the realities of parenthood, and their accompanying frustrations, worries and disappointments.

The imbalance is never more poignant than for the parents of an infant prematurely removed from mother's womb and sustained in an artificial place somewhere between the womb and birth. The beginnings are truly awful.

Inner world processes to do with a new mother's identity with her own mother are affected by prematurity

In pregnancy, a woman's rivalry with her mother is heightened. There may be anger with her mother for making her a woman, ambivalently coupled with gratitude to her mother for her womanhood and a great desire to emulate her. Past conflicts with her mother that are unresolved may return to affect the balance, but when there is prematurity and real danger, the balance is truly lost.

For the new young mother of the premature infant, there is a fear of not having her good internal mother's love and support; there is an unconscious fear that her internal mother will take her baby in revengeful reprisal for anger experienced towards her mother during pregnancy or adolescence or any other time during childhood (Pines 1982). For the new mother, the birth of a healthy infant has a massive impact on her identity with her own mother, and she sees herself as another healthy and capable child-bearer. It is her final step of separating out from her mother as she is herself now a successful mother. If her baby is in any way damaged or ill, she struggles with a sense of being inferior to her mother, of failing to measure up to her, of somehow even failing to measure up to womanhood or motherhood in general. Internal conflicts become exaggerated and seem to be the cause of her infant's illness (Lax 1972):

> I was alone. My mother came in when I called her and said, 'They want to take the baby now, and it will probably be born dead'. My mother cried and I cried too.
>
> I only have half a womb and I was born like that. My mother caused it, and it caused the prematurity. It's like I have to suffer for something she did to me for the whole of my life. No! Feelings are not very friendly between us to say the least.

For this grandmother, it was also a time of distress:

> I couldn't help blaming my daughter. 'What had she done?', I kept thinking, holding her responsible, blaming her. She was always a bit of a ratbag. 'I could have done it better than her' kept running through my head. These were awful thoughts and I was ashamed of having them but they were there.

The new father

For the new father, it is no less terrifying. In pregnancy, a woman needs internally to accept the fetus as a representation of her sexual partner, both physically and mentally. When something goes wrong, she does not present him with a healthy narcissistic image of himself but with a mirroring of his own fears of being damaged. His terrifying internal imagos of a punishing father are also alive and disturbing at this time. Any guilts from childhood about sexuality are reawakened. All sorts of convoluted patterns may appear. If the infant is impaired in any way or there is a threat to their life, the father's protective capacity is challenged. He may identify with their infant as weak, vulnerable and hurting. He may feel angry with the infant for showing up his deficiencies. His own confusion about what to do, and having to place his family in the care of specialists, can further add to his sense of failure. He particularly suffers from the fact that the focus of the world is all too often sympathetic towards the mother and he is expected to cope regardless:

There was something dangerous about the whole situation. The baby was not getting enough oxygen. I asked the doctor whether it was the baby or my wife. He was quite open, he said, 'It's your wife'. Of course, I was thinking the worst. I had been thinking negatively anyhow. If something went wrong, they were both at risk, but now it was my wife who was the higher risk. I held my wife's hand while the doctor got the baby out. She had an epidural. I was actually watching him pulling out the baby by the feet and his head was still stuck in there. It looked like the head was getting in a bit of trouble, and I was caught between looking down at my wife and looking up to see what the doctor was doing with my son. He came out so blue and I remember thinking, 'No one told me! Are babies born blue?'.

My wife gave birth at seven months – her blood pressure was extremely high. There was some disappointment with doctors and the medical system, my own self as well: I was very disappointed I didn't read the signs a bit earlier. My wife had some swelling, but we always thought and had been told it was quite a normal thing in pregnancy. The swelling increased over the next weekend to a point where, I would say, she wasn't recognisable. They admitted her to our own hospital then rushed her to this specialist hospital for pregnant women that same night. Everybody got a shock. I think the biggest shock was how could things happen so fast. I started questioning the system, whether a person in her situation should have been examined a bit more often, or whether just some freakish situation happened to my wife. My immediate feelings then were a fear for both my wife and my child. To be quite honest, I was really worried, wondering whether one of them would not survive this extreme situation.

So often with a premature infant, the father's role changes considerably. If the premature baby is in a different hospital from the mother, the father will be the one to keep close and direct contact with the baby. He has the burden of supporting and emotionally carrying his wife. He has the discussions with doctors and hospital staff. He has the preoccupation with the survival of his infant. During this crisis, there can be an intense sense of ownership, of bonding by the father. The mother may be too terrified to bond with an infant who may die, or she may experience the infant as also having failed her. The father has to be available for her feelings to the sacrifice of his own.

A maternally sensitive period fractured by prematurity

Winnicott (1956) formulated the term 'primary maternal preoccupation' to describe the mother's intense involvement during the early days before birth and the weeks after birth: 'It gradually develops and becomes a state of heightened sensitivity during and especially towards the end of pregnancy. It lasts for a few weeks after the birth of the child'. The term 'sensitive period' generally implies that an individual's characteristics can be more strongly influenced by a single event at one stage of development than at any other stage (Bateson 1979). One aspect of a sensitive period is that it is a time of rapid organisation, when a developing individual is more easily de-established by deprivation or disturbance of any kind. We feel that this concept is central to our thesis and that such a normally sensitive period is made much worse with the crisis and trauma of prematurity.

Primary maternal preoccupation in the mother provides a protective shield around the infant to hold them from overstimulation resulting from external world impingements, overstimulation caused by his/her own excitation at the workings of his/her own body, and overstimulation from being exposed to the mother's inner world emotionality. This shield is fractured when the mother feels that she has failed to carry her infant to full term (James 1960). When there is trauma associated with a premature birth and the infant is admitted to a neonatal ward with a fear of death or damage, all the mother's preoccupation about protecting her infant from harm, from pain, from discomfort and from destructiveness seems to her to have failed. She seems incapable of being the protector of her infant and may well feel that she is 'bad' for her baby. Sometimes she carries the guilt for her normal negative ambivalence and feels that she has caused this. Her preoccupation becomes fixated or avoided and denied, and her contact with her infant is severely affected.

Stern writes of the mother's need to transform and reorganise her self-identity in the new constellation of motherhood. In essence, the new mother must shift her centre of identity from daughter to mother, from wife to parent, from careerist to matron, from one generation to the subsequent one. Some mothers of premature infants whom we saw seemed to be overinvested and involved or even settled in these identity tasks, but to our surprise this did not hold.

Alia heroically struggled to establish feeding and seemed certain to continue once she did so. However, without external reason, she just decided to give up and overnight put her baby on the bottle. When the interviewer gently asked what had prompted her to do this, she seemed not to know. A little later she seemed unable to separate from her infant at all and had him by her bedside at night and with her in the same room all day. Suddenly, she told the interviewer that she was going back to work 'next Monday': her mother would mind the baby and 'would do it much better'. When Alia had a full-term infant a year later, she telephoned the interviewer saying, 'I'm staying home with this one'. Why had she become pregnant straight away when she could not take care of this baby, or did she fantasise that she did not have it? This is only surmising, but this cut-out, which reminds one of the 'infants with insecure attachment' in attachment research (see, for example Ainsworth et al 1978, Main and Weston 1982), seemed to be present in the mothers.

Jane, who could not even go to the toilet without her baby, left her at eight weeks and went back to work, to her husband's amazement and displeasure. The older mother, who had seemed so thrilled after years of infertility, went back to full-time familiar work almost immediately. In contrast, the mothers of the full-term infants struggled and discussed and worked out with great difficulty whether to stay home and for how long. All the mothers of the premature infants had begun work, either full or part time, by the time the infants were six weeks old. Were they repeating the dislocation occurring at birth? Was this part of the psychic split experienced by the trauma? Had something important to do with their confidence been seriously dislocated? Were they too angry to bond satisfactorily? Was the price they paid for being a mother too high? Did they flee from being too close and risk losing? Did they have no faith in themselves as mothers and feel that others could do it better? Were they punishing the infant, or in their fantasy saving him or her from themselves? I could not properly answer this multitude of questions. Although this is such a small sample, it fitted the experiences of the ward social workers and my own previous experiences over the years, and certainly demonstrated the dislocation of the preoccupation, with a flight into reality.

Depression, mourning and melancholia in the mother

Klein (1948) presented the dynamic of a constant struggle between an irrepressible urge to destroy one's objects and a desire to preserve them. Prematurity affects a mother's belief that her 'life-giving' capacity may not be as great as her capacity to destroy. Such a fantasy is terrifying to the mother. She fears that her own destructiveness has made the infant ill or has come from outside herself as a punishment for her sexuality or rivalry with her mother. As early as 1953, Bibring gave a definition of depression as being:

> due to an intrapsychic, systemic (that is, tension caused in the ego itself) ego conflict, which occurs whenever the ego experiences a shocking awareness of its helplessness in regard to its aspirations.

A mother may think that the infant demonstrates to the outside world her own inferiority as a mother.

The loss of healthy narcissism at such an early stage is a critical blow. The impaired infant represents the mother's infantile damaged self. The mother feels that the infant she has created is an image of what she most fears she herself is, that is, sick and damaged. She seeks answers to unanswerable questions such as, 'What have I done to deserve this?', 'What is wrong with me to have given birth to an infant like this?' and 'What did I do to cause it?'. In the unconscious, there is a forbidden wish to have an infant with the father, a wish to be a boy and not a girl, a hatred towards the mother for depriving her by making her a woman. All of these may awaken as living proof of her guilt. The premature infant's instinctive equipment for fixing on the mother and locating her is absent or impaired so he/she cannot hold out any evidence of health through his/her responsiveness to his/her mother in these early days. The mother's own responses are dealt a severe blow through having inadequate physical contact with the infant.

'When the infant feels he exists in the mother's mind then together they can explore and discover the world' (Reid 1990). Many of the mothers of premature infants we initially interviewed seemed 'mindless' of their infants. For a woman, birth is a paradox of dependency and power. The baby is a woman's gift to her partner and their parents. This gift acknowledges her partner's contribution to her fulfilment as a mother. How devastating it must be for her to see her gift as impaired and to feel herself as having brought grief instead of joy. Pregnant women have fantasies of the baby they wish to deliver. These include the wish for a perfect child and the fear of having a damaged child (Solnit and Stark 1961).

Mourning the loss of the 'perfect' baby takes a lifetime, the parents being compensated by the presence of a 'good enough' one. This compensation is markedly delayed when the baby is in intensive care and the issue is one of survival rather than being good enough. Kaplan and Mason (1960) describe four very distinct stages through which a mother needs to go in order to recover from a premature baby in crisis:

1. anticipatory grief linked to anticipating the fear that the infant may die;
2. a feeling of having failed;
3. a resumption of the process of relating to the infant;
4. an understanding of the needs of very low birthweight infants.

Kaplan and Mason's study of parents' reactions to the birth of preterm infants suggests that the absence of grief rather than high grief may be an ominous sign of impending family disorganisation and conflict.

Affect of prematurity on normal maternal and paternal narcissism

The mother and father's acute awareness of their incapacity and helplessness, caused by the illness of their infant, results in a partial or complete collapse of their positively cathected self-image.

Lax (1972) writes that the severity of the depressive reaction in the mother depends on the extent to which the mother unconsciously perceives her child as an externalisation of her defective self. Lax further states that the overprotective and oversolicitous smothering of the infant or the neglectful indifferent attitude is the opposite means that a mother uses to cope with the hostile and frequently murderous impulses that are harboured towards the 'defective' infant. This in turn reflects unconscious feelings of self-hatred, which are projected onto the infant as an unconscious negatively cathected self-image representation. Guilt may be a result of this. Since the unconscious maternal attitude is introjected into the infant's sense of self, such a beginning may well be crucial to the unconscious nucleus of the infant's basic personality. It is further documented that depressed mothers are more likely to behave insensitively towards their infants, in a hostile and intrusive manner or with detached withdrawal (Cohn et al 1986).

Developmental outcomes for children with unresponsive and depressed mothers have been found to be disturbed in the cognitive and affective domains (Cox et al 1987). This is a matter of special concern for children who may already be at developmental risk from biological conditions.

Depression is not an uncommon state in mothers experiencing difficult life events or postpartum endocrinological changes. Untoward events associated with the child's birth may also have an impact on the quality of the mother–infant interaction. This was demonstrated by Field et al (1985), who also found associations between mothers' depression and their interaction with their infants. Mothers and infants who have experienced serious perinatal complications are often at cumulative risks of a compromise to normal development. The interactions of these mothers of atypical infants may be influenced by depressive symptoms (Field et al 1988). In most studies, the mother's responsiveness to her infant was more strongly associated with the mother's self-rapport or depression than with either the child's degree of risk or maternal cognitive skills. Depressive symptoms were the only variable to have an independent negative effect on the mother's interaction.

The survival of the mother–infant couple in prematurity

Perhaps the greatest threat to the health of the mother–infant coupling is the distortion of the normal psychic events of this early birth stage to do with fusion and individuation. Margaret Little has developed the idea of basic unity – 'primary total undifferentiatedness' – occurring between

mother and infant in the first few weeks of an infant's life. She gives
clinical evidence of adults who cannot in any circumstances take survival
for granted if this basic unity has been disrupted. In their unconscious
exists what she defines as terror of annihilation.

Bion (1962) writes that there has in many cases been, in early infancy,
some actual threat to life, such as illness in the infant or mother, hostility
in the environment or psychological catastrophe or disaster. There is a
constant need for both mother and infant to return to basic unity even
though there is also a fear of being immersed or lost in the other. The
boundaries of self and non-self are blurred in the earliest post-birth states.
The infant continues a postnatal existence that, through his mother's
protective care, is very much a continuation of the prenatal situation.
Premature psychological birth constitutes a catastrophe. Oceanic feelings
from the womb linger on after birth. If these early oceanic illusions are
prematurely interrupted, or if the physical birth has been a difficult one,
the psychological birth may also be disrupted (Tustin 1981a, Field et al
1988, Als 1989).

Margaret Mahler writes about how the vulnerable infant, after birth, is
readily thrown into affectomotor storm rage reactions that, if not relieved
by the mother's ministrations, may result in a state of organismic distress
of a most dreadful kind. As a result of this homoeostatic insufficiency, the
young infant may exhaust their life energy and lapse into a kind of semi-
stupor reminiscent of their fetal existence. Tustin adds quite clearly,
'Landmarks of fragmentation of the ego are traumatisations through
sickness or separation'. The intrusions in neonatal intensive care, with all
the equipment and all the tests, seem to fit this kind of description. This is
indeed a dismal image.

The work of Heidi Als (1997) and Tiffany Field (1996) gives testimony
to the need to consider the comfort and homeostasis of the infant at this
time. Mahler clearly defines how bodily contact with the mother, such as
cuddling, is an integral prerequisite to the demarcation of the body ego
from the non-self within the range of somatopsychic symbiosis of the
mother–infant unity. The ward staff's capacity to involve the mother and
father obviouly plays a significant role here.

References

Ainsworth DMS, Blehar MC, Waters E, Walls W (1978) Patterns of Attachment: A
    Psychological Study of the Strange Situation. Hillsdale, NJ: Lawrence Erlbaum
    Associates.
Als H (1989) Neurobiology of early infant behaviour. In Von Euler Fonsberglagercrantz
    (Ed.) Continuity and Consequences of Behaviour in Preterm Infants. Stockholm:
    Stockholm Press/Macmillan.

Bateson P (1979) How do senstitive periods arise and what are they for? Animal Behaviour 27: 470–86.

Benedek T (1952) Psychosexual Functions in Women. New York: Ronald Press.

Benedek T (1959) Parenthood as a developmental phase. Journal of the American Psychoanalytic Association 7: 3898–417.

Bibring E (1953) The mechanism of depression. In Greenacre P (Ed.) Affective Disorders. New York: International Universities Press.

Bibring GL (1959) Some considerations of the psychological processes in pregnancy. In Eissler RS, Freud A, Hartmann H et al (Eds) The Psychoanalytical Study of the Child, Volume 14. New York: International Universities Press.

Bibring GL, Dwyer TF, Huntington DS, Valenstein AF (1961) A study of the psychological processes in pregnancy and of the earliest mother–child relationship. I: Some propositions and comments. II: Methodological considerations. In Eissler RS, Freud A, Hartmann H et al (Eds) Psychoanalytic Study of the Child, Volume 16. New York: International Universities Press.

Bion WR (1962) Learning from Experience. London: Heinemann.

Bion WR (1963) Elements of Psychoanalysis. London: Heinemann.

Cohn J, Matias R, Tronick E, Connell D, Lyons-Ruth K (1986) Face-to-face interactions of depressed mothers and their infants. In Tronick E, Field T (Eds) Maternal Depression and Infant Disturbance: New Directions for Child Development, Volume 36. San Francisco: Jossey-Bass.

Cox AD, Puckering C, Pound A et al (1987) The impact of maternal depression in young children. Journal of Child Psychology and Psychiatry 28: 917–28.

Field T, Sandberg D, Garcia R, Vega-Lahr N, Goldstein S, Guy L (1985) Pregnancy problems, postpartum depression and early mother–infant interactions. Developmental Psychology 21: 1152–6.

Field T, Healy B, Goldstein S et al (1988) Infants of depressed mothers show 'depressed' behaviour even with non-depressed adults. Child Development 59: 1569–79.

James M (1960) Premature ego development: some observations on disturbances in the first three months of life. International Journal of Psychoanalysis 41: 222–94.

Kaplan DM, Mason EA (1960) Maternal reaction to premature birth viewed as an acute emotional disorder. American Journal of Orthopsychiatry 30: 539–52.

Klein M (1948) On the Theory of Anxiety and Guilt, and Envy and Gratitude and Other Works 1946–1963 (1975 edition). London: Hogarth Press/Institute of Psychoanalysis.

Lax RF (1972) Some aspects of the interaction between mother and impaired child; mother's narcissistic trauma. International Journal of Psychoanalysis 53: 339–45.

Lewis E (1976) The atmosphere in the labour ward. Journal of Child Psychotherapy 21(2): 89–92.

Mahler MS (1958) Autism and symbiosis: two extreme disturbances of identity. International Journal of Psychoanalysis 39: 77–83.

Main M, Weston DR (1982) Avoidance of the attachment figure in infancy: descriptions and interpretations. In Parkes CM, Stevenson-Hinde J (Eds) The Place of Attachment in Human Behaviour. New York: Basic Books.

Meltzer D (1987) On aesthetic reciprocity. Journal of Child Psychotherapy 13(2): 3–15.

Menzies-Lyth I (1976) Thoughts on maternal role in contemporary society. Journal of Child Psychotherapy 12(1): 5–14.

Pines D (1982) The relevance of early psychic development to pregnancy and abortion. International Journal of Psychoanalysis 63: 311–19.

Reid S (1990) The importance of beauty in the psychoanalytic experience. Journal of Child Psychotherapy 16(1): 29–51.

Solnit AJ, Stark MH (1961) Mourning the death of a defective child. In Eissler RS, Freud A, Hartmann H et al (Eds) Psychoanalytic Study of the Child, Volume 16. New York: International Universities Press.

Stern DN(1995) The Motherhood Constellation. New York: Basic Books.

Trowell J (1982) Effects of obstetric management on the mother–child relationship. In Parkes CM, Stevenson-Hinde J (Eds) The Place of Attachment in Human Behaviour. London: Tavistock.

Tustin F (1981a) Psychological birth and psychological catastrophe. In Grotstein JS (Ed.) Dare I Disturb the Universe? (1983 edition) London: Caesura Press.

Tustin F (1983) Psychological birth and psychological catastrophe. In Grotstein J (Ed.) Do I Dare Disturb the Universe? London: Marsefield Reprints.

Winnicott DW (1949) Birth memories, birth trauma and anxiety. In Collected Papers: Through Paediatrics to Psychoanalysis. London: Hogarth Press/Institute of Psychoanalysis. London.

Winnicott DW (1956) Primary maternal preoccupation. In Collected Papers: Through Paediatrics to Psychoanalysis. London: Hogarth Press/Tavistock Institute of Psychoanalysis.

Chapter 5
Narrative of a mother of a premature infant

NORMA TRACEY, PETER BLAKE, PAM SHEIN,
BEULAH WARREN, SYLVIA ENFIELD AND HELEN HARDY

This chapter asks, 'What happens in a mother's inner world when her infant is in an incubator instead of in her womb?'. For a mother with an infant in neonatal intensive care, there is a continuous struggle towards motherhood. While the survival of her infant is a remarkable medical achievement, there are serious interruptions to her maternal preoccupation with her infant. This chapter presents what we observed happening in the inner world of one mother – Deedie – while her baby was in a humidicrib.

The group of professionals working with parents and infants met for two hours each fortnight for 18 months listening to Deedie's nine audiotaped interviews. Because of limitations of space, only pertinent sections of each of the nine interviews are included here.

These nine interviews with Deedie initially took place weekly after her baby was born, and later fortnightly, the final interview being one month after that. The baby was 12 weeks old and at home by the time of the last interview.

The interviewer knows that Deedie is married and has a baby girl born at 24 weeks, weighing 642 g. The reason for the early birth is purposely unknown to the interviewer; she will learn it from Deedie. She knows that Deedie is a diabetic and that the infant is likely to do well. Here is Deedie's own narrative, along with a discussion of its content.

Interview 1

From the start I was pretty excited because I had a miscarriage about twelve months ago and I was hoping that everything would go all right with this baby. I've had some pretty terrible experiences over the last three weeks before the baby was born.

I came into the hospital for a couple of days because I started having pains and they stopped of their own accord and I was discharged, and then two days later I was readmitted because I contracted pneumonia and I couldn't breathe properly or anything. I was downstairs on Hunter 6 South [a hospital ward]. From there I progressively got worse and the antibiotics were not working, so they took me across the road to the main hospital for intensive care treatment in ICU. I was there for three days and then they brought me back to acute care in the maternity wing in Duncan 7 West for one shift of eight hours and I was just slowly getting worse and worse, so they took me back over to the Intensive Care Unit and I was there for a few hours, and that's when the doctor turned up and decided to do the emergency caesarean. That was on the 26th August about 5.00 pm.

From there, after the operation, they took me straight back to intensive care, and they expected me to be on the ventilation machine for three weeks. I was lucky that I recovered so quickly and was only on it for two days. For the first couple of days I was pretty much out of it and unconscious for about the first 36 hours. I really didn't wake up until Saturday morning; that's when they removed the ventilation and feeding tube. That Saturday they trolleyed me over the road to here so I could see my baby for the first time in the nursery. Bill came over on the Thursday night and had seen her. I was then moved to Brighton 10 East and this is where I am now.

Deedie is short, shaky and breathless. As she talks, her whole body is involuntarily tremulous. The interviewer experiences her as unemotional, cut off and monotonally dull. It seems paradoxical that she seems deadened but her whole body is shaking and she has difficulty breathing. In our group discussion, we think about her clinging to facts and about how her language is in a strange way like a doctor's report on ward round. It is as if she is reporting on someone else. We ask, 'Is she in a fragmented state and so holding desperately to facts, like a false skin?'. Perhaps, in her traumatised mind, language has no emotional meaning for her.

This phenomenon of reporting facts in detail and without affect, as if reporting someone else's story, was obvious in the first interview with each mother of a premature infant in the project. In every case, the language was stilted, was not syntonic with themselves and had an identical ring to it regardless of culture.

The interviewer documented immediately after Deedie's first session that she felt Deedie could not 'find her baby'. The group asks, 'Had the mother in her mind not yet had a baby? Or perhaps not re-found it after birth? Or was she fused with the baby?'. One of the group gives us the thought that maybe Deedie is the baby, and shows how much her absolute dependence mirrors exactly the plight of the newborn in the humidicrib. Like the newborn, she is dependent on others for her life. She has been 'near death', she shakes like a newborn and is having trouble ventilating. (Her infant was on a ventilator just as she has been.)

In our discussion, we wondered about the strength of the denial in her saying 'really good'. Her baby still weighs 624 g and is far from over the worst. Deedie has idealised and projected life into her baby. The deadness is in her. Like the other mothers interviewed, Deedie seems not to have a 'real' concept of her infant. There is a feeling that the baby has come out of nowhere and does not belong to her.

Bill's mother died three years ago, but in his family there is five of them. His mother was a sick lady. I never actually met her, I never met him till after she had passed away. She had life pretty hard. His father died when Bill was 14 and he went out to work to help support the family. As for my parents, my father died when I was 16. I have got a mother but I don't see her any more. We fell out about four years ago and I haven't spoken to her since. We had a big argument. I'm pretty hot-headed and we just don't speak any more [Deedie laughs]. We really have no family – it's just us and Bubby.

Bill's brothers – you wouldn't class them as brothers – they sort of want to take a lend of you all the time. I suppose the situation is Bill's been a pretty lonely sort of a person before I met him. He lived by himself for about eleven years. He's been married previously and his eldest child is 28 now. She has two children and she lives down in Kilburn, and we don't see her. It's a bit hard on him, but I think he's really happy to have a new daughter that he knows he can be a real father to for the next 30 or 40 years. Our family situation is not real good but we are just happy with the way we are, just having our few close friends.

For Deedie, the theme is loss, all the losses of her life. They present like a litany – her mother-in-law, her father, her own mother no longer available to her, Bill's dead marriage, his lost children. On one hand there is the mourning, on the other overinflated hope: 'father for next 30 or 40 years'. Deedie seems to be denying that her infant could die. Was such a thought unthinkable, we wondered?

Actually, before I had the baby I really felt ill, I felt like death warmed up; I couldn't breathe, I couldn't eat, I couldn't do anything. I just used to lay there like a shag on a rock [defined in the *Macquaie Dictionary Australia* as meaning alone, deserted and forlorn]. I couldn't do anything to help myself, I relied on the nurses all the time. ICU was really good. The first day or two after I come out of the anaesthetic I wasn't feeling 100 per cent but I knew I was on the mend. When they took the ventilation out, I was feeling much better and knew I was going to be all right. I was just still worried about my baby and how small she was.

She was only 625 g, which is only one and a half pounds. There's not very much of her. I know she will grow and get stronger, and I know the staff in the nursery are looking after her. She's a little fighter like her mother, so she will fight on and end up a nice strong person like her parents. When she starts school I might go back to work; until then I want to stay at home and look after her. I don't want anyone to mind her, I want to be a full-time mum myself. As far as work's concerned, I think you should stay at home and look after your baby; that's what you bring them into the world for!

We saw Deedie as living either in the past or in the future, as if she has no present. She says she will be a good mother in the future, perhaps not daring to ask whether she will be a mother at all in the present. We pondered whether she dare not have memory or desire as reality has been too harsh for her.

We wondered about her own dependence, how much a 'shag on a rock' was her internal representation of herself, like a blob – unformulated, a fetal-like object without personification. Is she a 'shag on a rock', abandoned, alone, unreaching and unreachable to herself or to her baby? There is a feeling of 'unintegration' here. Deedie moves from this to give an image of her true internal deprivation.

> I'm bored, real bored with this place, I am. I go to the nursery twice a day. I bore really easily. I can't do nothing with her, just watch her. Sometimes I like to sit there and look at her. She moves and wiggles and worms and tries to take the nasal prongs out of her nose. I know that she's breathing because she was crying today, so I know she's getting better.
>
> I just get bored so easily, because at home you can do what you want, you can shop or visit your friends, but in hospital you can't have your home comforts. Funny how I haven't got postnatally depressed. I know I'm getting better and she's doing all right. I know it's just going to take time for her to grow up.

We think that Deedie's boredom may be because she is not connected to her internal world or to her baby's life. Her baby does not yet have an emotional meaning for her, so attachment and preoccupation cannot occur. If she had an internal baby, she would not be bored.

Interview 2

Deedie and her husband are visiting their baby.

> I made some notes last week about things that I thought about for this session, like about during my pregnancy.
>
> I went into St Edward's Hospital because I was getting pains, and I ended up signing myself out. That's how I ended up in here; they were damn useless in there. When I had a hypo attack because I'm a diabetic, the Sister said to Bill, 'What do you do when her sugar's so low?'. That's not very good nursing staff as far as we're concerned! That was in their High Risk Pregnancy Unit.
>
> When I complained about the staff, my doctor, he told Bill that I needed physciatric [sic] help. So that proves what sort of a silly old fool he is! I actually

got cranky at the time but now I think it's funny! I think he might have been all right once, but the old fool's past it now, and he should retire before he does some real damage. I think if I still had have been under him with all the trouble that I had, I don't think I would have been here today. I don't think me or the baby would have survived the big trauma that I went through. I think if I hadn't had this hospital here, I wouldn't have been here today.

The group discussed the primitive, simplistic level of splitting here. This splitting phenomenon was present in all research subjects. The group wondered, with this lack of certainty where good and bad and life and death are so close, whether splitting and projecting out is the main defence against going mad. They questioned whether Deedie had projected onto the doctor her sense of failure at preserving life. Was she 'past it'? Was she afraid that her good objects were not enough to support life? She seemed to be telling us that she felt full of badness – diabetes, high blood pressure, pneumonia and now, according to this doctor, 'madness'. The concept of 'if I had stayed with him I would have died' gives the notion that only 'one' can live, the other dies.

Between the first and second session, the father has taken a picture of the baby to the cemetery. He laid it against his mother's gravestone, took a picture of the two, framed it and hung it in their dining room. Deedie thought this was good. We wondered whether the father's good internal mother was being asked to preserve his infant's life.

> We nursed her the other day. That was an experience for me because there's not much to hang onto because she's so little. She didn't even weigh as much as a loaf of bread. The sheepskin was heavier than the baby. I was hanging on to her and there was hardly nothing there. If she was five pound or something, you might be able to feel her. But I suppose it was nice just to have her sitting in my arms. You actually think that she is a baby, not just a little thing laying in an incubator, that you know that there is actually a baby attached to all those cords.

The group is aware of Deedie's fragile attachment to her baby because of the statements 'The sheepskin was heavier than the baby' and 'There's not much to hang onto'. (Feeling the weight of the infant was significant for attachment in all the research mothers interviewed.) We wondered whether Deedie was bewildered or distressed by the infant's smallness, as if there were only a slender cord between life and death. Does Deedie feel unsure that she has a baby rather than a 'thing'?

> The hospital doesn't feel like a strange place because the nursing staff are all friendly. It's just when you're in hospital you feel so confined, and after you get over being really sick you feel like you just want to run down the street like a raving lunatic. Just to break loose from everything and yell and scream and

stamp your feet and carry on like a crazy man. You feel like you need a good night out on the town or a couple of drinks because you need a real big release. I don't know what else you could do. I suppose you could stand in the middle of the road and stamp your feet and hope you don't get run over by a truck. Something like that just to let all your tensions go.

At this point, we wondered how much Deedie was identifying with her infant being closed up in the womb and with the awesome 'closed in' confinement of her dependence when in hospital. Deedie seemed to us to be expressing a release from dependency, but she has moved to manic triumph and the release leads to a crazy independence rather than a holding one. This pattern persists throughout her narrative.

Interview 3

This week's been pretty busy. We've been to the hospital nearly every day this week [Deedie laughs]. She's going well and she's been moved out of the intensive care section of the nursery, and she's on the other side. She hasn't got her nasal prongs any more or any drips or anything. She has got a 'thing' in because she has a bit of an infection, but they haven't located it yet and they have been giving her antibiotics for that, and she still has her feeder tube. She's doing really well and being a little smarty pants like her mother was. She hates being disturbed, she hates being rolled over. We had a nurse of her today when we went in and she cried because we moved her.

The interviewer feels that the mother is avoiding the smallness and continuing near-death state of her infant. However, the group feels that this is normal on a premature infants' ward. An atmosphere of denial pervades. We wondered about the collusion between parents and staff in order to avoid the fear of death. The baby does not like 'being disturbed'. We had a fantasy that the infant was still in the mother's womb and, when they move the baby, it really impinges on both the mother and the baby.

On the other hand, Deedie is trying to find out, 'Whose baby is this? Look! she is ours. She has our colours!'.

The next thing I suppose will be to get out the feeder tube and try to get her on the breast when she's well enough in a couple more weeks. I suppose they can detach her from her little bits and pieces and see how she goes when she's breathing all right and doesn't need any oxygen. The breast milk is a bit of a dry argument. Yesterday and the day before I was as dry as the Sahara Desert. I'm only getting between 15 ml and 20 ml each time, which isn't enough to feed her anyway.

The idea of not enough breast milk supply linked into the father's interview that day. He was very worried that his income was not enough to keep the family. Many mothers interviewed in this research saw their milk as the single most important link with their baby; they were very anxious about its amount and the supply.

Interview 4

As is customary, the interviewer rang to confirm the appointment time. Either Deedie or her husband changed it twice. The second time the husband said that he was mowing the lawn and Deedie was out shopping, and that the interviewer would have to wait until they were ready. The interviewer described a strong feeling of the whole research being threatened with termination. On the way to their home, she felt quite depressed, with a sense of aloneness and of being in a totally defenceless position. She became aware of how intensely dependent on them she was. They were not my patients; they could terminate at will. She found herself wondering about the loneliness that such an intensely dependent infant must feel. Did Deedie also feel like this, she wondered.

> She wiggles a lot. She seems to wiggle a lot more than others do. She always seems to be moving her arms or kicking her legs or something. I moved her hand away so it would be better for her to breathe and she got cranky with me. She got the poos and pulled her arm away from my finger. She ranted and raved and got the shits with me and put her hand back up there. I give up in the end. On Wednesday I was there for an hour and I sat there and looked at her and looked at her, and just when I was getting ready to leave she woke up. She used to kick like crazy and now that she's out of the womb she still kicks like crazy. I've got all the furniture out of her room. It's not the spare room any more – it's bubby's room now. I don't want to set my hopes too high in case it's longer if something goes wrong. They all love her in there and even the doctors reckon she's cute.

The interviewer asks, 'Is Deedie beginning to bond with her baby?'. The group asks, 'Has she imagined her angry emotions to be her baby's emotions? Could this be the beginning of Deedie's infantile rage? Could Deedie think that her infant was angry with her because of the premature birth and the humidicrib?'. We had no answers.

> I'm just happy she's in the best place and that we both survived it. I couldn't imagine Bill having her and not me, because he couldn't look after a baby and that. And I couldn't imagine us being together and not having her either now after four weeks.
>   I think that if she had died, I think that would have been the hardest thing I had to deal with. I didn't really get upset when I miscarried, because I was nine weeks when I lost that one. I didn't feel like I was pregnant. With bubby I felt I was pregnant because I was seven months and getting the kicks in the stomach.

I knew she was inside me, whereas before with the pregnancy I lost I didn't. I suppose it is the first time I've felt lucky. Lucky that we're both here. We are lucky that we had good doctors. Thank heavens for that.

This is the first time that Deedie has presented material in a sad and serious voice. It is the first time that she has mentioned death or her possibly dying. In remembering the miscarriage, she speaks again of not feeling. We thought that perhaps death can only be considered and mentioned when it is no longer a possibility.

The interviewer tells the group that the father spent his interview speaking angrily of a Lebanese friend down the road who had promised to help them move from the 'dump of a house' they were living in to a much more cared-for one, and that the friend had failed them. (It should be noted here that the interviewer is of Lebanese descent.) 'Some friend! Came after it was all over with some lame excuse and asked could he help now! "Too late, mate!", I said. Carried it all on my own, didn't I? Did my back in doing it on my own, didn't I?'. We wondered whether Bill was saying that he carried everything from 'death' to 'life' with no help. He is angry with the interviewer ('mother?') for not being there then. Now it was too late.

As Bill saw the interviewer to the door, Deedie raced up the hall: 'The door is locked. You'll need me to let you out'. As she unlocked the door, she said, 'You know why we lock the door? It is to keep the thievin' Lebanese out'. Her husband nudged her in the back. 'Deedie, don't say that. Mrs Tracey might be Lebanese'. 'Oh she is,' said Deedie happily. 'I can tell! – You aren't the same as them though! They're bad'.

The group wonders what Deedie's fantasies might be. Had she stolen this baby from her mother and her punishment was to have a damaged baby? Was she afraid that the interviewer might steal her baby from her? Was the 'thief' the hospital or the surgeon who took the baby out?

Interview 5

My baby's wonderful! She's doing really good! She's 1210 g now, so she's put on lots of weight. The next hurdle is to get the oxygen level down. She's on about 28 per cent to 30 per cent oxygen. All the nurses love her, they do. She doesn't cry or anything. All the other babies cry, and she just sleeps and wiggles around. I'm a bit disappointed I can't feed her myself. I'm disappointed about it because they reckon if you breastfeed, you have a closer bonding with your baby. I can't do it, so there's not much I can do about it.

This mad doctor at the hospital informed me that in the next couple of years I will be on kidney dialysis. I was not very impressed with that statement, so I asked the blood pressure specialist about it. He said, 'Not in the near future. It could be ten or 15 years time'. I know for a fact that there is some damage in the kidneys from being a diabetic so long.

Mostly in ICU they were good, except for the bloke that put the central line in. I had a bit of disagreement with him. He tried in both arms and couldn't get it in. Because of the pneumonia I couldn't lay down, but he had a hard time and ended up putting it in my chest with local anaesthetic. He finally got it in and then they stitch them in. I had four stitches. I went to hell and back! Never again! No more babies!

The worst thing that happened was that I was terrified that he was going to lay me down because I knew that I couldn't breathe when I was flat on my back. And when they used to take the blood gases – because they have to take them out of the artery – I was bruised from my wrist to my elbow on both arms. Sometimes they were doing them three and four times a day. It really hurts because the arteries are just under the skin.

On that day I got more and more discomforted and in the end I couldn't breathe at all. 'Get her out! Get her out!', I screamed at Brian [the doctor]. 'Get her out before we both die!' I knew I would not be able to breathe with her pushing against my chest. Then he come up and said to me, 'I've decided to listen to you and take her out!' Bill was pretty choked up. I thought in my own mind that once he took the baby, I would be all right. Naturally that's what happened. None of the doctors can explain why it happened the way it did.

When I was in last time they asked if I would like to have a nurse. I was able to nurse her for about half an hour. Usually they only let you nurse for five or ten minutes, but they went to morning tea and forgot I still had her. Because she had all the leads on, it makes it really hard to get her back in the incubator. I was watching her monitor to make sure she had enough oxygen. She actually woke up for me the other day. I couldn't believe it.

It seems to the group that the danger has had to pass before it can be thought about. The interviewer felt that she was the trusted recipient of this material. 'Where was I? What happened to me?' – it was like an emotional awakening of her 'I'.

The group asked whether the doctor who brought her the bad news about her kidneys could, in Deedie's mind, be trying to make her dependent and entrapped, tied to a machine, even as her infant is dependent and tied to the machine. One group member felt that the doctor who could not insert the drip properly and the mother who could not bear her infant full term might be the same in Deedie's mind. There seems to be an issue of guilt and punishment: bad mothers bringing illness; a mother and an infant vying with each other for survival; who is to blame for what? Pneumonia at a metaphorical level seems to have a lot to do with spirit and loss of spirit, and breathing and loss of breath. It is as if the baby is taking all the breath; there is not enough breath for both. What is missing is the concept of sharing. One takes it from the other. They cannot survive together.

The interviewer is aware of the blackest depression during this interview. On a more conscious level, Deedie was more 'real' and sad. There is a background of deprivation and acting out in her past. Does trauma emphasise the basic template and take the sufferer back to it?

Between interviews 5 and 6, Deedie rang the interviewer at home. 'I'm really upset', she said. 'You know what they've done? They've put someone else's blood in our baby and they didn't even think we were important enough to tell us!'. She had telephoned the ward as usual that morning and Sister had said, 'We've just given her a top-up'. Deedie said, 'But she's drinking too much already!'. The Sister replied, 'Not milk, blood!'.

Interview 6

Deedie was awaiting the interviewer's arrival. 'I hope your recorder can take it,' she said, 'because I'm so upset and so mad angry!'

> The first time it happened, I think they discussed it on their ward rounds and they said she needed blood: could I come in and donate some. Of course, I said yes. We went in at 7.00 the next morning and the Sister told me they had transfused her overnight, and never rang us to tell us. I had said to the Sister that I didn't want her to have blood from the blood bank, only from myself, Bill or one of our friends. This time I said to the Sister, 'I told them before I didn't want her to have blood from the blood bank or without us being notified'. I got really shirty because I think, as the parents, she's my daughter, she's not their daughter. I think we should be notified if anything as drastic as a blood transfusion is needed.
>
> I got very upset, so upset they paged the doctor. An hour later I was still waiting. I thought no one was going to turn up because no one wants to take the blame for it. He explained how something in the bone marrow helps pump the oxygen around her body, and she didn't have enough. I thought that's a fair enough reason, but it only takes a minute to ring up and get the okay over the 'phone. He said, 'We do it automatically because there's no use delaying it. We would be on the 'phone all the time if we had to ring every parent about a blood transfusion'. Does 'neonatal' mean they have all rights over our baby? I'm furious. I rang again about 7.30 at night and I felt like getting in the car and driving in there and abusing the shit out of everyone. As parents you have to know. If I get a bill for a blood transfusion, I'm not going to pay it. That will teach them to let the parents know in advance.
>
> In other ways, the care is excellent. They started giving her a bottle the other day, but they told Bill she only took two sucks and wasn't interested. She's still only tiny, but three and a half pounds is better than one and a half. Some parents don't speak up – they just sit there like a shag on a rock. Someone's got to speak up so it may as well be me. They are wrong – it's your child. You have to look after them for the next 20 or 25 years before they leave home. If you sit back and don't say anything, the hospital and the doctors will keep making the same mistakes.

The group struggled with the idea of what not telephoning her meant to Deedie. Our ideas were: she feels that they have taken her identity as a mother from her, they are 'thoughtless' of her and she is not in their minds. We thought that, in trauma, one becomes 'brain dead' (Deedie's words in a previous session). Is Deedie struggling with giving emotional meaning to herself as mother and to her infant as baby? She has lost her place in the drama and, one group member suggested, has no existence as a mother in her own mind. Could the emphasis on 'getting my permission' be part of her feeling that all these terrible things have happened without her emotional presence or permission?

There is a quality of primitive envy here: 'They can keep the baby alive with their transfusions and I can't keep it alive with mine'. Her blood is no good, and it was her feeding by blood in the womb that in the end did not work. The baby has Bill's blood, not hers. Is he also stealing the baby from her? We decide that her initial confusion between blood and milk is caused by both being nourishing and life-giving, and she cannot give either. They are both transfusions. A baby is fed from blood in the womb – blood-feeding is more fetal, more primitive. Deedie ought still to be feeding her baby with her blood, and this is the narcissistic blow to Deedie.

The paradox of the transfusion is that it can either give life or destroy life by giving AIDS. Is this Deedie's quandary – to know whether she is a life-giver or a destroyer? Is the hospital a life-giver or a destroyer? She has lost the power of life and death over her infant. In the battle of 'Whose baby is this?', the possessiveness becomes a powerful force in her recovering her normal narcissistic maternal role. As her infant thrives, a mother becomes more assured of her own right to her baby. If her baby thrives as a result of another's care, this can be a threat to her.

Interview 7

She was nine weeks yesterday, so she is nine weeks and one day. It's just past 5 o'clock, so she is exactly nine weeks and one day and a few minutes. I was bathing Katherine, and the Head Sister of the nursery said, 'She's a cranky little thing. When she wants to be fed, she wants to be fed'. I thought she's a baby, not a 30-year-old adult that can do what they want for themselves. Naturally a baby wants to be fed when they want to be fed. I got pissed off about that. I came home and cried. I told Bill and he got pissed off about it too.

So I didn't know which paediatrician to talk to because I was going to push to get her transferred to our hospital near home here. I rang up my gyny to ask him for some help. I told him what had happened and I said, 'I think a few of the staff in the nursery were upset with me because I had a bit of a shot at them about the blood transfusions'. He said, 'Do you feel uncomfortable going into the nursery?' And I said, 'Yeah of course I do. I feel like I'm a shag on a rock!'.

He was going to speak to the head doctor in the nursery about getting her transferred. She is doing really well. I went in this morning and bathed her. I got sprung with the first dirty nappy today; that didn't worry me either. One nurse in there is absolutely hopeless. I have bathed her now about half a dozen times and she was there fussing around and she wouldn't let me dress her, and she has to wrap her up when you put her back in the cot and all this sort of rubbish. It's my child and I am quite capable of looking after her.

This dopey ass of a Sister put the tube in and nearly choked her. Another Sister actually showed me how to take it out myself. You take the tape off her mouth and pinch it so doesn't run down the back of her throat, because that will make her choke, and then give it a steady pull and pull it out. This old grandma one said, 'You can start feeding her'. I said, 'Is it all right if I take her feeder tube out?' and old grandma grizzle guts said, 'I'll do it!'. And when she did, Katherine started choking on it again. I was biting my tongue. I tell you what, I was going to grab her and punch her and put her head through the wall. I felt like saying, 'If you looked after your children like that they must be bloody useless now, because you are not going to look after my baby like that'.

I feel well in myself but I just feel like I get more depressed now than what I was before. I just want to get her home, I just want her home here. I'm sick of all those old fiddle farts in there.

We were aware of how many times in the early interviews Deedie saw the ward as 'the best place for her'. As she started to become well and the baby was improving, she was less and less convinced that it was the best place. She denigrated it, rubbished their care and held up her capacity to care for her baby. They were the fools, not her. Yet in her mind, she was the fool who couldn't even hold a baby. Instead of mercilessly blaming herself, she blamed the staff. We asked, 'Does the mother rival a mother inside her – a bad mother?'. A powerful primitive possessiveness had come to life in Deedie.

Interview 8

What's happened over the last two weeks? Getting the shits with the doctors, which is nothing unusual. They are a big bunch of hypocritical, egotistical bastards as far as I'm concerned. They don't worry about anyone but themselves. This doctor, an intern, came in and said, 'I've been speaking to Katherine's paediatrician, and she won't be home by Christmas'. I got all upset and I was throwing things around, kicking, swearing, cursing and carrying on, because they think that they own her and they want to keep her there for their own benefit, rather than me being the mother and me looking after her. It's not like they own her and we have to buy her off them.

I went to the hospital and I said, 'I want her transferred and I'm a private patient. I have the right to take her out of the hospital and put her into another one'. The doctor came in and said, 'We will transfer her but we were very concerned about her having the bradycardias.' She said a few things, and make sure you get your follow-up appointments and all this garbage, which I am not taking her to anyway. She's not going into that hospital ever again. She is going to her paediatrician in Hilton Hospital and that's it. Since she's been in Hilton Hospital there has not been one problem with her. She hasn't had a brady-cardia. They are very good in the nursery up there.

We asked whether Deedie was now empowered by taking control, by bringing her baby to her hospital. When her baby is doing well, she is freed to 'own' her, to claim her as her own. A member of the group wondered whether Deedie was now re-enacting her birth trauma. Perhaps in Deedie's mind the hospital is a bad mother who cannot look after a baby, who cannot keep a baby alive, who is neglectful and misunderstanding of the baby. In the new narrative, Deedie and Bill become the rescuers. Far from being powerless, they are the ones in control.

Interview 9

The first day we came home she was good, new environment and everything. We had no problems with her at all. She fed really well and we went and picked up our new car, which was good. Then we took her shopping at Woolworths and Bill carried her around in the harness, and she just layed there asleep with not a worry in the world. She couldn't care less where she was. She's been pretty good. Sometimes she will sleep the four hours and sometimes it will be only three or three and a half.

The doctor said, before she come home, she had gone 13 days without a bradycardia or an apnoea. If I am doing something, about 15 minutes is the longest stretch before I walk in to check on her. She lays there so still sometimes I think, 'Oh my God is she breathing?'. My heart starts to pound and I put my hand gently on her chest, and her little heart is beating away and I think, 'Thank God for that!' I'm a real big panic merchant! It just worries you because she rolls around and kicks so much, but when she is really quiet, you think is she all right? I don't think I could ask for a better baby – she feeds well, she was drinking between 60 ml and 90 ml when she was in hospital, and now she is going between 90 and 120 ml for milk each time.

I've been pretty good I suppose; I'm just happy that she is home. It's a joy to have her home and not having to organise your day around going to the hospital, and coming home and trying to do all the other things that you normally do anyway. I just bundle her up and put her in the car and away we go, and it's no great major hassle to do anything.

The doctor said to me the other day, 'You're doing a good job!' I took that as a compliment. Yeah, she is going great guns!

After the interview was over, the interviewer said, 'Deedie, you have talked about Katherine for the whole forty-five minutes!' 'Well, she is my daughter!', Deedie replied. She and her husband then took pictures of the interviewer with the baby: 'We want to remember you!', they said.

Conclusion: effect on inner world imagos and dynamics and on the identity of self as mother

We suggest that the premature birth of Deedie's infant in 'life-and-death' circumstances for both Deedie and her baby, and her baby being kept alive by others in a humidicrib, severely affected Deedie's inner world dynamics. We surmise that the trauma vastly altered her capacity to process these experiences. We see this trauma as having seriously interfered with her internal perception of herself as a mother, and her infant as her baby. There seemed confusion in the beginning over who was the mother and who was the baby, who had done what to whom. It seemed as though death and destruction were present, but by whom and to whom? Was this baby even born in her mind, and was it hers or the ward's?

We came to understand, by the end of our study of Deedie and her baby, how the trauma of an early birth and the terror of death would overload a mother psychically. We see her as having cut off from her emotions to protect herself, becoming affectless, regressed and dependent. We propose that, when this happens, a primitive archaic defence of denial takes over from normal repression. Her emotions cannot be felt in the sense that the experience cannot be 'thought about' or symbolised. Deedie's emotions remained in a primitive, raw and paranoid unprocessed state at one level, while at another level she was in an autistic-like, affectless state. Deedie's loss of confidence in her good internal mother and her capacity to protect her left her undernourished emotionally. She did not seem to us to have a safe space in which to go 'mad' and experience her chaos.

When the 'madness' broke through and Deedie awakened from the denial, her inner world characters took on a life of their own, with no centre to hold or separate external reality from internal fantasy. Deedie became paranoid about the ownership of the baby. She was possessive of it and furious with the care-takers, whom she saw as robbing her of her baby. She centred all these angry feelings on the blood transfusion, but we think that they were deeper and less circumspect than this. She had been intruded on physically and emotionally in an extraordinary way and experienced rage at the assault, at the robbery.

The loss of control over her life and death affected her concept of 'two' living together. She screamed, 'Get it out before we both die'. There is a fantasy of the infant robbing her of the very breath of life. The 'sharing' she initially allows to the neonatal intensive care team later also breaks down. The infant is hers, not theirs. They were trying to keep her baby for 'their own use and purposes'. In her mind, they were trying to rob her of her baby. At this stage, her inner world had taken over. She re-enacts the original drama with her in a different role. She removes the baby from 'their womb/hospital ward' never to return there, and puts her baby in 'her womb/hospital ward' and then in the womb of her home.

In the replay of this drama Deedie was the capable one, the staff the stupid ones. She had the power and the control; they had lost it. Projective identification plays an important part here: Deedie becomes the life-giver. Her internal 'madness' becomes external and aggressive. To us, Deedie's problems seemed to be in evidence long before this trauma. We see the trauma as exposing, for each traumatised person, the basic template of her personality functioning.

But what of Deedie and her partner as a couple? We do not have space to discuss this adequately here; we can only surmise that her partner seemed fused with her feelings and emotions. They seemed as one in their war against the 'enemy' hospital. Their separateness was submerged; even their the words of criticism were the same. This fusion seemed present in every research couple with a premature infant.

And what of Deedie's baby? We dared not surmise how much such beginnings might affect her internal world and her future, nor how reparable such a harsh separation might be. Her life narrative has had awful beginnings.

For the mother of a premature infant, there is a serious interruption to her idealised image of a full-term baby. It is substituted by a 'scrap of humanity' in a machine, with no experience of birth to confirm her as mother. The balance of love and hate, and murderousness and protectiveness, is severely disrupted. The mother is proved more than a failure: she is proved a murderer in the sense that the baby would have died had it been left inside her. Our image of what may have happened in Deedie's internal world is that this anger she has with herself for being a failure is unbearable. She sees the ward and the hospital as having substituted their collective womb for her own, which has been found to be full of bad things (sickness, 'unholding' and inadequacy). By projecting, she clears the way for her repossession of her infant and her right to mother.

Mothers of full-term infants cannot think, as they gather up the fragmented parts, of themselves in the new state of motherhood. This is so much harder for the mother of a premature baby. A harsh biological confrontation such as premature birth, and a preceding severe illness, interferes with and interrupts her internal perception of her fetal infant. It intrudes on her autonomous space with her infant by introducing reality too harshly or prematurely into the delicate balance of the inner world processes of pregnancy. Fantasy life at first freezes and then grows rife. The struggle to mother becomes a difficult and hazardous journey.

References

Bion WR (1962) Learning from Experience. London: Heinemann.
Tracey N (1991) The psychic space in trauma. Journal of Child Psychotherapy 17(2): 29–45.
Tustin E (1994) Autistic children who are assessed as non-brain-damaged. Journal of Child Psychotherapy 20(1): 103–33.

Chapter 6
The premature infant in the mind of the mother

BEULAH WARREN

Although infants born prematurely or very sick would not survive without advances in technology, there does seem to be a cost to the infant's development and to the parent–infant relationship. For healthy survival, the growing fetus and newborn needs to be held in the mind of another human being, so that the adult, preferably the mother, will have times of reverie about the baby, a time of thinking with the baby and for the baby (Fonegy et al 1991). This adult will ponder on the infant's perspective (Stern 1990) and be the focus of the infant's earliest self-regulation (Sander 1997).

This chapter is an examination of the baby in the mind of the mother, in this case the mother of a premature infant. It is an exploration of the mother's perceptions of her baby and the baby's behaviour as revealed in interviews over the first four months of the baby's life. Parents' perceptions of their baby's behaviour are likely to shape their handling of their baby. The chapter will explore how perceptions change over time and how the baby's behaviour may be a reflection of the mother's internal processes.

Neonatal intensive care has advanced considerably over the past 5–10 years, with a subsequent decline in mortality, especially for very low birth-weight infants. However, the rate of moderate-to-severe handicap has remained relatively stable at around 10 per cent, while other neurodevelopmental conditions occur more frequently (Paneth et al 1994).

Thompson et al (1994) found that psychosocial stress in the mother influenced the developmental outcome of the infant over and above the biological risk that the infant had experienced (measured by Neurobiological Risk Score [NBRS]) over the first two years of the child's life. Preterm infants, like all infants of the human species, are psychobiologically social (Als et al 1996) and expect the security of three inherited environments – their mother's womb, their parents' bodies and their family's social group – to support their development (Hofer 1987). Thus, the parents' role as the infant's primary nurturers is fundamental to the survival and growth of the premature infant and has to be protected and reinforced. Three questions come to mind:

1. What is the impact on the interaction between mother and baby of the trauma of premature birth?
2. What is the impact on the infant's and the family's interactive or inter-subjective development of this traumatic event?
3. Is it possible for the neonatal intensive care unit (NICU) to be both life-saving and emotionally nurturing of all involved – infant, family and staff?

The premature birth

For the parents

The event of a baby arriving prematurely means that there is also prematurity of the parents' developmental process of becoming parents: they are being 'hurled' into parenthood. Much work is done within the psyche of parents during pregnancy as they progress from a concept of themselves as individual people to the new concept of self as parent. The pregnant parents fantasise about the baby in the womb, what amazing attributes he/she will have, what characteristics? Towards the end of the pregnancy, the fantasies become even more focused on just what this baby inside will be like. Will everything be all right?

Norma Tracey (Tracey et al 1995) talks of the premature birth causing a serious interruption of the mother's preoccupation with her infant. With premature birth, the mother loses her sensory contact with her infant, that which kept her involved with her infant and rewarded her. Her baby is not able to suck on the breast, but the mother must express her milk using a machine. She is recovering from the trauma of the birth, often a caesarean section. The father, too, has often experienced trauma – his wife suddenly having to be hospitalised, or going in to premature labour. Is she, as well as the infant, in a life-and-death situation?

Tracey interviewed 12 couples who had just had their first baby, inter-viewing each parent nine times over the first four months of their child's life. Seven of the couples had given birth to a baby weighing less than 2000 g and equal to or less than 33 weeks' gestational age. Tracey's summary of the experience for those parents whose baby was born prematurely was that they were initially in affectless shock. They roused from this to feelings that were primitive and chaotic, sensing the impossibility of forming a relationship with the infant at the same time as experiencing constant fear that the infant might die. There was a feeling of powerlessness because there was no sense of control of the circumstances surrounding their infant's care. The machine – not the parents – is the life-giver, and the staff are the primary care-givers. The parents often feel that they have failed as life-giving parents. So where is the premature baby in all this? Is the baby at least being held in the mind of the parents, if not within the mother's body?

For the infant

Prematurity separates the infant from the ideal protective environment for his/her growth and development – the mother's womb. How can one estimate the effect on the developing nervous system of moving too early, 'from the relative equilibrium of the intrauturine aquatic econiche of the mother, to the extrauturine terrestrial environment of the NICU, by-passing the "on body" phase of early nurturance?' (Alberts and Cramer 1988, quoted in Als and Gilkerson 1995, p 3).

The approach to neonatal care that addresses this concern, and is gaining momentum in the USA and Australia, is a model that is family centred and developmentally supportive of the infant. It is a family and professional alliance that supports and fosters the parents' preoccupation with their infant and the infant's neurobiologically based expectations of nurturance (Als 1993). This approach acknowledges that the infant's needs for an optimal developmental outcome are a continuation of the contact with the parents' bodies and the family's social group. It was with this framework in mind that I examined the nine interviews.

One mother's experience

Interview 1

The tapes I examined were of the interviews with a mother of a premature baby, born by caesarean section at 33 weeks' gestational age and weighing 1940 g at birth. When this mother, Rowena (a pseudonym), was first interviewed by Tracey, her baby was two weeks of age and had been in the intensive care nursery for just under a week when he was transferred to the special care nursery. Relatively speaking, this baby was of little concern to staff at the time of the interview. He was not receiving oxygen, was off the monitor and was being tube fed; in addition, his mother was breast-feeding him twice a day.

Despite this, the first interview contains many examples of anxiety and distress when Rowena speaks about her baby. She appears preoccupied with the distress that the experience has caused her and the baby's father, and about her uncertainty about the baby's being 'normal'. Not until the end of the interview do we hear this mother say, 'we'll get there. I'm getting more confident with him.' Only once in the hour does Rowena refer to her baby by name, and not once is there mention of joy or excitement. The sentences containing a reference to the baby comprise four pages, whereas the transcript of this first interview runs to 21. This is very unusual: with the mothers of full-term babies, the reverse would be true. We have to be persistent in our search to 'find' this baby.

Below is an account of the first few minutes of the interview:

OK, well where do I start?

Interviewer: Wherever you like.

What do you want me to tell you? Just about the birth?

Int.: Yes.

Well, the whole thing was a bit of a shock, because I only found out the day before that I was going to have the baby, 'cause my blood pressure was not being controlled and so it wasn't the obstetrician that decided.

I didn't really have any fears that the baby wouldn't be normal, because I didn't know anything about premature babies.

Int.: Right. Something you knew nothing about.

Yeah. I was in hospital for two weeks, and I thought I'd probably be in there for quite a few more weeks and they'd control my blood pressure, but it didn't work out that way. So I had the caesarean and it wasn't until the neonatal doctor kept coming up to me, to see me every day in hospital to tell me how the baby was progressing, I thought there could be problems, and I don't think there will be and hopefully there won't. But then I started expressing milk which was a real drama because it was every four hours, so I wasn't getting any sleep.

So that was quite stressful and my blood pressure didn't come down after the birth, like they said it probably would. And they cut my tablets down and then I just wasn't getting any sleep, I was so I was worried about myself and worried about the baby – but the Sisters were fabulous. There was, in the nurseries and on the ward where I was, there was no problems there, and so doctors decided I'd be better off at home, probably get more rest there. And now I'm just racing backwards and forwards to the hospital every day. We were going once a day, now we're going twice 'cause I'm breastfeeding him twice, and then I'll get up to three breastfeeds a day and then four. Then I might have to room in for a few days, so I can feed him every four hours.

But he's doing really well, but it's a terrible time. I had a bit of postnatal depression, and I think it was just exacerbated by the circumstances. But now I think I'm more in control of my feelings, but you still worry. You go in there and you see them, all those babies in the cribs, but I don't think there's any problems with our baby at the moment. He seems to be getting along all right.

They don't really tell you much.

It was more not being in control of your feelings, and I think it was just made worse because I wasn't that well. Recovered from the caesar, no problems; the physical side wasn't a problem, but I was worried about my blood pressure and they kept saying it should come down and it didn't, and then the postnatal depression, you can't describe it. You're just in tears all the time for no reason. And of course when I saw the baby I'd be in tears; when he cried I'd be in tears. I think if it had have been a normal birth, I probably would have had a bit of depression for a few days and that would have been it. This continued for well, ten days or so, so it was quite severe. But I did a bit better when I came home and my husband's very supportive, so that was OK.

The baby is embedded in Rowena's preoccupation with her experience and subsequent illness. The preoccupation with the baby is competing with Rowena's preoccupation with her blood pressure. The baby is being organised 'around' her trauma. Further quotes illustrate how Rowena's mind is full of the trauma of her own illness rather than full of her baby:

But going into the hospital now, I'm more in control. When I see the baby, I'm more confident with him and feel that he's doing quite well so I'm not so upset, but it's still very stressful, all those things. And I don't think the staff realise the pressure on you as far as the breastfeeding. They say can you come back more times a day. It's not that you don't want to, it's that it's awful being there, 'cause I found it was upsetting me to be there. But as time goes on, it's gonna be a lot better, and also I can see, they haven't actually said when he's coming home, but I can see a time. It's not too far away, it's only a few weeks.

And it's funny – a lot of people say he's in the best place and it will give you time to do the nursery and all those sorts of things, but no-one realises. I think people with children realise to a small degree, but nothing like this. It's really very emotional.

But you really can't do much about it; it affects people differently I think. And a lot of my friends haven't had any depression at all after a birth, and then you're made to feel a bit abnormal [laughing] by it. I don't know what else I can say about it; it's just a very, very hard time.

I think my husband – he's more practical, not emotional, and of course he hasn't given birth to the baby so he doesn't have all those hormones running round his body, 'cause that's half the problem, all the hormones. So it's great he's like that, 'cause he gives me a lot of support in that regard. If we were both like that, we'd be terrible.

But I think that's all I can say about it. It's just the first few weeks are really dreadful, but in our case it won't go on for too long. Then there's the fear of bringing him home – and he's so little and all that sort of thing – then there'll be more worries, but it will be a different type of worry I think. But a big shock to the system.

I think when you rang me, I'd had about three hours sleep in two days, because the staff were at me continually. I had a couple of problems with the nursery. They were ringing me up for milk and there was milk in the freezer down there. They rang at 4 o'clock in the morning, and I was up there, I had expressed and I was just putting it into the fridge on the floor that I was on, and one of the Sisters came in and said, 'The nursery's on the 'phone, they need more milk'. I said, 'You know that's ridiculous because there's milk down there', and she checked and there was. So that happened a couple of times, a few mix-ups there. So that put on even more stress, because I wasn't getting much at the beginning, and trying to keep ahead of him, I was only four hours in front.

The blood pressure was going sky high, and they were taking my blood pressure four times a day, which made it worse. Every time the machine came in I got tense, and then every time I went to the nursery I'd miss the doctor. Either the blood pressure doctor or my obstetrician would come in to see me and I wasn't there. And then visitors were coming in and I was having something like nine 'phone calls a day. My husband was telling people not to ring me and it got too much; I was so glad to get out of there. I can't really fault it for anything, but you just really don't get any rest in hospital.

The biggest fear is that because he's premature, he could be more prone to cot death than other babies. That's something I've thought about a lot. I know I'll be paranoid when I bring him home, probably won't put him down to sleep, and so I'll have to learn to control myself about that. But that's probably the biggest fear.

It's good that I haven't had any problems with the milk, and the support was good in hospital – it's great for the lactation team. I didn't expect anything like that, so the support there is good. But the demands, there are a lot of demands and you don't know whether you're spending long enough in the hospital either, seeing your baby. The baby's asleep most of the time, and we got into a little bit of trouble one day 'cause we had him out of the crib for too long and he got cold. We were told to unwrap him to breastfeed and then we didn't wrap him properly back up, and Steven nursed him for an hour and his temperature went right down and he couldn't have a bath. So I was in tears then [laughing], but I don't think they realised that. 'Cause you don't know anything about a baby unless you've had one before, or you've been exposed to babies.

Where is the baby?

In the interview we have just read, we are looking for baby Harry. Where is he? – 'in the space between'. In discussing the case, Mary Sue Moore, American clinical psychologist and psychotherapist (personal correspondence, August 1998), said that she had a sense of the baby being on a 'detour': the baby was stuck somewhere, the 'baby had been derailed'.

The premature birth was a terrible experience for Rowena. The process of carrying her baby was catastrophically interrupted. The situation was unpredictable, and it did not feel safe for Rowena. Initially, Rowena was still with the baby in her mind, a robust, healthy baby. The reality of the risks to the newborn became apparent to Rowena after the baby was born, when the staff kept telling her that her baby was progressing well. Rowena talks of the distress arising from her baby's early arrival and her anxiety with regard to whether or not he will have problems, in particular any increased risk of cot death. Rowena and her partner do not know this baby; the staff know him. The parents feel guilt and shame that they do not meet the expectations of staff when they are thrown into a situation and expected to know what to do.

Was it that Rowena had found it difficult to take in the instructions of the staff on how to care for this baby? Do staff expect too much knowledge of new parents confronted with a baby who does not match the baby in their mind? Also, do staff take into account the new parents' reduced capacity to learn while stressed? Little bursts of release from the anxiety and distress come with comments of it 'being nice' to be wheeled down to see her baby from the theatre, on an operating bed, and it being 'fantastic' to be allowed to hold him. However, it seemed that Rowena had to be grateful to these people. How unnatural that one should be in a position of obligation because of being 'allowed' to see and hold one's own baby.

Rowena gave several examples of feeling misunderstood, of nursery staff, family and friends not being aware of her sense of the baby being 'derailed'. Rowena expressed this in her ambivalence about just what was the best place for her baby. Well-meaning friends said that he was in 'the best place', but within herself Rowena knew that, for both herself and her baby, nothing would replace his remaining within her until term.

Stress for the parents

How vulnerable the reconnecting of the parents with their baby is. Within a few days, Rowena and Steven were told that they could hold their baby as often as they wished. How excited yet apprehensive they were at the prospect, Rowena saying she felt he was much more comfortable 'in there', referring to the crib. But was she referring to her womb? Her arms are reluctant to do what her uterus could not do. She has lost her sense of agency and feels impotent.

We can feel their shame as they were reprimanded because, in their eagerness to hold and reconnect with their baby Harry, they did not keep an eye on his temperature or wrap him correctly. This is confirmation that they do not know this baby. There is a paralysis in relation to this baby. This is not the baby Rowena is familiar with, the baby of her thoughts. She does not know this baby. There is inner conflict because in some ways she is still hanging on to the baby in her mind, who is not the baby in her arms. More than that, however, this baby is better known and better understood by others. The staff know about the baby's vulnerability to temperature. In not knowing her baby, Rowena experiences shame, which leads to impotence. Mother has been left out in relation to this baby, and she cannot get it right. Her actions in relation to this baby are inappropriate and irrelevant.

Stress for the baby

Perry (1995) has written of how infants manage stress. The human body, when confronted with a life-threatening experience, has the protective capacity of fight, flight and freeze. What is the premature infant able to do in the initial period after birth? Does the infant freeze, to survive? As the infant cuts out the stimuli, does the mother experience this as not being able to reach her baby, of not knowing her baby? Is this why she cannot speak of her feelings or even behave emotionally towards her newborn baby? In the last trimester of a full-term pregnancy, mothers fantasise about their infant. They talk about the characteristics of which they have become aware as their baby grows inside them. The reality of a baby, born out there and at risk, is in conflict with the fantasy of the baby's potential.

For the baby in the uterus, the last few weeks are spent becoming familiar with their environment. We know that from 30 weeks' gestation, the infant can habituate to various stimuli (Hepper 1996). The fetus can learn to associate two stimuli together (Feijoo 1975, 1981, in Hepper 1996) and is able to recognise their mother's voice and even acoustic cues and music. The baby is beginning to regulate his/her states, with a cycle of deep sleep, light sleep, wakefulness, active periods and periods of quiet alertness (Brazelton and Cramer 1990). At birth, the right side of the brain is fully functioning, ready to process the affect experience with the care-taker (Schore 1996).

Harry, however, is born into a situation where his natural processes are interrupted. Most handling is associated with discomfort, is not carried out by someone with whom he is familiar, and does not occur in response to his initiation. Harry is missing out on gaining a more intimate knowledge of his mother. He is fed on a schedule rather than when he is feeling hungry. Touch, which is critical for the healthy development of the newborn (Mahler et al 1975, Field et al 1986), is associated with unpleas-antness. This is classical conditioned learning, and an additional challenge for the parents and staff is to decondition the baby.

Interview 2

Harry is still in hospital at the time of the second interview. He is around 36 weeks corrected age, or three weeks of age from birth. We are looking for descriptions of the interaction between Rowena and Harry. In this interview, Rowena expresses the roller-coaster emotions that she is experiencing:

> I think it's all the traipsing back to the hospital, it wears you down a bit. You think you're getting closer to bringing the baby home and then you really don't

know because they don't tell you. They can't say until things are established, like feeding and temperature control and things like that, but baby's had a few choking fits when he's been eating as well, which is worrying [laughing]. But the nurses up there know exactly what to do and they tell you it's pretty normal. You know he's just gulping too much, but when you don't know what to do, you panic.

Steven's very much in control so he sort of took over and everything was OK. But it could be another ten days or two weeks even before we bring him home, and just going back and forth all the time really gets you down. And some days you feel optimistic, and then other days you feel depressed, which is stupid because you're getting closer to the time. Well you think you are anyway, but it's just very tiring and wearing.

But I've finally set the nursery up, which is encouraging [laughing].

Rowena speaks of being worn out by visiting the hospital, of the uncertainty of knowing when they will bring the baby home, of optimism when she thinks of her baby coming home and of how she has created a space for him. There is further confirmation of her not knowing this baby and how to care for him as she recounts the choking episode, and she ponders over how she will manage that at home. A little later, Rowena speaks of not being able to take the baby out in the cold and says:

I didn't realise all that; they will be a normal baby but there's just that bit of extra care that you've gotta take when you first bring them home. It's just a bit hard, I didn't think about that before, and keep people away who've got colds and things like that.

In this interview, we see Rowena struggling with understanding the particular vulnerabilities of her premature baby and desperately searching for evidence of progress being made. Progress relates to Harry taking three breastfeeds a day and a bottle the night before, 'which is good 'cause that means he had four suckings in 24 hours'. Progress is also identified as Harry sleeping in an open cot and gaining weight. However, Harry's progress is not related to Rowena. She does not feel responsible or even involved in his progress. There is a sadness as she speaks of it:

It's funny 'cause you don't really feel encouraged, even by the weight gain. It's good and everything, and you think he might be closer to coming home, but it doesn't seem like another step forward. It's the same thing every day you know – it's just a real drag. But it'll be good to tell him all about this in years to come.

The challenge for the newborn is to establish homeostasis (Sander 1962, Sroufe 1979, Greenspan 1981), to be able to have one's basic nutritional needs met, to control one's temperature and to have stability of states and smooth movement between states. The newborn infant is reliant on the mother as a container, modulator and shaper of affective experiences (Lieberman and Slade 1997). For Rowena, however, her baby is regulating independently of her, and when they are together it is a fumbling process. Here she recounts another choking episode while she was bathing Harry, and the anxiety of not knowing how to nurture and protect her baby.

> Yeah, I am worn out. I think 'cause today's been a bad day. And with the baby choking like that last night and today, it just sort of hit me, 'cause today when he did it he wasn't feeding. I'd just bathed him but I hadn't dressed him – I was just about to. I think I'd put on his nappy and I laid him down on his back in the cot, and he just started coughing and spluttering and then I said, 'He's choking', and one of the nurses picked him up and I don't know what she did, it happened so quick, and she said, 'Oh, he's OK'. There was nothing there, but I should have, well I was dressing him so I couldn't put him on his side, but it might have been that water up the ... he was crying a lot when I put him in the water, and he might have regurgitated a bit of the milk from this morning. It's probably his digestive system's not 100 per cent yet. He's doing quite well because he's putting on weight, but he'll probably take a couple of weeks to catch up.

Harry is attempting to cope with his bodily processes while simultaneously engaging and learning about the world outside himself, and he needs to feel the containment of the other. It is difficult to imagine Harry experiencing containment as Rowena expresses her anxiety:

> That was very stressful. I felt my blood pressure go right up then, I was flushed in the cheeks and my head was banging. Then I fed him and it didn't calm me down, so it's just those little tensions. I suppose all new mothers have the worries and upsets. And it's fear I suppose, fear of, well, not knowing. Not being confident in caring for the baby and things like that. I don't know if it would have been different if he was full term.

Almost at the end of this second interview, Rowena speaks of Harry's progress in interacting with herself and Steven, how Harry is reconnecting with them, and how breastfeeding has been a slim thread onto which they have both hung.

> *Int.*: He's in K7 West?
>
> Yeah, for two weeks now. He's just fattening up. And he actually looks better now, his skin's not so papery. He's still got no bottom at all, no fat on his bottom, but his face looks better, and his eyes – when he's awake he's more aware and with it, and his eyes actually look bigger. He seems to be focusing more, and when I go to breastfeed him, he looks at me a lot, and then if Steven says something he tries to turn his head to have a look. It's really marvellous, 'cause he knows us and that's a really nice feeling. Sometimes he's so hungry that he just latches on straight away, but sometimes he looks around for a

couple of minutes and then he starts feeding. That's when he's awake. So that's really good. So I imagine that'll just improve and improve.

Int: Are you enjoying the feeding, Rowena?

Yeah, I do enjoy the feeding. I don't relax enough. Sometimes I feel really relaxed, depends what's on my mind, but it's great. That's one thing I'm glad I can do, 'cause I've got friends who just couldn't do it at all, and maybe it's been a bit easier because I'm expressing and you don't get sore initially. A lot of women get sore straight away and that hasn't happened.

We're gonna have him with us in our room for a while. I said to Steven, 'I'll have to get up to change him in the other room, so there's gonna be the lights on and stuff', and he said, 'That's all right'. So I'll see how long Steven can stand it – he'll be off [work] for a little while anyway, so it won't be too bad. But it'll be nice to have the baby in with us. Some people say it's not a good idea because babies make lots of noises and you never get any sleep, but I probably wouldn't get much sleep if he was in the other room anyway. So we'll see how that goes. I feel exhausted.

We can recognise Rowena's efforts to accelerate the process of getting to know her baby by having his bassinet in their room. She cannot imagine herself sleeping away from him. In this way, Rowena's intended availability and responsiveness will provide the scaffolding that will enable Harry to get into his own rhythm of feeding, sleeping and quiet alertness, that is, to establish self-regulation, which is the developmental challenge of the newborn.

Interview 3

The next week, when the third interview was recorded, Harry was at home. Rowena spoke of being told that they might be able to take Harry home in a week, but it was in fact two days later. 'It was a major shock' as there were still things to organise. As they left the hospital, Rowena said that she had a weird feeling: 'it was leaving the security behind'.

The staff were reassuring but this did not allay her anxiety, for this interview is about Rowena's anxiety at home: how she or Steven stayed with the bassinet all the time for fear of the cats jumping into the crib, how they kept taking Harry's temperature, how they did not sleep at night because of the noises that Harry made, of a telephone call to the hospital nursery in the early hours of the morning because his temperature had dropped. The visit of the discharge nurse two days after leaving the hospital gave a boost to Rowena's confidence as the nurse took Rowena through the practicalities of bathing Harry and different breastfeeding positions for greater efficiency.

Rowena is still looking for her baby: at one point she comments that 'he is such a lovely little boy', yet it is still three weeks prior to due date. She then drifts into how it is working out for them and into managing bath time that morning. We are not informed of the qualities that identify Harry as 'gorgeous':

> 'Cause he's such a lovely little boy, it's gorgeous.
> So it's all worked out I think; it seems to be coming together. Lots of support and everything. And of course as time goes, I'll probably relax more with him. I'm not worried about him any more; I'm not taking his temperature, that's a good thing. I don't think I've taken it at all today, which is amazing [laughing].
> I was bathing him today; he screamed and it's the most I've heard him cry for ages. He used to cry a little bit in the nursery when they bathed him but nothing like that, and I got a little bit tense 'cause everyone was watching me 'cause we had the nurse here, and also she brought a trainee midwife with her who looked after me on my first day after the caesar, which is really nice, and she's a lovely girl. And Steven was here, he was filming me bath him, and so I got a little bit tense 'cause he was crying so much – once he's in the water he's OK. When you take his clothes off, and I was a little bit disorganised 'cause I had things in the bathroom, things up there and things here. But it was [a] good place to do it, and she said I don't have to bath him every day, just maybe every two or three days is enough. There's no need to do it all the time. And 'specially when it's cold.

Rowena speaks of the blur of the past weeks and of now wanting life to return to normal, although she realises that it will be different as they are 'a family now'. She has a 'funny feeling' when she thinks of the fact that she has 'a little person to take care of'. For the first time, Rowena mentions that her mother also had a premature baby, and although a visit is spoken about, Rowena does not speak of her mother as being supportive of her. In fact, her mother lets her know that Rowena is better off than she had been when she had taken Rowena's sister home. Rowena does not feel held by her mother, nor does Rowena feel held by her partner as he struggles to get to know his son.

Although there is some dissatisfaction expressed in terms of not being able to get out of the house, in this interview Rowena is pleased to be home, not to have to go running back and forth to the hospital, but admits to being very anxious about leaving Harry alone and only having done so since they installed a monitor.

Subsequent interviews at home

In the remaining interviews at home, we are still looking for Harry. When Rowena speaks of Harry, she once again speaks of him being 'a good baby', in a routine. We are not told how she feels about Harry or how Harry might be feeling, about Harry the person. There is much about 'doing':

Harry's fine. I think that was a wind pain, 'cause apparently new babies smile at six weeks but premature babies don't smile for another six weeks or seven weeks on top of that. I don't know how true that is, but hopefully I'll be able to tell the difference between a wind smile and a happy smile. But he's a good baby, he's in quite a routine and he's doing really well. The only thing is I haven't been allowed to take him out yet. So I've been stuck in the house for two weeks which is a real pain. And Steven's had two days off so I could get out and about a bit, but I want him to have about a week off, but he's so busy at work it's almost impossible. So I've had various friends come over for an hour or two and I've gone out, and the nurse said today that after his original birth day, I'll be able to start taking him out a bit. So [I'll] be able to go for walks and things but still not to expose him to too many people – all I want to do is take him out and show him off, but you can't. That's probably been the hardest part.

And a little later:

I just think about Harry and getting bigger and looking forward to getting out with our friends and things like that – that's what I'm really looking forward to.

The tapes are predominantly of this mother's struggle to become a mother. She is preoccupied with her own illnesses. She talks at length of high blood pressure, a breast lump, kidney cysts and a narrowing of a tube leading from the kidney. In her mind, the baby organises around her experience – how she will manage to breastfeed when she has to go into hospital to have the narrowed tube opened. It seems that Rowena is desperate for someone to take care of her. Was there a message in her family of origin that being sick was how one gained the attention to which one was entitled? Perhaps the fragile premature sister had taken all of her mother's attention and energy.

With such a focus on illness, it is not surprising that Harry continued to 'choke' and that, after one episode, he was rushed to the children's hospital in the middle of the night. The family was hospitalised for four days and Harry given a diagnosis of 'marked reflux'. We could ask whether Harry, with his frequent choking episodes, is feeling safe, or whether he is feeling panic. As Hardy (1988) has stated, 'Everything a baby does is communicating'. We could surmise that Harry is not feeling integrated as he struggles to co-ordinate his breathing, sucking and swallowing. The baby will have difficulty regulating if he is not first contained by the mother, if she is unable to contain her own hyperarousal. Winnicott (1965) states that 'The baby's experience of bodily processes is intricately connected with the mothering experience'.

I haven't really enjoyed the last few weeks at all. I feel a bit guilty about that, because I think that I should be really enjoying motherhood, but it's a very a strange start to it and hopefully things will get better. I'm sure they will. I'll start to be able to enjoy it, but at the moment it's just I feel like you lose your identity. You just feel like you could stay inside for ever and the whole world passes by, and it's just an awful feeling, I can't explain it. But it won't be forever; it's only been for a few weeks but it feels like it's been about months and months [laughing].

That's another thing, he's not sleeping through the night and I don't expect that to happen for a while. But there are no rewards; he's just started to smile now and it's just so hard with it. I never thought it would be this hard, but you don't get anything back from them for quite a few months, and that's what this girl with this premmie baby was saying yesterday, that her baby's still like a little baby. And I said, 'Well so is he, still like a little baby'.

There are two topics to which Rowena keeps returning throughout these interviews: having another baby and when to return to work:

I don't know whether I'll like staying home full time; I think I look forward to going back to work in maybe six months' time. I don't know, maybe I might be enjoying it a bit more by then. At the moment I can't see it and just to have that bit of independence.

I had to see my obstetrician today, and we had a really good talk about having another baby 'cause he just asked me about contraception. And I said, 'Well I definitely don't want another baby' and he said, 'I shouldn't think like that', and a lot of women who have problems with their first baby just immediately think they can't have another one or they won't because they're worried about the problems that could happen again, and he said I shouldn't even worry about that.

And from interview number 7:

It's taken a while but it is getting much better, and I think we're both going to get a lot of enjoyment out of that baby, and I'm even thinking it'd be nice maybe [in] a year to try and have another one, and my doctor said it's OK. But then I think, oh I'm lucky to have him and I should maybe just stick with one. Think myself lucky that everything's OK with him. I don't know, see how I do [laughing]. See how I feel in about a year's time.

The frequent revisiting of these two topics gives an indication of how difficult it is for Rowena to stay with the day-to-day issues of baby Harry and his needs – the task of 'holding the baby in mind'. There is a hope that the stressful experiences of the past and present weeks can be replaced with a full-term healthy pregnancy and baby, a baby which is not continually threatening to die, or that the stress can be lessened by having the mind taken up with work.

Self-regulation theory

Self-regulation has been identified as an essential organising principle, 'if not a fundamental mechanism of the development of dynamic living systems' (Schore 1996). As stated earlier, the growing fetus and newborn requires, for their survival, another human being to hold them in mind, and for an adult, preferably the mother, to have times of reverie about the baby, times of thinking with the baby and for the baby (Fonegy et al 1991), in short an adult who is able to take the infant's perspective (Stern 1990). The baby's need is for their mother, from the very beginning, to be an organiser of experiences, to help them to meet the challenge of learning to regulate themself, through the hundreds of interactions they have with one other.

Harry is struggling to regulate himself in relation to one of the basic functions, that of breathing while sucking and swallowing – an issue of survival. In a parallel process, it seems that he is also struggling to be held in the mind of his mother, competing with her dilemma of having another baby, of whether or not to go back to work, and with her preoccupation with her own health.

It is now understood that the infant brain is a self-organising system and that the self-organisation of the developing brain occurs in the context of a relationship with another self, another brain (Schore 1996). When an infant is not held in the mind of their mother, when the mother does not act as an effective 'external psychobiological regulator', the infant's frontal lobe development is limited (Schore 1996).

Conclusion

In the final interview, the listener is encouraged by the evidence of positive affect between mother, father and infant. Harry is now 17 weeks, or nine weeks corrected age:

> He's just gorgeous. And just the last few days amazing things have happened with him, all of a sudden. The smiling is laughing now, giggling, and Steven thinks it's probably 'cause we're interacting more with him as well. And in the mornings, or any time actually when he wakes up, middle of the night, you go in and he smiles straight at you. And today when we were at the doctor's, he was asleep when I got there and woke up a few minutes later, and oh he was just gorgeous for about 20 minutes, just smiling and cooing, and it's just really been in the last few days it's all happened. He's been smiling for a couple of weeks but not near as much as he has been lately.
>
> And he seems to know who you are, he just looks at you – you just melt. He looks at you, and I mean he can change dramatically from that to screaming, but

that's a lot due to the reflux and I think if he didn't have reflux he'd be a very, very happy baby. I went to my mother's group today, a lot of those little babies are crying all the time I was there and he's great, he really is a gorgeous baby.

And I'm getting so much more enjoyment out of him now. When he cries now, I don't worry about it. He used to cry all day a few weeks back; I was having a really hard time, and by the time Steven got home from work I was so fed up and I wasn't getting any enjoyment at all, and part of that I suppose was this reflux, but also because he wasn't doing anything either and the lack of sleep. He's still not sleeping really well; he's sleeping longer periods but he's awake. He seems to have a bit of a pattern between probably 6 'til midnight. I should go to bed earlier but I never do, and then he'll wake up and then he'll probably go back to sleep about 1 'til about 5 or 6. So that's quite good.

Rowena says that he 'seems to know who you are, he just looks at you' as well as smiling and laughing. His father believes that it is because they are interacting with him more. It would seem that there is an increasing amount of time during which Harry and his mother and father are participating in a 'reciprocal reward system' (Schwartz 1990), increasing the opportunity for pleasurable states and heightened interest, that is affect attunement (Stern 1985).

This expanding positive affective relationship is also influencing Harry's bodily states and his movement between states, as he is reported to be 'not so demanding; now when he is hungry he can wait a little bit'.

Perhaps, after the weeks of separation in the nursery and the heightened anxiety in the early weeks at home, Rowena and Harry are at last experiencing increasing periods of mutually positive affect and interest. It is such experiences that specifically influence the 'ontogeny of homeostatic self-regulatory and attachment systems' (Greenspan 1981). There is evidence of Harry regulating himself, of Rowena being less anxious and more confident as she reads his signals more successfully, and of both Rowena and Steven becoming sensitive to their position in the mind of Harry as they are holding Harry in their minds. A quote by Sander (1975) seems appropriate here:

> One of the features most idiosyncratic during the first three months is the extent to which the infant is helped or compromised in beginning to determine aspects of his own regulation ... (and the mother's) feeling of confidence that she knows her baby's needs and can specifically meet them.

But how deep are the scars for these parents? How does such a traumatic period influence a couple's attempt to have another baby, and what of the first baby when the second arrives? In correspondence to Norma Tracey while preparing this chapter, Rowena wrote, 'we have a lovely baby girl named Ellen born on 9 September. After three miscarriages and a difficult pregnancy, she really is a miracle! Harry is well and keeps us very busy with his constant chattering'. With the reparative full-term daughter, Rowena may feel that she has the family she spoke of wistfully in the second interview so long ago. Meanwhile, Harry has found a way to keep himself in his parents' focus!

References

Alberts JR, Cramer CP (1988) Ecology and experience: sources of means and meaning of developmental change. In Blass ME (Ed.), Handbook of Behavioral Neurobiology: Developmental Psychology and Behavioral Ecology. New York: Plenum Press.

Als H (1993) Data from the National Collaborative Research Institute. Conference presentation, Contemporary Forums Developmental Interventions in Neonatal Care Conference, San Francisco, December.

Als H, Gilkerson L (1995) Developmentally supportive care in the neonatal intensive care unit. Zero to Three 15(6): 1–10.

Als H, Duffy FH, McAnulty GB (1996) Effectiveness of individualised neurodevelopmental care in the newborn intensive care unit (NICU). Acta Paediatrica (Supplement) 416: 21–30.

Brazelton TB, Cramer BG (1990) The Earliest Relationship: Parents, Infants and the Drama of Early Attachment. Reading, MA: Addison-Wesley.

Field TM, Schanberg SM, Scafidi F et al (1986) Tactile/kinesthetic stimulation effects on preterm neonates. Pediatrics 77: 654–8.

Fonegy P, Steele M, Steele H, Moran GS, Higgitt AC (1991) The capacity for understanding mental states: the reflective self in parent and child and its significance for security of attachment. Infant Mental Health Journal 12(3): 201–8.

Greenspan SI (1981) Psychopathology and Adaptation in Infancy and Early Childhood: Principles of Clinical Diagnosis and Preventive Intervention. New York: International Universities Press.

Hardy H (1988) Paper presented at the workship 'Defining and Treating the Trauma of Parents and Their Infants in Neonatal Intensive Care, at the AAIMHI conference 'With no Language but a Cry – Trauma in Infancy', Sydney, September.

Hepper PG (1996) Fetal memory: Does it exist? What does it do? Acta Paediatrica (Supplement) 416: 16–20.

Hofer MA (1987) Early social relationships: a psychobiologist's view. Child Development 58: 633–47.

Lieberman AF, Slade A (1997) The first year of life. In Noshpitz JD (Ed.) Handbook of Child and Adolescent Psychiatry. Volume 1: Infants and Preschoolers: Development and Syndromes. New York: John Wiley & Sons.

Mahler M, Pine F, Bergman A (1975) The Psychological Birth of the Human Infant. New York: Basic Books.

Paneth N, Rudelli R, Kazam L, Monte W (1994) Brain damage in the preterm infant. Clinics in Developmental Medicine No. 131. London: MacKeith Press/Cambridge University Press.

Perry B (1995) Childhood trauma, adaptation and the use-dependent development of the brain: how 'states' become 'traits'. Infant Mental Health Journal 16(4): 271–91.

Sander LW (1962) Issues in early mother–child interaction. Journal of the American Academy of Child Psychiatry 1: 141–66.

Sander LW (1975) Infant and caretaking environment: investigation and conceptualisation of adaptive behavior in a system of increasing complexity. In Anthony EJ (Ed.) Explorations in Child Psychiatry. New York: Plenum Press.

Sander LW (1997) Paradox and resolution from the beginning. In Noshpitz JD (Ed.) Handbook of Child and Adolescent Psychiatry. Volume 1: Infants and Preschoolers: Developmental and Syndromes. New York: John Wiley & Sons.

Schore AN (1996) The experience-dependent maturation of a regulatory system in the orbital prefrontal cortex and the origin of developmental psychopathology. Development and Psychopathology 8: 59–87.

Schwartz GE (1990) Psychobiology of repression and health: a systems approach. In Singer JL (Ed.) Repression and Dissociation. Chicago: University of Chicago Press.

Sroufe LA (1979) The coherence of individual development. American Psychologist 34: 834–41.

Stern DN (1985) The Interpersonal World of the Infant. New York: Basic Books.

Stern DN (1990) Diary of a Baby. New York: Basic Books.

Thompson RJ, Goldstein RF, Oehler JM, Gustafson KE, Catlett AT, Brazy JE (1994) Developmental outcome of very low birth weight infants as a function of biological risk and psychosocial risk. Developmental and Behavioral Pediatrics 15: 232–8.

Tracey N, Blake P, Warren B, Hardy H, Enfield S, Schein P (1995) A mother's narrative of premature birth. Journal of Child Psychotherapy 21(1): 43–64.

Winnicott DW (1965) The Maturational Process and the Facilitating Environment. New York: International Universities Press.

Chapter 7
Two mothers without mothers

FRANCES THOMSON SALO

This chapter will explore the unique stories of two women whose mothers had died, in order to show how they began the process of refinding a good mother within themselves. Both women had lost their mothers in tragic circumstances, and such a loss creates vulnerability for a woman as she faces motherhood. As Freud (1915) said of the experience of the loss of a loved one, 'the shadow of the object fell upon the ego'.

The excerpts below are taken from the audiotaped narrations of two mothers: Karen (a full-term mother) and Liz (a neonatal intensive care unit [NICU] mother). The aim is draw out how difficulties of coming to terms with the loss of a mother's mother can have an overridingly powerful effect during this time of maternal preoccupation. Whereas Liz had to manage the stress of having an infant in NICU for two months, Karen brought more overt vulnerability to becoming a mother. She experienced overwhelming sadness in reliving the loss of her mother. I hope to show that, in the context of a caring relationship with another, be it a professional or a friend, much of the sadness from the past can be eased in quite a short space of time.

This chapter is about how both these mothers found their 'good internal mothers' again. The term 'good object' is used to refer to an internal mind representation, a way of talking about a child's live inner experience of her mother. The mother's loving and caring for the child becomes an integral part of the way the child feels about herself. Good experiences increase this sense of self-worth; bad experiences take from it. The feelings of loss and depression that affected Karen and Liz eased as their identification with what they experienced as a damaged or dead internal mother lessened. They were able to experience a more alive mother within themselves, as they could experience a more alive baby in their external world. The gradual elation with regard to the baby, and the sense of her having a mind of her own, helped to give these mothers hope.

Dreaming played an important part in these mothers' recovery. Karen brought two dreams to Norma Tracey, the interviewer, and Liz brought one. The creativity in these dreams was very important to the working through of the primary maternal preoccupation stage. Dreaming acts as a way of recovering the internal good object. Their dreaming helped the two mothers to achieve a more coherent narrative of their personal past and the place of their mothers in it.

Mothers need mothers. External support is crucial in helping a mother to regain the sense of an internal good mother if this has become fragile after her baby's birth. Both Karen and Liz acknowledged the help that they received from their partners, hospital staff and friends. Mothers who have lost their mothers will at times desperately miss their own mother just being present to know about their daughter's feelings. Liz and Karen felt mothered by the interviewer's interest, and this helped towards their regaining a sense of inner well-being.

Their interviews allow us to consider in detail the different adjustments that they have to make. It highlights the need for staff to be open to hearing what the mothers bring from their past, and to balance this with the events that they are experiencing in the present.

Introducing the two mothers

Karen is in the control group of mothers with a full-term baby. She had suffered considerable pain throughout her pregnancy, with nausea, sciatica and pre-eclampsia. She underwent a caesarean section and had high blood pressure for several weeks after the birth. She subsequently became extremely sad at times, yet her daughter was a thriving, beautiful baby, a poignant counterpoint to her mother's unhappiness. When Karen was two years old, her mother was diagnosed with breast cancer. She was late in her pregnancy with Karen's younger sister and died three years later. Karen's father then married a woman who dealt with her own difficulties by an outward harshness to her three little stepdaughters.

Liz had severe toxaemia and, because of the risk to her own life and that of her daughter, underwent an emergency caesarean section when her daughter was 26 weeks gestation. The baby weighed 850 g and needed oxygen and the full support of NICU, where she lived for two months. Liz's mother, who had a long history of manic-depressive illness, had committed suicide five years before Liz's daughter was born. Liz was pregnant at the time of her mother's suicide and miscarried a month later.

There were a number of similarities between Karen and Liz. They were both in their thirties and were tertiary-educated women who had developed careers for themselves. They had both had difficulty with their anger: Liz had considerable anxiety about expressing hers; Karen had idealised her mother, giving her so much 'goodness' that it depleted Karen of any sense of her own goodness.

Karen's narration: 'Telling these stories about my life'

As Karen describes her mother's life and the time that she shared with her, she is often overcome with grief, and her sobbing punctuates the interviews.

Interview 1

In her first interview, Karen says of her daughter:

> I find myself just crying at the thought that she's here. I love her so much and fear that I might lose her because I don't think I've ever cared so much about anyone else. I've always been healthy but my mother was sick when I was little. She died of cancer when I was five, so which is, you know, well it's not something that upsets me greatly these days. I've had 30 years to get used to it, but it's still, it is part of my life.

At this point, Karen became slightly incoherent as she was overcome with emotion. Here we see the ghosts of the past rising up to haunt her.

Now let us continue Karen's story:

> I can remember when I was pregnant about halfway through, really I had quite a tearful emotional sort of pregnancy. But it struck me one night that here was me about to become a mother and I'd never really had a mother. It also hit me what my mother must have felt. She had three babies when she died, my little sister was three and I was five and my older sister was seven. She had to leave us, and it had never struck me before just how traumatic this must have been for her – not just to face death herself but to know her babies weren't going to be looked after.
>
> And we weren't well looked after. My father married again and my stepmother wasn't a happy person, and we were abused, an emotional sort of thing. I've forgiven her now, but there's still some resentment that that happened. And I think it's also terrifying that not only could your baby die but you could die, and the same terrible things could happen and no one could protect her. And I mean that's – Oh, God, I can't breathe – that was something that hit me while I was still pregnant and I suppose that's still there in the background.

In fact, it is in the foreground. We see how Karen has become confused between her mother, her baby and herself. When she is describing her sisters' ages, it is as though she has become a child again. When she cannot breathe, she is having a psychosomatic reaction similar to her mother's illness.

Karen spends the rest of her interviews working through this area.

Interview 2

Karen talks, in her second interview, of mourning the loss of the couple relationship with her partner and then about the mothering she has had:

> My grandmother looked after us when my mother was ill. In fact we had quite a few other mothers; my mother's sister looked after us a lot, so she was a kind of second mother. She only died earlier this year which was like losing another mother, and then there's my stepmother. I've got really bad mothering models: my mother who dies and a stepmother who neglected us. I can remember thinking when I was about 20, I couldn't remember a single happy day, and it's only at times like this when I look back on my childhood and feel really sad about what happened, but most of the time I'm OK about it.

Karen talks of another loss – of her culture – and in doing so regains some of it:

> I have a sense of loss that my child won't have that richness of culture. I'm sad that I don't have a babushka in the house to look after my child like my parents did. But Poppy the Greek woman from next door brought me over a beautiful Madonna icon to protect the baby. We'll just give her other things instead of that heritage. Because everyone I know does have their mother to come around and babysit, and I'll never have that.
>
> My mother was a kind of fairy princess, she was brilliant and beautiful and had the best clothes. This meant we grew up under her shadow, but it meant for my stepmother she could never be good enough. I think at heart she was a good person but it meant she was living up to the impossible ideal of the beautiful Marilyn Joy.

Karen adds: 'Not having a mother is at the heart of why I'm sad now'.

When any mother does not have a sense of an internal mother who accompanies her, she will keep looking to find her in the real external world, and Karen describes this here:

> Part of the problem of letting go of the hospital was having a woman obstetrician and always having that kind of bond with older women who look after me, and for me it slotted straight into the absent mother thing.

Interview 3

Karen had found breastfeeding difficult with painful nipples. It had a life-or-death quality, as it had for her mother, whose life had been claimed by breast cancer after breastfeeding. In the third interview, Karen says:

I've given up breastfeeding. I'm sad but not dramatically so. She's thriving. One of the things that was stopping me sleeping was looking at her in fear thinking, 'It's my body and nipples that she's dependent on and if I don't survive she doesn't survive', and it was putting a really strong pressure on me when I'm probably the weakest physically I've ever been.

It's not just my body coming back, it's my life coming back. I realise even taking it one feed at a time was terrifying; I was really hanging on the edge. I just didn't feel that I had it in me. I know people didn't die any more because of pre-eclampsia, but the fact that it could have happened in the past is quite scary when illness has the kind of emotional stuff that it does for me because of my mother. I felt breastfeeding was something I could be good at like all the other things I tried as a child to be good at to make up to my father for my mother dying.

Here the ghosts from the past are dramatically operative, casting a long shadow over the present.

As Karen begins to do this linking of the present to the past, nurturant features reappear: 'I made generous food. I suddenly felt, if I can cook and enjoy food, everything's OK. In hospital it's like eating dead things'. Some hope is rekindled; she is moving from eating 'dead things' to alive food that she, as the alive mother, can prepare and enjoy. I saw this as being linked to her infant's progress as her next sentence was, 'Now the baby's getting bigger and happier and being awake more, and she's cute'.

Interview 4

During the fourth interview, Karen talks of the pleasures multiplying. Here we see the infant's contribution in pulling the mother forward. Karen describes intermittent waves of grief and says that if the baby were not settled and she was without a supportive partner, she would find it harder to get out of the pit of despair. Regaining the couple relationship is particularly important for a mother who has lost her own mother.

One of the things that makes it difficult for Karen is that 'I've got no idea about "why" to anything about this baby'. If she had a sense that the baby has a mind of her own, it would help to reassure her of her daughter's resilience and add to her hope. In fact, we see that she is actually getting to know her baby better – she says that as her baby looks in her face 'you start to feel she's really looking at you and there are some signs of recognition'. In turn, Karen feels more confident and says she is starting to enjoy her.

Interview 5

Karen says in the fifth interview, 'It's days and days since I cried'. Again, this is linked to her infant's progress: 'She's starting to be a bit more responsive. There's days when I sit there staring at her thinking how beautiful she is'. I think possibly she reminds Karen of looking at her own mother. 'It's the being able to look after myself part of me that's starting to come back. I feel I can not only look after her, I can look after myself, and both of us will be all right.' Karen has an alive mother and an alive baby in her internal world now:

> And that's important for my self-confidence, which disappeared during the birth because I didn't do any of it by myself. All of pregnancy and birth took me back emotionally to my own childhood, to the loss and fear of loss. I hope me getting sick and the drugs I was on haven't harmed her, that's something's that going to haunt me all my life. I gave up breastfeeding very close to all the other sadnesses, so all of it's confused in my mind and memory.

In the light of feeling alive and well, Karen can now look back to days when there was a fear of damage to both mother and infant.

When Karen is now asked about her mother, she is now able to talk without tears:

> My mother used to take me to work with her – teaching. There's not a day in my life before motherhood when I wouldn't refer back to my mother, and it makes me sadder about things, although at stressful times like the first weeks of having a baby it was swamping me, but what's happening to me now, I understand it a bit better in relation to what happened to me before; there's a sense of things fit together now. I suppose your life's a pattern of falling apart and coming back together, and this week I'm in one of the times when I feel a bit wholer.

Karen conveys with an almost poetic clarity the feelings of chaos and loss of order that are linked with of the early days of motherhood.

Interview 6

In this next interview, Karen felt sad and anxious as her husband had to be away with work and a cousin was diagnosed with breast cancer. Karen found it 'threatening that breast cancer is sitting there in wait for all of us, possibly for my daughter ... anyway I went and had a massage'. This could be Karen's way of unconsciously regaining a sense of her mother's hands caring for her. She links her sadness with:

> grief about my mother, panic sitting there under the surface just waiting to come out, and my sister and I talked about ways that we'd coped with losing our mother when we were little. I just keep thinking of her dying knowing she was leaving the three of us with only my father and her sister, and I don't know how I'd bear it; I couldn't leave a baby but she had to.

The empathy with her mother's sense of loss of her child now forms an important link in her mind with, and her own sense of loss of, her mother.

These are important links in her mind at this point. Until this time, Karen seemed to be reliving her experience of being the child who was left; now the identification with her dying mother is clearer.

Karen brought the first of her two dreams to this interview. It appears that she had 'come together' enough to realise fully that the interviewer, who had in some way filled the place of a mother for her, would be leaving soon. The dream was the result of that sadness and the need to revisit some unfinished business with the interviewer as the mother before she leaves her. Until this time, Karen has only referred to having nightmares that she attributes to the blood pressure medication. This dream is different:

> I keep having this dream that I find old photos of our mother and of us when we're little, and they fill in all the gaps. Then I wake up and there aren't any photos. I don't know what it means. It has nothing to do with baby; she's just triggered it off. I think I had it again last night.
>
> There's so little that we know about our mother and we couldn't ask our father because he wouldn't ever talk about any of it, and our stepmother threw out our mother's clothes. It made it harder for us because there was so little to know about her as we were growing up. In the dream we find photos and somehow what we didn't know becomes known – maybe that's what's happening.

Karen seems to have redreamt the dream for the interviewer to hear. It is almost as if she is a child again. This dream for the interviewer has an important function of recognising a wish that cannot be fulfilled and the need to move on past this. Karen is more right than she knows about the baby triggering it off – Karen needs to get the sense of being mothered in order to mother her own child.

By now, Karen has become less tearful. She then talks of her baby's progress and says, 'We're starting to get feedback now; it's like we're dealing with a person now so she's completely beautiful'. Here the joy of knowing her baby gives her hope of being an alive mother to that baby.

With the dream, Karen goes on to make links so that she does come to 'know more':

> She was a shadowy figure in a nightie we visited in hospital, and I had three years of her being in hospital. She supported my father through university. It wouldn't have helped her general health, to keep working and having children, it was terrible stress, and the abortion before they married. My mother's mother had nothing to do with us because she disapproved of my father. She talked my mother into having a termination – a terrible thing for a mother to do to her daughter, nightmarish. She was a horrible woman. She was never there for us. So mothering is a fairly traumatic experience for all of us. But I suspect that there was this strong mothering that I got in the little bit of time that I did get to spend with my own mother.

In talking about her grandmother, we meet a terrible internal mother but also see Karen's identification with her mother's strengths.

The relevance of a mother for a mother at this time is shown in the amount of interview time spent not on Karen and the baby, but on her mother and her as her mother's child.

Interview 7

By the seventh interview, Karen is aware she has been stuck but does not realise that the dream she brings the interviewer this week is about her underground wellspring of tears:

> Telling those stories about my life will probably always reduce me to tears no matter how much I come to terms with it. The sadness is not interfering with anything; when I need to be happy to play with the baby I can do that. I have to deal with the way I feel before I can move on.

The dream Karen is about to recount will help:

> I had a dream that I went to Moscow. We arrived on a tour bus, and things were frozen and there were people going about their daily work in the street, scenes you'd see out of a bus window, but they were all encased in ice. The whole city was like that apart from one bit outside the city where it was like a river bank but it had all been silted up, polluted with dirty water. I don't know what it means, it was one of those vivid dreams; it seemed important.

The dream concerns how something was frozen as a result of her mother's death but could be more integrated as Karen takes responsibility for her conflicting emotions. In the dream, touring foreign places indicates the hope of a more playful life.

Interview 8

Karen says, 'I'm feeling so much more accepting of things. It was wonderful to spend time with my sister and my niece, who completely adores her cousin; she pretends Alexi is her sister'. Here Karen begins to name her daughter; she now has more of a presence. 'I've had a lot of sadness in my own childhood that being a parent has brought up for me, but I'm starting to think that there are a lot of positive things that I wouldn't have thought about if I hadn't had a child.' By talking about her mother, Karen is able to mourn her mother's death more fully; she is able to feel that her mother has given to her and not just left her with an empty aching void.

Interview 9

In the last interview, Karen says:

I'm emotionally in a completely different space. There are longer periods between the falling apart, and even when I'm still really distressed, I know it's gonna come to an end. We spent some time with my younger sister and she fell in love with the baby. I think the fact that Alexi always was a lovely natured baby, very smiley and playful, won over my sister. It was nice for me to have some family admiring my daughter. It's so much fun seeing her changing each day.

Liz's experience

Liz does not convey the same degree of sadness that Karen does; the needy infant is more evident in Karen than in Liz. What Liz says is often punctuated by laughter. It seems probable that, until Liz can take her baby home from NICU, she has to shut down. However, she has had a sense early on of her baby's personality and mind, which may give the hope she needs to carry her through. Liz calls her baby by her name early and often. She only mentions her mother directly in four interviews, but it is possible to see her shadow behind much of what Liz says.

Interview 1

In this first interview, Liz says, 'I produced this wonderful little girl and I feel really close to her now. It was great being able to hold her and pick her up, so little, little, little'. But the joy is muted, and Liz soon talks of her anxiety about her mother's psychiatric history. She was concerned about postnatal depression because:

> my mother who is no longer with us, I was told sort of had postnatal depression and so I thought oh well, what happened to your mother it might happen to me, and so I've been looking; don't look, you know if you look too hard you're gonna find these things, but I'm glad I'm busy at the moment so I've got plenty to do.

Here we see the wish to avoid anxiety by moving quickly away from the topic and being busy, avoiding contact with the internal mother who is felt to be damaged and dead. The words are fast and confused as if many voices are talking.

Interview 2

In this interview, Liz says of her daughter Rosie, 'I look in her little eyes and they're still sort of a bit skew-whiff and I think are you gonna be regular and normal?'. For Liz and her baby, the absent mother cannot provide her loving, assuring gaze. This would have helped to hold Liz, for as she talks about her mother she becomes less articulate and presents almost as a motherless waif. In her frequent use of the phrase 'you know', there is a wish for a mother who would just know without needing to be told.

> I notice that a lot of the ladies have their mothers around, and I go to a mater-
> nity shop and some mothers are saying, 'Look at this, darling', and I think
> 'Where's my mother?'. And there's certain people that have taken up a similar
> role and but I don't know if it's because I send out message of 'Gee, I'm
> motherless at the moment'.
>
> My mother actually killed herself, and I wasn't OK for a long time. But I'm
> OK now because you know that's a decision that she made for herself, and it
> was really unusual, the day after Mother's Day, so it's just like she hung out for
> Mother's Day and then she did it the next day. It was really strange because I
> was actually pregnant at the time, and I lost that child and I didn't know I was
> pregnant then, but it was about four weeks later that it just didn't get off the
> ground.
>
> I do sound pretty detached at the moment, but I went to see a counsellor
> and I'm glad I did. There's things that come into my head at the moment
> because my mother was mentally ill. She had manic-depressive psychosis, and
> you know it has been mentioned that you know there's a higher incidence of
> this recurring, and actually I hadn't thought directly about that but it's troubling
> because it can't be really predicted, it just pops out later in life. My father
> mentioned it when I miscarried; he says, 'Oh, it might be for the best'. [Laughs]
> I'll kill him.
>
> ... So Mum's, my mother's not around, and I wish she was but she isn't. I've
> got a half sister who really likes little babies and she's been helpful, and I've got
> a pretty extensive support network. And it was five years ago, my mother was
> 66, and it's been a big adjustment.

Interview 3

By the third interview, Liz, like Karen, had had a massage: 'It was nice'. Again, it appears that Liz could be trying unconsciously to recreate the sense of her mother's hands caring for her. Liz talks of having fun with her daughter, caressing her with her hands. She continues:

> Having a baby around can arouse all sorts of issues about one's own upbringing
> and whether we felt deprived or nurtured. I really feel very fortunate that I've
> got my husband, who's so understanding and totally non-judgemental, but I'm
> learning not be so hard on myself.

Liz has not yet made the link between how hard she is on herself and her mother's high expectations of her, but this is foreshadowed: 'I'm sure there's things floating around in my head which I still haven't acknowl-edged properly and one I touched on maybe just today'. This was whether she would judge her daughter in the same way that she is hard on herself.

Liz goes on to recount her dream:

There's a lady from work whom I talk to quite a bit and we went to this place to find clothes, and there was this woman in a wheelchair and she was looking at all these clothes, and I saw this little jacket with all these autumn tones and I said 'Oh, Rosie would look really good in that. If that lady in the wheelchair puts down that jacket then maybe I can get it for Rosie'. Then this lady picked up this large dressing gown for an eight-year-old and said, 'Oh that would look good on my daughter Rosie' and I first thought to myself in this dream, 'Oh, what a coincidence'. I didn't think there were that many Rosies around.

It could be that, although Liz did not realise it, the 'lady from work' she talked to was the interviewer. Liz said about the dream:

It shocked me, and I thought what's the wheelchair connection and is it putting myself in that particular position in the wheelchair because – now I'm describing it to you I'm getting more of a connection – I was put in that wheelchair going up to the nursery and I'd never considered myself wheelchair material.

Liz wondered:

is Rosie going to be intellectually in the normal range? I know me, the high achiever, what if she's going to be just struggling and having learning difficulties. I don't want to think about it. When she connects with my eyes all those fears get dispelled.

Liz interprets one of the dream's meanings for herself. She is also working out thoughts and feelings about her damaged mother. The wheelchair mother and the autumnal tones stand for the damaged mother. Children whose parents have committed suicide feel that it is an aggressive act and feel guilty about their anger with their parent. The three 'Oh's' convey Liz's sense of shock at what has happened to her and her loss of feeling special. One of her central questions is whether she and Rosie can escape being in a wheelchair themselves, and lead fulfilled lives.

Liz finishes the interview in a more integrated state. She muses:

Is there a nice way to replenish that feeling that something has been taken away? So I think my next thing is opening up and integrating and allowing space, and I guess I haven't thought about a lot of things.

Some of these may be whether she damaged her mother and will in turn be damaged, the damage being revisited down through the generations on to her daughter in terms of the psychosis.

Interview 4

In the next interview, Liz explores her 'darker side' with its split-off anger and how she punishes herself. This seems to be the last piece of 'work' she needs to do before making the link in the subsequent interview with her mother's difficulties. She starts with an observation that shows she is getting to know her daughter:

> She seems to want to feed and she doesn't get all stressed. So that's really reinforcing me as a new mother, thinking I've got all this nourishment here. I've been tapping on the humidicrib and she seems to follow.
>   ... We poor parents are really torturing ourselves and it's just our fantasies. I look around at other mothers and they want to throw their babies out of the window. I've just got to keep coming back to – be kind to yourself, Liz. But I'm wondering about the real me; my darker side's the one that worries me. And I think what am I going to do when Rosie's driving me crazy, when she's three and says no all the time; I have all these awful visions.

Is Liz wondering whether she is allowed to have a live good baby, rather than one who goes through the window, when she has a mother who did not survive? The hate is safely attributed to the other mothers, although there is an integrity in Liz's struggle to own her feelings.

When Liz arrived late at the hospital, the nurses had fed Rosie and Liz felt a failure:

> If I'm observing my behaviour and it's not what I say I'm going to do, I've got to change the behaviour or the words in order to have a bit more harmony, otherwise I keep on whipping myself. I guess it's the way I've been brought up. I can learn so much from Rosie.

Here we see how Liz could be depressed as her mother was and observe Liz's attempt to make it better for her daughter than it was for herself. The idealising projection that Rosie has the necessary knowledge plays a useful function in rescuing Liz from criticising herself.

Interview 5

The fifth interview is the turning point:

> Today I just held her and she fell asleep in an upright position, like a little koala that hangs onto a gum tree. Really the first cuddle was today, and she just seemed so much more baby-like, and it was really great because she was content, she made a few little sounds.

Now Liz's baby is holding her and indicating that she wants her.

> My father's going to be my major daytime support person. It's not that I just want another woman around that's been through the same situation. My father will store things up till he can't take it any longer and there's this big volcano comes out. If I feel angry, I try and talk myself out of it till I defuse it all away. I still have this fear of anger.

Although Liz denies wanting another woman who is a mother, lying behind her comment is, one can suggest, a longing for the good mother who could have helped with her fear of anger. This is what now breaks through with the re-emergence of a traumatic memory and being able to re-experience a childhood fear in the holding presence of a benign adult.

> I remember when I was young I used to have these passionate feelings of rage. And I don't know who couldn't cope with it in my family, but it was probably my mother, and I used to get locked away in a bathroom and I couldn't come out till I was really peaceful. And I remember kicking all the paint off the door. I was about four; I had these fantasies that the bathroom window wasn't there, and I could get out and I could fly, and I didn't need to be trapped in this funny little room and kick all the paint off. And I've been thinking about that recently and then I remember my father saying, 'I never thought it was a good idea to lock you in the bathroom'. Jesus, well why didn't you do something about it?
>
> So it's probably why I don't get angry. Rosie will go off her brain because she's a baby, and they do go off their brains and, I'm getting sweaty palms just thinking about it. But I didn't realise until today, that it's probably that my mother couldn't handle my feelings of anger, she couldn't handle her own feelings of anger.

Liz is making a link here that she has not made before. That it is difficult can be seen from her sweaty palms. As a child, she could feel that her anger damaged her mother, who did not want to stay around an angry child. It explains why Liz has worked so hard to overcome her anger. The internal bad mother drove her to excel in the tasks she set herself. Liz does not want to carry this ghost into her daughter's nursery.

Liz continues: 'I talk myself out of anger, and feelings of deprivation I just discard'. However, she does have to confront anger coming from having an infant:

> I suppose it's an anger thing that I'm being rushed into things. There's a time, you know, I forget that I'm a mother. How does a mother know they're a mother? Because there's babies around.

Liz is propelled headlong into dealing with the past while trying to get to know her infant, whom she does not have physically present with her. Her mother, who knew she was a mother as she had two babies, gave up this knowing by taking her life.

Interview 6

By the sixth interview, Liz knows that Rosie will be coming home:

> I feel better. I am nervous. She's bright and alert and turning into a regular little baby. Rosie will be far more adaptable than me; she'll be everyone's friend. But

I'll be lenient on myself, establishing personal space. I've changed a lot in my estimate of mums, and I see it through a totally different light now. People think about their mothers and the way their mothers have been doing things. I don't have that situation but there's that good warm fuzzy thing inside.

But Liz is still scared she'll get it wrong 'like a kid'.

Interview 7

Rosie is home for the seventh interview:

Rosie rocks on as if 'Wow, it's really nice living here and it's nice having you around', like she thought this is totally no big deal and I can learn a lot from that, take one thing at a time, and I just look into her little face and it's just so immediate, and the moods, they're real. And she's such a cutey.

Interview 8

Liz says that the times when she does not understand why Rosie is distressed are when she probably comes closest to the anger that she feels she is being rushed into confronting:

I think if I try and squash away all these unownable feelings then they might get the better of me somehow. So I talk to her about it and I find it helps. She's got her good phases and her cranky phases just like everyone else. It's just a matter of us fitting into her rhythm and her fitting into ours. It just takes time, but it's been remarkably quick.

The feeling here is not that Liz is using the baby as a container but rather that, in talking about her anger, she is neutralising it and is then able to act as a container for her daughter.

Interview 9

By the final interview, Liz is reviewing where she has reached:

She seems to be a really social baby. I modify things gradually and Rosie responds well to that sort of repetition. Taking care of yourself is actually taking care of her. These are special times. I think her existence is enhanced by me being around and vice versa.

I feel really fortunate that I've got this special place in Rosie's life now, and I think one of my major achievements of my life is creating a relationship that works well. And I thanked her for letting me be my – her mother. Achieving success in this relationship is powerful but quiet – feeling happy walking the street or pushing a pram or making dinner, that's the important stuff. She's really the happiness, the real future.

... I haven't got my mum around like a lot of people I see but I'm so blessed in other ways. I have much more empathy for people. Mothers seem to connect with one another and there's eye contact when you pass them on the street; it's like 'I know what you're going through'. And that's wonderful and you don't have to say anything.

Liz's slip of the tongue when she refers to her mother when she means being the mother to her baby shows us that she is still somewhere preoccupied. However, we can also see that even if there are still difficulties for Liz in regaining an identification with a good mother, an integration provides firmer ground than continued splitting. As Liz feels she gets something back from Rosie, she feels mothered in turn. The love, hope and creativity indicate that there is now a more secure good internal mother.

Discussion

The following themes in Karen's and Liz's interviews convey their experience of the interwoven strands of primary maternal preoccupation and their emergence from this stage.

'The vivid present' (Auden 1958)

When a baby is born, the sense of lived time is altered: it goes into suspended infinity, as though time were standing still. As Karen said, 'Having a baby puts you in another world' – that of your own childhood past. Memories buried deep with a different time frame bring their own emotional colouring to the events and experiences of the neonatal period.

Norma Tracey writes vividly in Chapter 20 of the dead space at the heart of the traumatic experience. Both Liz and Karen experienced traumatic events. For Karen, two senses of time collided: the trauma of her mother's early death and the timelessness of primary maternal preoccupation. For Liz, there was also the trauma of the premature, anxiety-provoking birth. Above all, with a baby in NICU, there is no baby to hold in your arms and dream over timelessly. The two mothers bring their dreams to the interviewer for her to hear with them and to understand implicitly.

Reclaiming the joy

There is more elation in primary maternal preoccupation than Winnicott (1956) suggests, as well as a quieter kind of joy. We know so much about the exquisite capacities of newborns and the turn-taking that goes on between them and their mothers. Second by second, the mother influences the baby, and the baby influences the mother. There is pleasure in the mirroring of attunement. If the mother feels the baby acting on her, this is a kind of claiming that would connect the mother more closely to the infant, give her pleasure and confirm her as a mother. When all goes well for the mother, it means that her good internal mother is back and she feels loved and good, with a sense of her baby not just as a wanted baby but as a precious one. For a mother who is depressed or has a baby in NICU, joy becomes much more of an achievement to be gained.

Banishing the bad fairy godmother

For a new mother, there is always the possibility of a bad fairy godmother waiting in the wings, as with Sleeping Beauty, in the mother's anxiety that something bad will happen to her baby or she will be angry with the baby or the baby will die. There is ever-present guilt on her part, fearing that she has failed her child and not been perfect.

For Karen and Liz, such fears take longer to banish because of unfinished mourning, fears about their mothers' illnesses and fears for their infants' development. If mothers feel that their internal mother is fragile, it is as if they become small again, and the absence of the longed-for mother who could comfort them becomes so painful that it is as if they are being hurt. For the NICU mother, other more competent 'mothers' – the nurses – look after her baby, so she can easily feel not as good a mother as her own mother was, or as if she has a bad, rejecting internal mother.

The infant has a mind

The sense that her infant has a mind of her own and an inner world can help a mother to emerge from maternal preoccupation. The preoccupation is about losing herself in order to get to know her infant. The infant needs the mother to help to give her a sense of her physical and psychic skin. The recognition that she has a mind of her own signals a psychic separation of a new kind. But if the mother faces this, it means that the infant is becoming her own person, and is viable as a separate individual being. As the distorting projections, the idealising ones as well as the anxious ones, are given up for a more realistic view of the infant, this helps to consolidate an awareness of the infant's mind. Recognising this moves the mother towards relinquishing her total preoccupation with the infant. Recognising that the infant has a mind and a personality of her own helps to reinstall the good mother because there is some external confirmation that the baby's mother is a good mother. To contain for an infant means the return of the processing internal mother.

Liz saw her baby as having a personality and mind very early on, and one function of this is that it helped Liz to bridge the physical gap between them. Karen found it harder to let herself be in touch with her daughter's mind, but her own was preoccupied much of the time with her childhood losses.

The struggle to acknowledge the ambivalence

Whatever the hopeful emotions of joy and elation, there will also be anger, guilt and at times hate. The mother fears a loss of her sense of self, and at an unconscious level she feels that she is faced with a choice between her life and that of the infant. Joy over the infant and a sense that she has a mind of her own and can survive the mother's difficulties help to mitigate the ambivalence. When a mother can accept the different aspects in her relationship with her infant, she is able to be tolerant of her ambivalence. Being tolerant means that she is not deserted by her internal good mother, that if she had felt she had lost the internal mother when the baby was little, she is back securely in the mother's inner world.

Love, hope and creativity

When a mother begins to enjoy herself, she has found again an internal good mother who is caring. Both Karen and Liz became more able to care for themselves. Caring and having fun are in themselves creative activities. They are more quietly creative than the big creative acts but are nevertheless evidence of an enduring creativity. The new mother regains a perspective that time exists again; it exists with hope. Mothers can now contemplate taking a risk. The most basic psychic risk is to hope that their child will live and be happy.

Conclusion

Liz had to go through the usual time of primary maternal preoccupation without having looked after her baby much and had to work hard at making bridges to her. Karen, who had a full-term baby, felt devastated by the returning sadness and had to come through this. While having a premature baby obviously impinges on primary maternal preoccupation, as each woman's experience is unique we have also to look and see with what resilience or fragility she approaches having a baby.

We also have to consider the contribution that the baby makes towards pulling the mother into a live connection with her, and the nature of the support on which the mother can call. Karen and Liz were able to use the very special support offered through the interviewer's accompanying them, to feel that they and their babies were held.

As Karen said, 'It's always useful to talk, and people nearly always give you a new perspective on things if they've got time to, and professionals have time'. I think we need to make the time to remember the vulnerability of a mother who has lost her mother, and to listen.

References

Auden WH (1958) A Selection by the Author. London: Penguin.

Freud S (1915) Mourning and melancholia. In the Standard Edition of the Complete Psychological Works of Sigmund Freud (1914–1916). London: Hogarth Press/Institute of Psychoanalysis.

Winnicott DW (1956) Primary maternal preoccupation. In Collected Papers. Through Paediatrics to Psychoanalysis. London: Tavistock Publications.

PART 3
THE FATHERS

Chapter 8
Fathers of full-term infants

LORRAINE ROSE

In this chapter, we will look at the fathers of the newborns whose wives had a full-term pregnancy. We will collate the interview material from just after the birth, with a further look at 4–6 weeks, and finally one at 10–12 weeks.

After the birth

During this time, the fathers, like the mothers, were preoccupied with reviewing their own parenting and were being taken back to the previous generation, revisiting their own relationship with their father. They too felt much confusion over their role as a father, and held confused and mixed feelings in relation to their child. In contrast to their wives, however, they had a sense of being left out of the intense intimacy that occurs between the mother and baby, while wishing for and supporting the developing connection between their wife and their baby. While their wives were engrossed in their new offspring, the fathers carried the worry about the future of the family, particularly in relation to financial concerns.

Reviewing the past was something that almost all the fathers did as part of their working through of their transformation to fatherhood. Where this review did not take place, the father had greater difficulty in bonding with his child. As with the mother, revisiting the past was an important part of the process. Each father did this in his own way.

The husband of the woman who had lost her mother as a child was concerned with his own history and links the beginning of a new life with the end of another:

It's been harrowing. I am enjoying parenthood but I am scared. There were a lot of things in my childhood, with my parents divorcing and my father's mental illness, and my brother's mental illness. Later my father committed suicide. The strongest emotion I have ever felt was at his funeral and I was grieving. The only comparable feeling was the birth of our daughter – the labour was scary; it was harrowing. I was crying; I was so relieved the baby was alive – they wrapped her up and gave her to me.

Another man was concerned about how he was going to be as a father when his own father had been so absent. The anxieties about not having a good role model were clearly present for the fathers:

It is difficult for me to know how to be a father – my father was a very busy man; he felt it was the right thing to be spending time doing his work and was often not at home so I don't really have a good model for what it means to be a father. Also I am the youngest and I've never been in a situation where there's been a baby around.

For another father, it was a time to review how he wanted to be with this child and how he would like to be a father, as opposed to the fathering he received:

Basically we had a good upbringing, although I wasn't all that close to my Dad. One thing we didn't do was talk about things very much, and I would like that to be different – that we could discuss things more.

A lot of confusion was experienced by the fathers, as it was for the mothers. The fathers were able to articulate this state in a variety of ways. I feel it is best to let them speak about how it was for them and to experience with them their state of uncertainty in the face of such a new situation for themselves.

Talking about his wife and baby, one man said:

she wasn't feeling confident about her ability to be able to feed the baby, and I was trying to tell her that she was doing really well. The first day she was feeding the baby was very difficult. The baby's learning how to do it, and mum's learning how to do it, and the father feels as useful as pockets on a singlet.

Another was more explicit about the degree of confusion he was feeling and seemed unable to realise that the baby was also new to the situation: 'They're the baby and they know what to do, but we're really the babies because we don't know what to do'. This father was quite open about the confusion he felt and the range of feelings he experienced at the various points in the process of becoming a father:

It was a bit of a shock having a baby because it was only 12 months after our marriage and it was the result of failed contraception. I wanted more time together before having a baby. I was very unsure and a bit worried about how my feelings might be towards the baby when it was born. I didn't know if I would really love it, whether I'd genuinely have feelings for it, but I haven't had any

worries since it was born. It is just easy to love it and to care for it, and you really
go over the top worrying about it. I am glad I have genuine feelings for the baby.

Struggling with mixed feelings provoked by the birth are clearly
described by this father. The extract also indicates that it is a sensitive time
for the father too, as he goes through his trial-and-error process of finding
out how to handle his child:

> You're not sure what you are supposed to feel. Sometimes you feel great love
> when they snuggle into your neck, but if they continually scream then you
> understand how parents can accidentally squash or beat their child. It is
> confusing. It is difficult to describe my relationship to the child at the moment
> because he likes to be picked up by anybody.
>   I don't really know what I'm doing half the time so I start to panic a bit. I'm
> not really sure what is appropriate, and suddenly I get told that what I'm doing
> is not appropriate. I tend not to respond positively to being told things like
> that, so that can cause tension.

It is clearly not easy for the fathers at this point in time as they endeavour
to find their way into their new situation of fatherhood. Fathers can
experience great uncertainty at this time and similarly need time and
support to grow into being a parent.
    While happy about their new addition, the fathers felt, in varying
degrees, left out and on the outside of the experience. They do, however,
occupy a position that requires much generosity. Their support is greatly
needed, but it is needed to facilitate the growing relationship between the
mother and baby in the early weeks. This is not an easy task – to step aside
and support and foster the growing intimacy between their partner and
their child. As one father put it:

> I was excited when I found out about the pregnancy. I was supportive of my wife
> – just watching it grow. You're not living it like they are, in that respect you are a
> bit left out. After the birth, you can participate more but the baby is so time-
> consuming for my wife – he is a perpetual feeder and she is on edge all the time.

Both sides of the picture – wanting to support the mother and baby
and the implications of that – are clearly discussed by this father:

> We are not doing much together and we need to look at that. I was a bit worried
> at first because Gay seemed a bit distant and offhand when the baby first came. I
> was worried the first couple of days that the whole thing was going to be a bit of
> a failure. Rather than the child being what she wanted it, could be just another
> problem that would need to be sorted out. However, he seems to have won her
> heart now.
>   You can understand how people could become very jealous of the child. I
> was watching Gay just prior to feeding him the other night, lying on the bed
> looking at him with the sort of eyes that every man would like to be looked at

with, just stroking him gently and just pure love coming out of her, but I am
glad he is here.

I felt for the fathers who experienced this struggle of feeling left out at a
time when they themselves had needs of their own. While the mother
entered, in varying degrees, into her maternal preoccupation, the fathers
were holding the concern for the whole family. This usually manifested
itself in relation to concerns of having enough money and what the future
would bring. As one husband, who worked in the finance sector, said, 'I
worry about all the costs, because of my job, I think, financially. We should
be OK but it doesn't stop you worrying'.

Financial concerns were frequently accompanied by a concern that
related to current study commitments that many of the fathers had and
about the future of the relationship with the child:

I am worried financially, and I worry about the future, mainly in terms of my
study now and how I will relate to our child as we get older. I worry about how
I will get my study done and at the same time be more available to the baby than
my father was.

To conclude, listening to the fathers at this early stage gave me the
opportunity to experience how difficult it is to be in that role. The father's
relationship to the baby is not as immediate, and this creates a sense of his
being a little behind where his partner is in her connection to the baby
growing inside her. It is as if he has to keep catching up. On the other
hand, the father does not experience the intensity of the connection in the
same way but needs to find his own sense of involvement based on finding
his own role rather than replicating that of the mother. I could feel that
this was a genuinely difficult struggle for the fathers, although they did
grapple with being involved. It is harder for the father to see how critical
he is in the process when his role is less immediately obvious. That the
father was an important part of the development of the mother's capacity
to mother was very clear, but it was difficult for the fathers to conceptu-
alise this important task in such a direct way. Their task was clearly a
different one from the mother's maternal preoccupation and was more a
protective, mediating one with the outside world, which left the mother
freer to engage in the relationship with her baby.

4–6 weeks

In this section, we will, as we did for the mothers in Chapter 2, follow each
father and assess the development of his relationship with the baby.

The first father, who partnered the mother who found a great deal of
joy in her baby, is equally thrilled about his new offspring and is genuinely

interested in the emerging little personality of his baby girl. He speaks in glowing terms of his wife in her capacity as a mother:

> This little baby is developing into something more than a vegetable at last. You notice changes: she has a lot more control over her limbs and she's a lot more animated in her movements. She is obviously developing a sense of what she likes and what she wants – if she doesn't want the bottle now she pushes it away, or won't let you put it into her mouth, or if she wants it she hangs on to your hand until you can't move it, and holds you.
>
> She gets up in the mornings at 6 so we throw her into bed with us and generally we play fathers and daughters. You find an hour later that you're still lying there with her and it's time you got up and went to work. I am always interested to find out what she's done when I come home, and I always rush home to find out what she has been doing. I like having a girl. She seems to focus on funny little things and you wish you could understand what she is thinking [laughs].
>
> Pam is a very proud mother. I keep saying how tolerant she is, how I'm continually amazed at the length and breadth of her tolerance. She's just one of those women with a natural flair; she's really blossomed. She looks good and feels good in herself. She still says I am the major thing in her life and I don't doubt that, but there's another one now that's very high on her list of important things.

The father with the unexpected pregnancy, the couple having just begun to live together around the time of the birth, was having difficulty adjusting to having a wife as well as a baby and to some extent counting the cost, at this point, of all the changes in his life. He was also perhaps trying to control his circumstances, and the baby, when they seemed to be taking over his life:

> In the past two weeks his behaviour has improved, particularly at night. Cate went to Possum Cottage and they gave her some pointers. [At this point, the father itemised all the costs of the baby so far, which, including photos and formula milk, came to nearly Australian $7000]. I'm not badly off on my salary but I don't know how people with two other children on a lower salary can afford it and can continue to feed and clothe their children and themselves.
>
> The more I get to understand about how babies operate, 'normal' is a very broad term. A common occurrence is for a baby to feed and have play time, then wiggle around and spit and cry a bit, that's for about one and a half hours, then they should go to sleep until the next feed. From 10 pm to 6 am they should sleep, except they may have one waking period when they need to be fed. It is not happening yet but he is getting there. My wife sleeps easily and worries about sleeping through his crying – I put ear plugs in. She gets behind with things and still insists on nursing him when she probably shouldn't. I'm not being critical of her but she has a sucker mentality; she has a very soft heart and obviously she is going to be soft-hearted around a child. I think she's making a rod for her own back in the future.

The next father was the father of the child whose controlled crying seemed to have disrupted the early rhythm that the baby and mother were attempting to establish. While more of the care had so far been his wife's responsibility, he was looking forward to a greater involvement with his son in the future as his wife returned to work:

At the moment I've got him asleep on my lap and stomach; he'll quieten down for a little bit now. He's my responsibility for the day so we'll see how that goes. I have to give him a couple of bottle feeds today as June is going out and it's his first time just with me as I have been back at University and studying. He's going along well and is bigger and heavier. He's definitely getting stronger and bigger lungs.

He still doesn't know how to fall asleep by himself. I think that is what is frustrating him – he gets tired and upset and then expresses himself by crying. When he sleeps he sleeps, when he doesn't he doesn't. He's unpredictable. Hopefully, he will be good today so I might be able to show June up a little bit there. He still falls asleep on her after a feed and he will fall asleep there, but as soon as she goes to put him down, he wakes up and starts crying again. He likes to be held and he likes the sling, I think it is the warmth and security. We're happy – we're finding he's actually a little more responsive and smiling a lot more these days, and giggling.

I think we are managing well, June more so because she is with him more now, but after Easter I will have him on Wednesdays and Fridays and a little bit on Mondays as well, and we'll share on the weekends. I think I will have a closer bond than a lot of fathers because they are working.

The next father is finding that the birth of a baby can precipitate a lot of development in the parent as he gets in touch with his baby:

He's started smiling especially with Rose when she's playing with him, tickling his tummy. Just seeing him smile has made her so happy and it was really good to see that. Over Easter, because I had been holding him and feeding him a bit more, he really smiled at me. He seems generally to be happy about things.

He's pretty active. Sometimes if he's a bit unsettled we just put him on the floor and give him his own space, and he likes that. He follows Rose now as she walks around the room, and he seems to be experimenting with sounds.

My mum came and she was thrilled, and I was pleased about that. She was really happy that things were going so well. I'm with the general medical unit — it's hard work but it is good. Things are going better than I expected. I thought I might be out of my depth this year but I am finding it quite satisfying as well as enjoyable.

It is difficult finding time to talk to Rose about things, my feelings and her feelings, what's happened and my course, things to do with the hospital and the baby. I'm more reserved than she is and I did close off my feelings, but with the baby my feelings tend to flow a bit more naturally towards him and he breaks down those barriers – you know he can't harm you. Rose also brings me out of my shell and gives me a sense of security – I can let it all hang out a bit more.

It does have an effect having a baby – even last night I played one of the records that I had as a child, you know, children's favourite songs – it has got 'Ugly Duckling' on it and 'This Old Man', and I was happy to sing along with him.

The father who had been away on business in the early weeks is struggling, at this point, to allow himself to be fully involved with his baby son. Having suffered the early disruption of their bonding process, it is perhaps harder for him to identify with his son having his own needs rather than just fitting in with their needs:

When I was away, Gay would hold the 'phone so I could hear him, but it was really her that I missed. And being away I got out of the swing of being a parent – it took me a few days to get back into it, but in general he has been really good.

He's good at picking up what is happening in the house – I had a test today and I was stressed last night, and he was fairly grumpy and took ages to get to sleep. He was lying on my stomach at half past one going, 'Dad, isn't it just great just spending time together?', and I'm thinking, 'Go to sleep'. I took most of the week trying to recover from that. Generally he is good; we are getting seven or eight hours sleep a night now. It helps daddy a lot because I've got to get on with a bit of study at last. I think we're pretty strong both on him and on ourselves about making sure that when we've put him in the cot and lights off and that means you will sleep, and you will really have to scream long and loud before we come in, and that seems to be fairly successful.

I think it is mainly because he's a very placid baby. Other people are still having three-hourly feeds, 24 hours a day no matter what. The baby tends to recognise Gay more and smile, but that may be more due to smell than sight. He has a smiley time, a couple of smiles are his quota for the day, but he tends to be better at frowns and surprised looks and those sorts of things. With me at times, when I pick him up, he looks at me as if to say, 'Oh you, you're not the one that feeds me, do I know you?'.

It's funny how you get into baby talk as a parent. I do really enjoy having him. I think it's almost as if I have to try and not get too attached so I keep my work going. I'm the one, when he starts crying at night, that wants to get up and pick him up, and Gay is going, 'No, we said we were going to try and teach him'. I worry – it is not an emotional attachment – it is not what I expected to feel, but it is like animalistic logic, he is my son therefore I need to be concerned about him. You like the babyness, it needs you and you want it but it's not really a human being.

The father and mother who had both experienced difficult early histories were doing the best they could within their resources to provide what nurturing they could. Without our own experience of being well nurtured, it is difficult, despite our best intentions, to provide for others what we have not had:

Our relationship is going through the usual strains associated with lack of sleep. You're expecting there to be lack of sleep but you are still surprised by the continuous nature of it.

One day last week, I had a feeling of being trapped. I was looking after the baby while Briony had a break and I was trying to do some work. What I should have done was forget work and gone for a walk with the baby, but there was a build-up of pressure.

We have certain disadvantages because we don't have our extended family around us. We can't afford to fly my mother up, and she is busy with her mother anyway. I can't help resenting somehow the demands being made on me. I know at the same time how important it is and how enjoyable it is to be at home. It will be hard when I am away, then later Briony will be back at work, and I will be looking after the baby a bit more. We are looking at some child-care to help.

We visited some colleagues of Briony and felt maybe that the parents didn't really have time to get to know the children so I took them to the park. I was thinking how important it was to get a balance for yourself but be available to them when you are home and not resent them and put up a barrier.

Maybe we have had some smiles – she just lies there and occasionally she moves her arms or legs. I guess she is encapsulated in her own thing.

These fathers were experiencing varying degrees of difficulty in becoming a father and all struggled in their own way. These partners, like the mothers, faced enormous changes in their lives at a time when the external world was making many demands on their time. These fathers had to keep selflessly holding the good of their new family in mind at a time when they felt that they had lost something from the primary relationship which was now being given to the new member of the family, that is, the time and attention of the mother. As the baby matured, it seemed more possible for them to make a contribution and develop their own relationship with the baby, and most were endeavouring to develop their own links in their own way.

10–12 weeks

At this stage, there were signs that each father was beginning to gather his wife and child into a family unit, and most were reconnecting to their partner and were beginning to become a threesome. Most fathers held concerns about the future but were gaining in their confidence in the family unit.

While most were co-operating well with each other around this time, one couple had not been able to connect to each other and find the time for this process to take place. As the father says:

In terms of our relationship, we are almost too busy again. It's not so much because of our boy, but with other work that I've been doing and the Church, and Gay doing things she hasn't been doing before. We're still getting to know each other and still talking quite a lot before we go to sleep, but we don't seem to have spent much time actually doing things together. I don't really see how it's going to change much at the moment – also with the amount of work that I've got to do and the amount of studying that I've got to do. We've tried to watch a video but it is usually impossible with a baby, and conjugal relationships, well things haven't moved much there.

Because of his early absence, this father had had difficulty making a connection to his son at an earlier stage, but he was now more bonded, albeit still ambivalent about his relationship and what future it might have. He says:

Whenever I am out I think, 'Where is he?' even though I know he is at home. At the supermarket, you see these two-year-olds that are really at the 'no' stage. I'm not sure I want him to get to that stage; it might be a hard adjustment to make.

Major shifts have occurred in the relationship that was precipitated by the pregnancy, the father commenting, 'Cate and I are going well. I really thought there would have been more adjustment than there is, but I do miss going to the movies together'. On the other hand, there are still disagreements about how to deal with their baby boy:

The housework is now getting done and I think that reflects on the fact that Cate is more comfortable with the baby. But I still think she picks him up too quickly. That's where our disagreements occur and I think they will continue to occur. I let him go. I check him to make sure he is all right. I don't think I am being cruel. It's draining on Cate.

The next couple's enjoyment is interlinked with the relationship between them and with their baby as they share the task of bringing him up:

I look after him a couple of days a week now that June is working. He loves the shower; we still do it as a tag team — it's either June in the shower or I'm in the shower, and whoever's out dries him off and dresses him. But he is growing all the time. I love him and my wife. We're both ecstatic about the baby – we wouldn't change anything for him. We're both growing as a unit and as a person as well.

Marriage and parenthood have also been good for the next couple:

It was our anniversary on Sunday and we went out on Saturday, and that was nice and very special. The family chipped in for it and it was good. It's been a year now we've been married – it doesn't seem like a year; things are still going really well between Rose and myself. In fact we've really drawn a lot closer in the last week. We've had some good talks, and I've definitely broken down a few barriers and I'm more open and honest about feelings. I'm not afraid to criticise her and to say there are some things that maybe I don't like or she could do better. I was always afraid to do that because I thought she was very fragile in her self-esteem. I think things will get even better. Now I realise there are problems and there are things to be worked out; this is not the perfect marriage but when you deal with the problems you love each other a lot more.

This father remains in touch with his son and is able to support the mother in her role: 'I like putting him to bed ... we're wondering about when he will go into the cot, in the next room. He's getting almost as long as his bassinet now, it will be hard for Rose'.

The couple who experienced a great deal of joy at the birth of their daughter continue to enjoy the process of becoming parents:

Our little daughter continues to grow into a very likeable little person. The baby is affecting us as a couple. It just draws us closer together. I can see how it could drive a wedge between a man and woman. The man feels that he's come off second best, which is silly, but you know it doesn't work rationally at times. We don't have many blues and don't get upset around the baby. I am not agitated at her crying as I sometimes was with the previous children; I think I must be happier and older and more temperate. My immediate concern is to stabilise us financially.

Finally, the couple who share a difficult history had found that the baby had brought them together. As the father states, 'I think the relationship with Briony is intensified as a result of having the baby. I certainly feel that, even though we get on each other's nerves at times'.

What seemed more difficult, however, was that the baby perhaps did have more needs than they could see and understand, and perhaps because of this the baby had adapted her demands to the situation. As this father puts it:

She can look after herself a lot if you're doing stuff around the house. You only need to keep an eye and ear out just to make sure that she's not crying or anything, but she'll happily play. She's quite happy to just play on her own there, whereas Ruby [another baby they occasionally mind] is a bit more inclined to feel a bit lonely.

I'll be looking after the baby most days when Briony is back at work. We think there will be some child-care but that probably won't start until next year at the earliest, just a couple of days a week.

When she plays, she is really concentrating so she doesn't need us there somehow. She needs to know we're around but she doesn't need us to be holding her or whatever. She is an easy baby and I am glad I don't have a more demanding one.

On the whole, these fathers are beginning to catch up with their partners in their relationship with the child and seem to be gathering their family unit together more. This would possibly involve re-establishing greater links with the marriage relationship as the mother came out of a period of preoccupation with her baby, but this was not really clear at this point.

Conclusion

In the main, these fathers are coping with the stresses and strains of parenthood. They are largely involved with their children and tend to take their cue about how to be with their babies from the mother. While many expressed concern in the initial interviews about their ability to be a father, most dealt with the changes in their lives and progressively became more engaged as the baby grew.

Reflecting on their own parenting in the past seemed to facilitate the bonding process for the fathers, the father who did not reminisce being perhaps the one father who made the least connection. On the other hand, those who had not received good parenting themselves found it hard to provide for the needs of another.

While the fathers initially had a less immediate connection to their newborn, this soon grew as the birth became more real to them, and it continued to grow. Confusion concerning their role was evident, particularly in the newborn phase, and it seemed unclear to them that their major role might be one of supporting the mother and baby during this early time. Most connected to their new babies in terms of doing things for them, for example changing nappies and knowing about their routines. This in itself is supportive of the mother. However, the clarity surrounding their major role of supporting the development of the relationship between the mother and baby was less clearly articulated.

These fathers did hold an overall and future-orientated concern about their families. This was expressed in their concern over finances in their role as the main provider for the family at this time. They also expressed more concern about their future relationship with the child than the mothers did; the mothers' preoccupation was focused very much more on the present.

The quality of the relationship with their baby was a protective one that held on to the broader perspective of the needs of the family. While in most cases the fathers certainly had a direct engagement and involvement with their infant, the language of intimacy and emotional connectedness in a more specific way still lay with the mother. This opens up for discussion the issue of 'maternal preoccupation' and who is best able to engage in this process. While individual men may in fact be able to fill this role on occasions, it may be that the mother is also 'hard-wired' to express this function in a way that is more difficult, although not impossible, for the male partner.

While not directly stated, most fathers had an intuitive sense of establishing the notion of 'family' once the shock of the newness of the situation receded and they gathered the members of their unit into a whole. What was less clear, and this is in part a function of the fact that the babies were only three months old at the time of the last interview, was whether the fathers felt confident to begin gradually to reclaim their primary relationship with the mother in order to create this family.

Chapter 9
A snapshot – a father's reaction to prematurity

PETER BLAKE

This chapter contains a 'snapshot' of a father's reaction to the premature birth of his son. This focus is clearly limited in its application and no generalisation can be made from it. However, having a detailed audiotape and transcript of the father's first interview after the birth, with no extra information, I was able to observe the content of the interview in a pure form. Thinking about the father's thoughts and comments from a psychodynamic perspective, it was possible to examine the underlying fantasies aroused by prematurity, and to think about the father's anxieties and his ways of coping with them. The chapter will follow the interviews of this father, Jack, in the sequence in which he gave them. The interviewer simply asked Jack to say what he felt about the experience of having a premature child.

Jack begins with a story of loss, not about this premature birth but recalling a miscarriage that had occurred 12 months before. From this beginning, I wondered if Jack might be experiencing this baby's premature arrival as another miscarriage, with the feeling that this baby too has not been properly born. Jack goes on to talk about his wife losing the baby after they began boasting to people that they were pregnant. This may give some hint of his fantasies, the causes of Jenny's past miscarriage and this premature birth: 'She didn't want to run the risk of it happening again 'cause we'd spruiked off to everybody about how she was pregnant!'. It seemed as if he saw the proud announcement as boastful and deserving of punishment. I wondered if in the child part of his mind he saw the pregnancy as a challenge to his own parents and especially to his father.

And so off she went into the theatre. This was about three and a half hours, three hours later, she went in the theatre, and I wasn't allowed in 'cause she was havin' a general. I was gonna be there if she just had a normal caesar, and the midwife, she was good, said, 'I'll be the first one out, I'll have the baby with me and we'll race it straight over to the other side over to where it can be cared for, with the humidicrib and that'. And she said that'd be 20 minutes, and after 20 minutes I was sorta waiting and waiting, and then another five minutes, nothing. It was about the longest half hour I've ever spent, just waiting for the kid to come in. And finally it came out; we raced it across, the little thing's cryin' and I'm waiting for it to die any second, and they got it hooked up, put some monitors on it and things, and by the way they were carrying on I sorta got the idea that it might be all right.

Jack talks in great detail about the timing, or rather mistiming, of the birth. He tells exactly when he was informed about his wife going into labour, how long it took him to get to the hospital, the time between contractions, how long he was waiting outside the operating theatre and every detail. His need accurately to account for the time appears to be an attempt to have some control over or knowledge of a process that was out of his control. Jack is preoccupied with time, and this is not surprising as it is time that has robbed him of a full-term, healthy baby. When an experience is overwhelming, as with Jack here, one always hears such a detailed story as if there were a need to cling to every detail to try to make it real.

The terrible tension and pain that Jack has suffered is obvious from the next quote:

Then I went back over to recovery to see Jenny – she don't remember any of that – and they wheeled her over to see the baby before it left. Saddest thing about that was I didn't get to hold him, thinking he was gonna die. He was wired up, God knows how many wires and tubes that went in. I left the hospital about 9, I couldn't talk to Jenny. I wanted to get home; I just didn't want to cry too much in front of her, 'cause it would really upset her.

Jack is worried about whom he should be looking after. Initially, he surrenders the hope that his baby may live and is concerned for the survival of his wife. However, he is torn between going with the baby and staying with his wife. His fathering function as protector of his wife and child was severely challenged when he was excluded from the operating theatre, and further threatened when, once the baby was born, he was immediately taken away and 'wired up'. 'The saddest thing was I didn't get to hold him.' For this father particularly, the opportunity to be a holding father was especially important because of the relationship with his own father. The chance to acknowledge and share this grief is impaired in this trauma as Jack feels that he must not cry in front of his wife as this would be failing in his male protective function.

Once home from the hospital, Jack cannot sleep and and goes to work at daybreak. This lack of sleep and continuing to work are in marked contrast to his description of his wife's confinement and her having nothing to do and no control over events. It is as if he is living for the two, or possibly the three, of them and is trying to be totally in control:

> So I just got home, hardly got any sleep that night, went to work at 5 am. Finished an hour early at 9 and went up to see Jenny. I had rung the hospital first thing to check he was alive. They said he was doing well. I started to think, maybe I am in with a chance with him. I went in still really scared and the nurse was really good and encouraging.

Here Jack describes the birth of his hope that his baby might survive. He says he begins to compare the size of his baby with that of other premature babies and feels that 'maybe mine's got a chance'. He comments that he is encouraged by the nurse who is on duty, although he struggles to trust her positive statements, saying, 'You don't know whether they are telling you the truth or not for your sake, whether they are just telling you to keep you happy. I don't know, I don't know what to think when they are telling me how he is doing'. In this traumatic time, it is hard to believe and trust in positive forces. This lack of trust in others may be related to Jack's doubts about his own goodness. I wondered whether, at a primitive level, the goodness of his sperm to be able to sustain life is brought into question with first the miscarriage and now this premature birth.

Jack's anxiety about losing his baby is countered when he goes on to talk about his videotape of his son. He filmed him the day after birth, saying that it was important to have a record of his son as well as to be able to show his wife this recording. It may be that with his wife still confined to bed, he feels that he must both observe and record this early period of his son's life, a function which in a full-term birth would be performed by the mother's watching and thinking about her baby. It must also be noted that Jack relates the camera to his own father, saying 'my dad always recorded everything that happened in our family with his camera. It means I've got everything through from when I was a baby, all my birthdays and every-thing, because of dad's camera'. I thought how much this positive identifi-cation with his own father clearly helped him in this period when the fragility of life was so pronounced.

Jack goes on to describe in even greater detail his need to protect and nurture his wife and baby. He tells about the dreams that he has been experiencing:

> Yeah! worry dreams, but then Jenny reckons she doesn't sleep because she's worried because I don't sleep, so that upsets me more. I keep trying to tell her that out of the three of us, I'm the least important at the moment. It's important that she keeps healthy for his sake, and it's important that he keeps healthy. If I

get sick, I'm all right, it doesn't matter about me, but that doesn't seem to sink
home with her. She seems more concerned about me than anything.

Jack clearly feels that his own health is not important as long as his wife
and child stay well. They must sleep and be peaceful while he will remain
awake and worried. This seems to be one of his strongest reactions to the
premature birth – to provide a peaceful continuity, free from impingements, so that life can continue. Jack says that when he falls asleep, he
begins to dream about his son and all his worries for him. This then
awakens him. It appears that the trauma keeps forcing Jack back into the
present, his dreams turning into nightmares.

Jack goes on to describe his confusion over which hospital it would be
best for his son to be in. He and his wife are advised that it is preferable for
the baby to stay in a large teaching hospital, KP, which is far away. However,
he and his wife were also told that the local community hospital would be
more appropriate. Jack says:

> At the start, when Kyle was in KP Hospital and Jenny was still in Community
> Hospital, they made us sort of feel as though Jenny had to be a patient in there
> at KP Hospital to recover. At Community Hospital they made us feel as though
> she had to be there to recover because they wouldn't look after her properly in
> at KP Hospital. So that sort of threw a spanner in our works; we didn't know
> what the hell to think! And the paediatrician here, he was very insistent that
> Kyle come back here as soon as possible, and at KP Hospital they make you feel
> as if he's better off there. So once again you don't know what to do. They make
> it feel as though it's sort of their patient and they wanna look after him until
> he's ready to come home, which might be true but you don't know. It makes
> better sense for us to have him back at Community, where we can see him as it
> is just up the road.

This makes Jack feel not only confused, but also angry that his son is no
longer his but a patient being fought over by different systems. The persecutory elements in the trauma come to the fore at this time. This inability
of the two hospital systems to work together may represent, at a deeper,
irrational level, Jack's fantasy that he and his wife did not work together
properly to produce a full-term, healthy baby. It also illustrates some of the
turmoil existing in his mind. Who is in control? Who is in charge?

Jack goes on to express his anger at the government for not supplying
more local hospitals, as well as at the hospital for not providing parents
and visitors with adequate parking. This is followed by a story in which he
feels angry on behalf of another father who is not given enough information about his premature son's condition.

> Such a hassle to get in there; wish the government would build the hospitals
> out west where it's easier to get to. The first time we went in there to see him,

we drove in the hospital grounds 'cause you can't get a b... car park on the streets. There's no room in there. Then they tell you there's a car park just down the road, so you get to the car park and you've got to have a $2 coin to get in. So of course I didn't have any coins on me; so then you gotta b... find a shop that'll give you change; then they won't give you change so you gotta buy something just to get a $2 coin; then you've got to get back in there and it took probably 20 minutes to find a shop to get a $2 coin and go in and see him.

Jack's grievances here might be an external expression of his internal situation – he feels that no-one wants to help him; everyone is putting up obstacles. I thought how, at this traumatic time, he is clearly identifying with his own son's powerlessness, and angry that he has not been given his full time in the womb. I wondered whether this anger at the outside world was a projection of his own 'badness' – that he, or even more primitively his sperm, was not giving enough of what was required. He might even have been angry with his wife that her egg and womb were not good enough to produce a full-term baby. Certainly, his baby didn't get an easy 'entry'. Jack's identification with his baby is also seen when he complains of not getting enough information about the development of premature babies. He feels he has not received enough 'facts and figures'. He is angry that he has had to 'ask questions, otherwise you won't get told anything'. This is like the situation with his son, who has to 'work' at staying alive.

At this point, Jack becomes very distressed, cries and asks the interviewer to turn off the tape.

He eventually is able to talk, and when he does, it is about his own parents. His emotions are intense. In any birth, especially that of the first child, the role of being a new parent reawakens many past issues concerning one's own parents. Jack is confronted with the question of whether he will be the kind of father to his son that his father was to him. The added pressure of being a first-time father to a very premature son places a great deal of strain on his earlier identification with his father. Jack already has to deal with the anxieties that he is not a good enough father as he has not supplied his own son with the perfect start.

Jack's parents have been separated for years. His mother came to see him half an hour after he had telephoned her: 'It was good to just have somebody around'. His need to be held while he is holding his wife and baby is evident. What becomes more evident is his need to feel held by his own father. Jack describes his attempts that first night to contact his father, who was out. He kept trying and trying to ring during the night, without success. He finally contacted his father the next morning:

Not the easiest of people to talk to, too much like his own father. If you wanted to see grandad, you had to go to him, he never came to you, and dad is sort of the same. He keeps very much to himself, very rarely rings – and I hope to God

I never end up like that! When I was younger I never really had a father. Sort of someone was there, but I never had the same sort of relationship with my father as other kids had with their dads. Now he is just a stranger and that's something I don't want to do to my son ... I thought he would be ecstatic, like his son had a son, but no it's just nothing; he just wanted to find out was he all right, but then that's him.

This quote powerfully demonstrates what this trauma of having a premature infant has stirred up in Jack. His concern that his infant has not been given sufficient time in the womb is like his own feeling that he was never given sufficient time with his father. Does he imagine that he is 'doing' to his son what he feels was done to him? His comments that his relationship with his father was different from that of other kids probably reflects his concern that his relationship with his son has already been interfered with by hospital and medical procedures, and will be different. Just as Jack is sad that his father is like a stranger to him, so he is anxious that the prematurity will disturb the development of an intimate relationship with his son. Is it hereditary?, he wonders, as he links the lack of intimacy back to his grandfather.

Jack sees his relationship with his mother as close and supportive – 'Mum's been great. Every night she says "Come down for tea"' – but he cannot keep away from the subject of his father, who has told him that he is too busy to see him. It is obvious how wounded Jack is by this. He tells the interviewer how his father will not take the time to drive Jack's grandmother to see her great-grandchild or even take her back home if Jack can get her there. Jack complains that his father is too busy to seem him, citing an example of his father asking Jack to pick up his grandmother so she can visit the hospital rather than doing this himself. Moreover, Jack is angry that his father is also reluctant to take his grandmother back home from the hospital. Does his description of his father as being uncaring and uncommitted to his own family arouse worries in Jack that he also is an uncaring father? Has his uncaringness created a premature baby? As Jack says:

I keep listening to the song 'Cat's in the Cradle' and I just think how true it is. How the father was always too busy to be bothered with his son, and then when his son grows up, he is too busy for his father. I just don't want that to happen this time round.

The interview ends around this issue, and Jack is left struggling to find a place for himself as a father to his son.

Some concluding thoughts

The early part of this interview highlights Jack's anxieties about his infant's survival and his wife's health. His initial reaction to the prematurity is to act as some sort of human humidicrib, trying to provide the continuity of care to his wife and child that the premature birth has disturbed. There is actually a surrendering of himself and his own needs in an attempt to give them life.

As the interview progresses, Jack becomes angry and resentful about being 'robbed'. He feels that his son has been taken over by the hospital medical system and is 'their patient' rather than his son. Most significantly, this sense of being robbed revives in him earlier childhood feelings of being 'robbed' of a father, by his father. The fragility of his son's life reminds Jack of how fragile the relationship with his own father was in the past and still is in the present. It further confronts him with the worry that this 'internal father' he carries inside him will hinder his great desire to be a supportive and available father to his own son.

So many of these ideas are thoughts for thinking, but a thinking space in the neonatal intensive care unit is necessary for the father's feelings if the resolution is to be meaningful. As stated at the beginning of this chapter, one must be careful when speculating on the limited material of one unstructured interview. Despite this qualification, I was amazed how this one interview highlighted, with such clarity and power, how much Jack's earlier relationship with his father affected his thinking in terms of his relationship with his newborn son. In Jack's case, he not only had to deal with the external trauma of whether his wife and child would survive, but was also now confronted with the earlier internal trauma of whether the relationship between his father and himself had ever truly been 'born'.

Chapter 10
Narrative of a father of a premature infant

NORMA TRACEY, PETER BLAKE, PAM SHEIN,
BEULAH WARREN, SYLVIA ENFIELD AND HELEN HARDY

This chapter is the narrative of a first-time father, Michael, whose son Timmy was born seven weeks early by caesarean section. Against the anxiety and the trauma of his infant's birth and his wife's illness, another inner darker drama is being relived. Michael shows all the wounds of a battered child. He asks two demanding questions: 'Will I be to my son as my father was to me?' and 'Will my son be to me as I was to my father?'. Fearful and at first unuttered as these questions are, the developing interviews give them a voice. We see in this chapter a sensitive revelation of Michael's being born inside himself anew as he makes contact with his real infant and his psychic infant within.

The authors of this chapter are all members of a parent–infant study group meeting regularly to discuss the interview material. They all work in the area of parent–infant relationships. While much of the discussion here is exploratory, we felt it valuable to present as it highlights thinking to do with intergenerational processes and the powerful primary preoccupation processes of a father's emotions at his infant's birth.

In the formal research project, there were 12 fathers from various age groups, social backgrounds and professions. Each father participated in nine interviews of 45 minutes' duration (108 interviews in total, all of which were audiotaped). The fathers were interviewed each week for the first month and then fortnightly for two months, the final session being a month after this. The research had concluded by the time each infant was four months old and at home.

The questions in our minds while listening to the audiotaped interviews with Michael were:

- What primitive unconscious emotions does a premature infant awaken in a father about his potency, his own father, his fathering of his son and who his son will be to him?
- Does a father whose infant struggles between life and death also struggle between his terror of destroying and his desire to rescue and save?

The initial work on which this chapter is based nominated Winnicott's (1956) concept of primary maternal preoccupation as being the focal area. Tracey (1994) wrote, 'For the father and the infant the process of Primary Maternal Preoccupation has immediate correlative parallels'. She proposed that the preoccupation exists not only to protect the infant from external impingements, or from the excessive excitation of his/her own internal needs, but also so that the parents can protect him/her from their own destructive impulses and their anger with the infant for 'being born' and separate.

Fraiberg et al (1975) gave us the classic notion of the 'ghosts' of the nursery, emphasising and adding to Freud's (1950) concept of the power of the past to repeat itself in present relationships. This Fraiberg et al understood not only as intergenerational relationship patterns, but also as a revivification. The intrusive power of the past in present new relationships with one's own infants was a force to be reckoned with.

It was Fonagy et al (1992) who gave a research basis to such a concept. Being one of the few researchers to concentrate on the father as well as the mother, Fonagy and his team, using Main et al's (1989) Adult Attachment Interview, were able to report that parental self-reflective capacity affected the development of self in the child. They demonstrated that the 'cross-generational' effects of self-reflective capacity could in fact be a predictor of security and attachment outcomes. The 'ghosts' of the nursery were alive and active. They found this to be no less so for the father than for the mother. Our research to date seems to give further confirmation of this. Michael's ghosts certainly returned to haunt him, as his narration reveals.

In the text below, discussions of Michael's narrative appear at the end of the interview extracts in order not to intrude on the reader's own thinking.

Michael's narrative

Interview 1

> Well I guess there's not much to say. The pregnancy happened perfectly as far
> as timing goes, and we'd been planning not to have children for a long time.
> When we decided that maybe we should, within a very short space of time
> Diane fell pregnant. It was maybe a little bit early, as we were planning an
> overseas trip. Diane came on the trip anyway, which was marvellous. Diane was
> a little bit concerned most of the holiday that it might affect the fetus in some
> way – the flying, altitude, pressure changes, time changes, late nights, dancing
> the night away.

We wondered about Michael's confusion over 'timing'. He told us that the
time was not right for his baby yet it was 'perfect timing'. We wondered
whether his confusion was caused by the shock of the premature birth: the
timing had, in reality, gone wrong. One of our group thought he might be
saying, 'Look, we did this with perfect planning! Look we didn't plan this
at all! ... We had a marvellous holiday. My wife was worried the whole
time'. Another of our group thought that Michael was eager to appear
cool, calm and in control of everything.

> I guess like most first-time fathers I didn't really tune in to the fact that there
> was a real person inside. We've got a neighbour with a couple of children. They
> were saying to us things like, 'Are you nesting?' And we'd sort of shun it and say,
> 'Oh yes. Sure!'. They spent time during the wife's pregnancy talking to this
> lump in her tummy. Well we couldn't, and I didn't really want to choose a name
> beforehand either. I wanted the baby to come out, look at me and I'd say,
> 'That's definitely a "Winston Churchill" or "Rumpelstiltskin" or whatever'.

We felt that Michael was anxious about the unknown. Would his baby be a
'prime minister' or a nasty fairy-tale character? Since Michael had not
wanted to have children and had then had a premature baby, we
wondered whether he would think, 'Have I caused this?'. We associated
Michael's word 'lump' with a tumour rather than a fetus. Did Michael have
a concept of a baby?

> Despite the fact that he was born seven weeks premature, I'm not worried,
> because I'm very, very practical. But I am concerned about Diane's health. The
> time that I spent in the hospital with Diane in the early stages before she gave
> birth, I'd been walking round greasing the door hinges, and I've fixed the tap in
> the nursery which didn't work, by cutting up a syringe and fitting it with wire to
> the tap and making a lever out of it. I can't contribute on emotional terms, or
> practically where the baby's concerned, so I do tend to feel a little bit outside of
> the circle ... So, anyway, the room that Diane was in is in pristine condition. I
> can assure you the doors don't squeak and the curtain hooks are well and truly
> fitted into the wall now, and it's all working.

Our group wondered about the 'fixing' of things. Is this a kind of lubricating to keep things going, to help them flow smoothly when things have gone anything but smoothly? Is Michael fixing elsewhere because the one thing he cannot sort out is his baby? We thought how sad it was that Michael could fix everything except his own baby and his own partner. Could the birth of his infant have awakened some important 'fixing' to do with the facing of an internal self and the shedding of a false self?

> When Diane went into hospital, I found that the thing that worried me was really her, not the condition of Timmy. Diane was admitted because of what they call HDP, Hypertensive Disease of Pregnancy, and which basically means she has high blood pressure. It's obvious that there's a mental link there. I've always known that Diane is more mortal that many of us. Her father died from cancer at a very early age, and her brother, of whom she was very fond, died from a drug overdose in his early thirties. So I think it's just put a lot of worry in her mind about health. So she was the real concern for me. I'm a very, very positive thinker and, besides, I hadn't associated with the baby all that much so I wasn't afraid for the baby's health because it was almost like somebody else's baby. I wasn't at all spun out.

We saw Michael as being detached and full of fear when he claimed to be a 'very, very positive thinker'. We were taken with the idiom 'spun out', seeing Michael as 'spun out' most of the time. Michael talked about the anxieties of his partner, and we wondered whether he was highlighting these in order not to have to see his own. Michael was unable to connect with his own anxiety, could not connect with Diane's, and indeed at this point seemed not to be connected with his infant.

> So, the caesar was performed and I didn't have any doubt that I was going to be there for that event. The staff were brilliant; they explained everything step by step. Mind you, I saw much of it from the position on my back, staring at the ceiling. I fainted!

The caesarean was such a cut! Perhaps Michael was trying to tell the interviewer that neither he nor Diane could cope with such a psychic cut as the caesarean section had been.

> It was the epidural that really did it for me. It's quite a large needle and it didn't work; they couldn't find the gap between the vertebrae. It's almost unimaginable that you can push a needle in between the vertebrae of the spine without killing somebody or giving them a stroke or something. He couldn't get it in the right place, and he'd take it out and then change the angle and push it back in again. I'm feeling sick just thinking about it. And then he'd push so hard that Diane would slide forward across the bed. Ah! I was thinking of the flesh, the muscle in that area being so bashed up by this needle going in and out, and that's when I fainted.

But within a minute or two I was back, and at that stage they'd decided to use a general anaesthetic. They asked me to leave and I didn't. I stood, as if I'd walked away, and hid between machines. They didn't even know I was there, they just got on with it. I saw a chair in a corner and sat on it. And I was quite close and I was able to watch the whole operation. Hardly any blood at all! Really remarkable! They perform the incision and then cauterise many of the vessels. That was really an education.

Nobody got into a panic and neither did I. They pulled Timmy out and he was clean, spotlessly clean, with a nice white film over his skin. There was none of the erky afterbirth and all the rest of it. I didn't know how big the baby should be, but he looked a perfectly normal-sized baby to me; he didn't seem that small. He cried instantly, and then stopped crying and then went into severe apnoea, which is lack of breathing, so they put a respirator on him straight away and started pumping it and prodding and shaking him. Two Sisters from intensive care put him in a crib and checked his pulse and his heartbeat, and fibrillated him, I think, to make him breathe, and then they said, 'You can have a look at him'. I knew he was going to be a boy.

Here we see Michael as being in a strange and fearful space. We thought about how worried he was, even as he was courageously trying to deny his fear. One of our group drew attention to Diane being 'so bashed up by this needle going in and out'. He wondered if Michael at this stage is aware of the violence of his sexuality – 'bashed ... going in and out'. On one level he is cool; on another there is a matter of life and death since the baby could die if he stops breathing.

At this point, the interviewer probed how Michael felt about the birth.

I think I have some kind of an emotional prohibition. My family was pretty large, five children; I'm in the middle. My mother was a very emotional sort of person but my father wasn't. He had a nasty temper and he was violent. Very violent. My father would never explain why you'd done something wrong, he'd just lash out. I always used to go round and see friends, after a good beating, and friends' mothers would say to me, 'God! That man! Are you all right son? Stay for dinner!', and I'd have one or two surrogate families. I used to say to my oldest sister, who left home as soon as she could, 'Don't worry about me. Don't think that just because I'm still living at home and dad's a lunatic that it bothers me'. But you never know, you question as you get older.

The step that I think I have been fearing is being a father myself. I have a temper with inanimate objects, not with people. I'll have a hammer in my hand and it doesn't seem to be putting the nail in right; the hammer has to go through something solid. But I'm afraid that I might have even the slightest element of my father's bad behaviour. Yeah! Really quite afraid of that, and so when I saw the baby for the first time on the ultrasound and he looked so small, that started me thinking, 'My goodness! I hope that I know myself well enough'. I can talk about it which is one thing. My father would not, never in his wildest dreams, talk about anything.

There was a confrontation eventually between myself and my father, and I overcame my father, so that then broke him. From there on I was the dominant male in the family, which is a tacky and revolting concept. I mean it was for my mother that I had to have that confrontation.

Anyway, one day he came back from one of his overseas holidays in Spain and we just weren't there any more. I'd got my mother out and my younger sister and brother out. Actually, we got them a council house. My father's since remarried and he's extremely happy. Turned into a lovely chap. The children of his present marriage all think a great deal of him, and my mother's a bitter and twisted woman. How's that for a sad ending? So, I'm so afraid that I'll have that temper like my father.

Michael is working 'at making sense of' how he was 'hammered' as a child. Here we saw a reversed Oedipal triangle resolution and wondered about the questions in his mind: 'Will I be to my son as my father was to me?', 'Will my son be to me as I was to my father?'. In a normal adolescent situation, the father wins over the son. How frightening it must be to think that you may be giving birth to the cause of your own eventual destruction. It is not surprising that Michael would be confused over whether having a son was a good or bad thing.

So that brings me back, I guess, to coming to Australia, because when the family were safe from him I left England. This is the best country in the world in my opinion. We don't have the awful violence and the terrible overriding peer pressure that the UK has. It's not going to last for ever, and we should enjoy it while it's here. What I'm really afraid of in Australia is race wars – the terrible violence that happens in Cabramatta between Vietnamese clans. Why on earth do they have to bring their fights over here? We're all pretty laid-back people. We'll have the Macedonians and the Greeks tearing each other apart here too. I'm wanting to be sure that there's a nice place for Timmy to grow up in here.

Has Timmy's birth awakened in Michael the family fights? We wondered whether Michael's 'best country' was now threatened with the migration of past conflicts: there was no 'nice place' for Michael to grow up in.

Interview 2

I got a panic call at work. I drove at a dangerous speed. So I took her into hospital and Diane's obstetrician said, 'Don't worry! We'll put you in bed and give you some drugs and you'll be OK'. And that's what they did! There were moments of panic, but, if there's something to worry about, let Diane do the worrying 'cause she'll do enough for everybody, nothing more certain.

We could see Michael denying his own panic behind a shell of false self. We discussed how many people who have been battered in their childhood seem to have the emotion 'battered out of them'; the feeling centre is frozen. We were aware of a very small premature self, a little like Michael's baby, beginning in Michael.

The operation was very simple, clean, and I didn't have a clue what to expect. I didn't know what the baby would look like; I don't know what a proper sized baby looks like. I don't believe that it's a failure on behalf of the woman to not carry a child to full term. Diane feels she is a failure. I try to reassure her. Timmy was on a CPAP, that's short for 'constant positive air pressure device', which is just two short tubes up into the nose, giving him assistance because his lungs hadn't fully developed and he didn't have the surfactants.

Because hypertension in pregnancy causes less blood to be fed to the child, it inhibits the growth of certain things in the child, and one of them is a surfactant in the lungs. Surfactant is a surface activating agent, I know that from chemistry anyway, and it generally makes modifications to surface tension. Without surfactant the tiny capillaries in the lungs can't expand to draw in the air. They try and expand but the surface tension is trying to compress them all the time. With enough surfactant coating the surface of these, capillaries can stretch and expand without that outer pressure keeping them down.

We felt that Michael had lost his way here and was behaving as though he were a 'professor of medicine'. Perhaps he has 'to know' in a space where he feels abandoned, unsupported and unknowing. Michael's processing mother is absent. He can know only about surfaces and not depth. It should be noted here that Michael is a company manager, and it is amazing how much of the language of the current situation he has absorbed.

The interviewer probes, inviting Michael to feel free to share some of his feelings about the birth with her.

Sure! But I'm not too sure that my emotional wires are all connected. And so I can't say for sure that what I felt is the same as anybody else would feel, but I'm very, very practical, and I can't help it, it's just the way I am.

So Timmy was lifted out of Diane, and that's weird. I think to see him come out of the vagina is much more natural than seeing him being lifted out of a cavity in a stomach, in the abdomen. But he was very small, much smaller than I really expected. He cried instantly.

We were surprised at how different Michael's story became: he was surprised at the smallness of his baby; it looked unnatural to him for the baby to be lifted out of the abdomen. This was the opposite of his previous narration; perhaps he was feeling more free to express some of his own real thoughts now.

So how did I feel? They carried Timmy over. I didn't immediately think, 'That's my baby, get your hands off him; give him to me, I want to look after him; I can do better than you can'. But I did feel protective and I was very much concerned. They put Timmy in a small crib and put tubes into his nose and into his mouth, so I watched what they were doing. He still hadn't breathed, so they were slapping him gently from side to side, and pinching his cheeks a little bit. They put a mask on to him and then he'd start breathing for a while, and whimpered a couple of times, but I really didn't have any feelings he wouldn't survive at all. I'd had absolute confidence that he was gonna make it. It would have been a tremendous shock if anything had gone wrong, because I never had any doubt.

He really did look very vulnerable and weak and they wheeled him away.

I didn't know where to go. I didn't know whether I should go with Timmy or stay with Diane. The anaesthetist said, 'Diane will be ages. Go with Timmy'. So I went with Timmy.

Michael acknowledges his confusion – lost in a space that was new, that he did not understand. It is as if he were himself newborn.

They started to do all sorts of maintenance things to him – checking pulse rate, his heart beat and checking over the skin surface and things. There were about five nurses there and they said, 'Look this will take a while, we'll call you when he's ready. Just go and sit in the waiting room'.

So I did that, and I started to flick through the magazine, and after a little time, suddenly it dawned on me. 'What the hell am I sitting here for reading a bloody magazine, and all the action is happening in there, and they've told me to get out of the way?' I threw the magazine down and I walked back in and just stood. They all turned as I walked in, and it was obvious from the look on my face that I was annoyed that I had even taken that advice and left the room in the first place.

They said again, 'Just make yourself a cup of tea and sit and wait', and I said, 'I'll be OK here'. And I carried on watching them with Timmy, and they finally attached all the tubes and monitors and things to him. They put a drip into his right arm, and the tubes up his nose, and a tube down into the stomach; it looked pretty grim. I really was quite upset to see all these tubes and things. The cat gets upset when I talk about this. [Michael's cat is jumping all over the place.]

Our group thought that Michael was now coming to life, claiming a place for himself and insisting on his role in the drama. However, he says the 'cat' gets upset. Michael is still having trouble facing his own 'upset'.

Diane's definitely more of a concern than Timmy. Yesterday he choked, and that was quite a scare because he went a very dark blue colour. But, as much as I was beginning to feel concerned, I had to give Diane the image of absolute non-concern, absolute confidence. I can say to Diane things like, 'What you're feeling is natural. You probably would want to wonder why, if you're not feeling these things. Each twinge that you go through in your body you wonder what the hell it is now, because they've pulled your core out and wrapped it around and put it back in again, so you're not gonna feel normal for a long time'.

It appears that Michael is now talking of himself: this interview has so much more feeling in it.

Interview 3

So, it's Tuesday today! Timmy has been home now since Saturday 2 o'clock-ish, so that's really three days. That's Sunday, Monday and Tuesday. But in that time, remarkably just in the last three days or so, his face has changed. When he came home his face hardly looked human, it was still so screwed up. But he's looking around now and he's looking at me, and he notices sounds. I can't believe the change that's occurred in that time.

On the Friday evening they said, 'Tomorrow morning, 9 o'clock'. I had to go and get one or two things that we felt we still needed, which was another heater and a thermometer, and some bonnets and other things to make sure Timmy was going to be warm. I forgot and I was at work until late. And Diane rang me and said, 'It's too late to go shopping now', and I was so angry with myself. Even now, with such an important issue, the needs of the office took over.

We sensed how terrified Michael must have been of the awesome responsibility of Timmy, and saw also how he seemed to be denying that he was about to have him home. Did he 'forget'? Or is Michael clinging to the old pattern, the familiar, as an avoidance of facing the new?

The first evening home with Timmy was eventful of course. We brought him home, and we took him out of the capsule and rushed him into the house, and we put an electric bar heater on. We put a 15 megajoule gas heater on full and an electric fan heater on full, a 2 kilowatt fan heater on full, and the furniture began to give off a strange odour, and we realised it was about to spontaneously combust if we didn't cool the room down a little bit.

We were sitting here with Timmy in his bassinet, wrapped up with his nappy on, sixteen layers of Damart thermal underwear, and woolly jumpers, mittens, boots and you name it. And Diane said, 'I still think he's cold'. She'd been told that if the baby is cold then wrapping him up in lots of woolly clothing isn't going to make him warm because it's going to insulate in the cold, because he doesn't have that brown fat that he can burn to create body heat and regulate it himself. So we were both poking this damn thermometer into him every five minutes to check and see if he was warm enough or not. We bought this electric digital thermometer and neither of us really knew whether the room should be hot or how hot.

When Diane gets really concerned then I begin to doubt, my assured attitude begins to fall apart. So we would unwrap him and I'd stick the thermometer in, and we got a reading of 36.4 and that worried us because they wouldn't let us bath Timmy if he was 36.4 in the nursery. It had to be 36.6 or above. So that meant hypothermia was next, obviously, if we didn't do something about it.

So we turned the heaters up as high as we could get them. Still when we measured him again, thirty-six seconds later, the temperature hadn't improved. So I started thinking about thermal dynamics and what was going on in the room, and I realised it's really hard when you're in a room for a long time to tell whether that room is hot or cold, because you can't relate your reading to anything else. You've got to have a relative reading. So I found that if I waved my hand about in the room that the air on the palm of the hand feels warm or cold to you, and even though you might be rugged up your hand would feel hot or cold. Timmy was in a bassinet on the carpet, and when I put my hand down close to the floor and waved my hand close to the floor it actually felt cold, and if you do that you can feel the difference between at waist level and at floor level. It's a lot colder down at the floor level and there were draughts blowing in at the doors and from the fireplace blowing along underneath us, we don't realise that. So I picked him up – he was grizzling and making snorting noises, strange sounds that concerned us. So we cleared the coffee table and put him on the coffee table. He went to sleep very quickly after that. I thought OK, we're on to something here, it's very hot up at head level and reasonably cold down low, so we could gradually then turn the heating down. We measured his temperature and it was coming up, and that was good. And then I thought I could measure the temperature in the folds at the back of the neck without being so intrusive and ripping all his clothes off.

That night was probably one of the hardest nights I've had because we took half an hour to set ourselves up for the night. I wheeled the bassinet into our bedroom and put the fan heater in our bedroom and the bar heater, the electric bar heater, in our bedroom, and had both on at warmth factor 16 to make sure the room was plenty hot enough. Neither of us could sleep a wink. Every time we heard him make a noise, and some of them sound awful like he's seriously choking, we'd just spring out of bed, run over to the bassinet, look at it, and he's lying there as peacefully as you like, and look at each other, roll our eyes and get back into bed. Then next thing Diane's tossing and turning because it's time to feed, and she gets very uncomfortable when it's time to feed him, and actually the bed sheets were soaking because she was leaking that much.

We haven't shown anybody more than Timmy's face. Not even his ears; they're covered by the bonnet, so he's tightly wrapped up all the time. This morning the Early Discharge Sister arrived and that was tremendous. Jenny said, 'You don't need all those heaters. What's comfortable for you is right for him. It's not really that necessary to let him be totally comatose right from hour 1 to hour 4 and then feed him from hour 4 to hour 8. It's quite OK to nurse him'. This evening I shall wrap him up around me and talk to him for a while.

Ah, but it is lovely to see he's recognising sounds and movement, and he's got these big eyes. It's a tremendous feeling. There is a feeling of, I guess, a reluctant love affair. Yeah, it's a strange feeling and yet there's the responsibility, total infatuation and obligation to this child. I wasn't thinking the first night what I'm thinking now. It was almost somebody else's baby and you're charged to look after him. But it gradually becomes your baby, and it's more than a responsibility all of a sudden; it is a reluctant love affair!

We were aware in this extract of the tremendous pull to get everything absolutely right. The awesome responsibility, the massive anxiety, the preoccupation, the terror of hanging between life and death, and the birth of 'he's ours' are all present for us here in Michael's narrative. We were sensitive to the fact that a premature infant considerably loads the parent's anxiety. All Michael's defences of knowing it all are no longer available to him. He is like a new infant himself. His preoccupation with temperature, as if Timmy were still in the womb, seemed to us a preoccupation with his own vulnerability. Michael is forced to confront his anxiety. We thought he was terrified that his inner destructiveness might be more powerful than his productiveness and creativity.

Interview 4

> I'm so used to working back really late. I've been working back late for ten years for the organisation. Now I intended to have time off as soon as Timmy got home, but unfortunately there's just been so much happening at work and so much that really hinges on me because I know the history. I'm really frustrated about it. The difficult thing at first is knowing (a) you don't know anything about this baby, you're scared to death about every noise he makes, and (b) feeding times tend to change – I don't know whether that's a good thing or a bad thing.
>
> I'm not spending anywhere near as much time with Timmy as I'd like to, even when I'm at home, 'cause he's asleep in bed. He's growing. After Diane's fed him a couple of times I've taken him in my lap and stayed just holding him for quite a long time. He's dreaming about breastfeeding, I know he is! Diane's still not very well; she still has a blood pressure problem. I'm fascinated how Diane seems to be in control now. She was feeding Timmy and he started to choke a little bit, but she didn't whisk him upright and put his head up the way she was doing originally. She just let him settle while he was still lying down on his side. She doesn't panic!
>
> Now, you see the cat; that cat's not getting the attention he's used to, so he's feeling a bit dejected. We've got a choice of making him feel a bit dejected and coping with it or putting him down, and the latter's a bit drastic.

Michael seems to be feeling left out with Diane's improved confidence in handling Timmy. Is he the cat?

> I noticed something when I went to the toilet and checked, and I'd got worms. I immediately took a pill that should kill the worms in one fell swoop, and we asked the parasite man at the Children's Hospital whether there was any risk to Timmy. And what are the long-term effects – I don't know. Does it mean in six months' time that his kidneys are irreparably damaged from the worms if he has caught them from us? Anything could happen! So we've all been wormed, including the cats.

The interviewer is aware of Michael feeling abnormally preoccupied. It is obvious to our group listening to the tape that much of the former jolliness has left his voice. We wonder whether he wants to say something about the darkness inside him, or perhaps he does not want to be seen in this highly anxious state. We think that the 'worms' are his terror of what he may have passed on to his son.

There are things that concern me that I would like to bring to this interview now. I still haven't written to my father to let him know that I've had a child. Now the rest of the family know – I rang my brother and my sisters, I rang my mother – but I haven't spoken to my father, and I'm still pretty much torn.

He wasn't a particularly nice chap when I was a child. My mother's bitter and twisted about things. I begin to think that maybe my mother created a lot of problems for dad but then I think, 'Bugger it! I'm not going to make the effort to communicate with him'. I don't know – maybe I'll be sorry later. It's almost as if all those crimes that he committed on the family, the terrible violence that we had to go through as children, didn't affect me. However, now, as I get a bit older, I'm thinking how unforgivable it all is. And he's never paid for it in any way. I mean, he had the upper hand all the way through and now he's married with another woman and having a great time.

Michael's escaping to work begins to make sense for us. He has been avoiding meeting his internal father. Michael is looking for his identity as a father, and to find it he has to deal with reawakened old conflicts. He is now confused about the damage done to him by his father. In one breath, he calls them 'crimes'. He is confused about the role his mother has played. Perhaps she is not as free of guilt as he had previously thought.

As the interviewer left after this interview, Michael insisted on accompanying her to her car, saying that the street was very dark and unsafe, and he did not want her to go alone. On the way he said, 'Norma, you are a psychotherapist as well as a researcher aren't you?' 'Yes I am,' she said. 'Norma! I look at Timmy and I think, "How could my father have done that to me? If he saw me like I see Timmy now, how could he have done that to me?"'. The two stood in the middle of the footpath and Michael cried.

Interview 5

Timmy's a matter of three days before his due date. To be born that is. And he's only just beginning to wake up at night and howl for a feed. I'm still trying to catch up at work so I'm bringing work home and doing it until quite late. I'll come to bed at 1 o'clock in the morning. Now Diane will not be ready to feed Timmy again until 2 o'clock or something, so I'm waking her up as I get into bed which is quite inconsiderate. Timmy's so tired and sleeps so much still that if I don't get home early I don't see him. It's like an eclipse – you're either outside and ready for it when it comes, or you miss it altogether.

It's going to be more fun as he gets stronger. I can see he's beginning to kick a bit more. He can actually lift his head up now, so it's not just a flopping appendage as it was before. That was really a scary thing the first time he did it. Suddenly his eyes widened and his head lifted forward, and I thought, '*The Exorcist* – you know, his head's gonna turn round three times'. And I thought, 'My goodness, where's he suddenly got this awful power from?'. And that really fazed me, I've got to tell you.

Here again is Michael's contradiction: on the one hand wanting Timmy to grow stronger, on the other being terrified of his growth, even referring to the film *The Exorcist*. Perhaps he wonders what he has given birth to. Is this a good power or a bad power? We do not believe that Michael knows yet whether the changes in Timmy and himself are good or bad – innocent and vulnerable, or monstrous and destructive.

> While Diane was out seeing the doctor, Timmy exhaled to the point that he'd gone extremely dusky. He was blue almost and he continued exhaling with this cry. I thought, 'He's going on me, CPR!, and I'm gonna have to start pumping some air into him'. It was going on and on and on and on, and I thought, 'God! this is it!'. And then suddenly he sort of just caught his breath and just breathed normally. Your fears go as soon as he stops 'cause he suddenly looks instantly well again. Certainly, I would be scared to death to be handling Timmy now without Diane. It would put the fear of God into me, in fact.

This is the first time that Michael has acknowledged his fear quite openly. He is now involved with his baby but has not yet found his place within the family. He does not know whether he is a valuable saviour or helpless and useless in the face of danger to his infant. He is increasingly in awe of his partner, with a growing respect for the mother–infant dyad and a respect for his partner's increased capacity and strength as a mother.

Interview 6

> Now, in the last couple of weeks there's definitely been some changes, and he's now demanding his food whenever he's hungry. It starts off with grunts and groans, and he wails when he's really hungry. Diane's certainly improved out of sight – she's almost completely got over the soft emotional stage where small things can prompt her to cry very easily.

Michael spent this session concentrating on Timmy and his growth. He has described the irritable hours of the evening. We think he is trying to tell us that Timmy is now a real presence. His involvement is now well established.

Interview 7

> Hello, good evening and welcome! Well, there have been a lot of changes in the last couple of weeks. Since I've been at work, Diane's learnt a few things about Timmy's temperament, about his schedule, about his needs. She's not handling him anywhere near as gingerly any more. He's 4 kilos now so he's resilient, anyway. He's the right sort of weight for a newborn. Timmy still seems to think that as soon as he's awake it's time to eat, and he's not finished feeding until he's asleep again.
>
> One of the interesting things that I noticed happening inside of me is definitely a greater identification with him. I can't describe what it is, but it's now dawned on me just why it's hard for a father to get that link with the baby.

I was looking for something inside me that already exists. When your wife is pregnant, you look for lights to come on that you have known before. And then he's born and none of the lights particularly light up because you're looking at the real baby, and it doesn't really mean a great deal to you. It's a gradual process of learning that none of those thirty connections that you're used to are going to come on. You see, there's other connections that you didn't know existed and they're the ones that are starting to light up. Things that you've never felt before are there and growing on me.

Also, having a child hasn't replaced any of the fulfilment that I got from my work. It's a totally different set of values, a totally different sensory fulfilment. But I can feel that there's something happening inside me that's actually quite alive. It's not what you perceive as love, but I'll be disappointed if I'm not discovering something new in myself after feeling this coming.

Michael is now coming to life as a father. The baby inside him is coming to life, and Michael is sensitively expressing the beginnings of new growth. Who gives life to whom, we begin to wonder? How relevant is the baby's role in giving life to the parent by surviving? Is it 'dawn' in Michael's recovery from the trauma of a premature infant?

I've mentioned that I don't have an extremely fond relationship with my father back in England, but he must have gone through the same things I'm going through with Timmy now. I think that my father's problem simply was that he couldn't relate, and in some respects I suppose I should be a little bit more understanding now of my father and make a bit of effort to communicate with him. I'm not really warm enough to that idea yet. As my relationship with Timmy grows, I'll see how the parallels reveal themselves and see if it helps me to feel a little bit more pity.

You don't grow up as a child and see that violence and not get affected by it in some way, and so I worried that I could end up like that somehow. He was very violent through most of my childhood and so I'm very disappointed in him. I don't think I can just let that go. I see now the terrible things that have happened to me.

Yeah! He can write to *me* if he wants to know about Timmy. I'd be interested to see how my feelings towards my father develop as my feelings towards Timmy develop, and I hope that I don't turn into some kind of person that'll throw a garden fork at him from the other side of the garden. That's something I'm really quite concerned about you know – that I'll turn into some kind of lunatic. I'm just worried that I'll get so fed up. But I'm sensible enough to walk outside and have a breath of fresh air and come back.

But there's another thing – and that is that I don't understand why he did it, and why he's never spoken to us about it. I want to prove to him that you can be a father and bring up a child without that, so that I can then say I have a ten-year-old child and I've never lifted a finger to him. I haven't beaten him black and blue, you know, and sent him to bed without anything to eat for a day and a half, and these kind of crazy things. And I've never poured boiling hot water on his mother either. These kind of things I hope I can say at a certain stage.

Our group felt that this material was a moving testament to Michael now facing what had occurred to him as a child. We saw it as Michael facing 'head on' his anxieties about what he would be to his son: how much would his childhood affect him? We were able to see how much a father affected his self-image when it came to becoming a father.

Interview 8

Beware all ye who follow me! The feelings that we're going through at the moment are, 'Oh my God! What have we done in having a child!' Timmy's now somewhere close to 14 weeks old – a bit further ahead, but almost at the stage of some of the newborn babies we've seen. He's awake a lot more, and he really does howl for his food now rather than whimper as he used to. We've only just had the odd smile here and there, so we're still not getting any real feedback. So we're giving everything and not getting anything back.

Now when I say we, there's no question that Diane's doing all the hard work. But even the moments where I've got dinner simmering and things seem under control, and then Diane will be beside herself and I'll take Timmy, and he's howling and twisting and turning and carrying on – it's hard work. The thought of having to pace around with Timmy for an hour when I've just got back from work when what I'd really like to do is immerse myself in the warmth and comfort and relaxation of being at home is a lot harder than staying at the office.

It's said that having a premature child is a traumatic period, that it puts a lot of strain on you. But this is now the hardest time for me, coming to terms with the fact that you're now expected to contribute quite a great deal of your own free time. The father doesn't come home and see this lovely thing curled up in a ball in the cot and give him a kiss on the cheek, and then go downstairs and start reading a book or put on the TV, and open a bottle of beer and relax. He'll come home and find the mother exasperated, this baby in her arms who just won't settle down. He's now got to put in a full effort!

You suddenly see all of the free time that you had disappear. You feel you'll never achieve what you want to achieve in your life anyway. And you start looking further ahead and you think, 'Well look, at what age is he not going to be demanding of every moment of our time?'. I think this is a culture shock and something that's very hard for parents. Humour is very important at this stage. We're constantly reminded that he's a premature baby, even now at 14 weeks, constantly reminded because he still has choking problems. He's got an under-developed epiglottis.

I haven't really drawn any more parallels between myself and my father recently with my relationship with Timmy and how that's going to develop. But I do think about it and wonder now how he was feeling when I was at this age. And how was he when I was going through what Timmy is going through now? I'm sure that he put in just as much effort, and cared just as much, and worried the same and comforted my mother the same way. Then I start to think that something went wrong somewhere. He lost it – why?

So maybe by having my own child I'm going to learn a hell of a lot more about my parents than they were ever able to tell me. And one thing is different

– I can talk about it. My father never could! He would never admit to anything about his own personal feelings. And I hope I can talk to Timmy about how I'm feeling about him and how he affects me. But it's all a complete change and you've got to learn how to deal with it. So I don't think we'll take him back and get our money back.

[To the interviewer] Norma, thank you for helping me put my feelings in perspective so I can think about what I'm doing. I wanted to say that because we won't see you for a month now, will we?

We could see the growth here of Michael coming to terms with the presence of his infant. He was facing more than ever before what might have happened for his father, and was always asking the same question: 'How did my father get to feel as brutally about me as he did?'. His transference with the interviewer is obvious to us here.

Interview 9

Timmy's four months old. With Timmy there's been a major change this week. He's beginning to show some ability to recognise us and smile a lot more when he sees us, to be able to lie back and just see moving objects and be entertained by them. [Michael is laughing heartily.] We tried beating it in to him but it didn't appear to do any good, so you know we just thought we'd let it happen naturally.

Instead of howling immediately when he wakes up, he now wakes up and has a look around and thinks, 'Well! I'm awake', rather than immediately, 'I must feed'. And he'll look around and grunt a bit and then manages to find his hand, and now he sucks his thumb and it's glorious to watch. It really is so good! We'll be lying in bed and you can just hear these sucking and smacking noises as he's trying to hold on to his hand. Every time he moves his arm, his hand comes out of his mouth. No one's explained to him why that is, and so you can hear him struggling trying to find his hand again.

I'm usually home at the moment around 6 to 6.30 instead of 7 to 7.30, so that's a positive thing. I still don't feel that I'm dying to get home to go up and change Timmy, and try and settle him down and stop him crying. I walk around with him for half an hour – I'm concerned about this. But he is fun to be around and he's really a pleasure, and you don't really think of him as a premature child except for the fact that you're still giving him Fergon and Pentavite.

I wrote a letter to my father; sent it off with some photographs of Timmy. I'm pleased that I've done it because it was a bit of a burden. I felt that not writing wasn't helping me to deal with things. And having written that offloads a bit of the guilt that you're feeling the way you are. It's a bit of a load off my mind and the ball's in his court.

Norma, thank you for the opportunity to participate in this thing; I think it's been a pleasure for us. We've enjoyed your company very much and it's kind of helped us a lot you know.

At this point, the interviewer commented to the group that she never stopped being amazed, with each of the subjects, how strong the transference became by her simply being there and listening. We could see that Michael had made some sort of a resolution towards his father. We felt that this was the infant beginnings of a long road towards understanding his own childhood and understanding his father.

Michael and Diane rang a few weeks after this final interview, at the time when another interview would have taken place. They wanted to say that Timmy was doing fine and smiling all the time. Diane's blood pressure was down and back to normal. Michael said, 'We miss you coming, you know'.

Final discussion

Michael and his narrative of his own fearful and precarious journey to fatherhood taught us all so much. His story is sometimes hidden in a powerful idiom of denial and a cloak of well-being; sometimes chinks show through the defensive edifice and we see his unconscious fears.

We came to view Michael's confusion, his helplessness and his apparent contradictions as part of a normal process created by the trauma of a premature birth, a sick infant and an ill wife, but the intrusions from his past clearly show the power of the internal representations of his father and the awakening of awful past internal dramas. These are normally awakened in pregnancy, but we saw them in awesome proportions with Michael because things had gone so wrong with the birth. We saw clearly Michael's fear of being towards his son as his father had been towards him. We saw too his fear of his son being a rival to him and being as he became to his father.

Michael's narrative is the story of how he no longer came to take flight from history but to make links, at first precarious and fear-ridden, and then moving towards a reluctant love affair, eventually being able to find pleasure in his newborn baby Timmy. We saw this as a sensitive unfolding story of a father coming to life with his real baby as he comes to terms with old conflicts with his father. We saw too a first-time father in the throes of primary paternal preoccupation. We wondered about his use of the research interviews and the researcher as the container of the powerful processes within him. This was similar to the experiences of infant observers and is in keeping with Winnicott's (1965) concept of space and boundary.

A father with an infant in neonatal intensive care lives in fear of his infant's death: his baby is in a machine instead of in the protection of his partner's womb; he has no sensory contact with his infant; and he has a seriously distressed partner to hold and support. The father of a premature infant has no space for his own feelings and needs, everything being focused on his wife and baby. These interviews seemed to give Michael that space.

Michael had been through a terrifying caesarean birth. He had had to communicate initially with the staff about his infant, and he may also have needed to sustain his position in the workplace. Rarely is the father's role in the drama seen as anything more than an adjunct to his wife. The research gave him a central position and, by its interest in him, restored his position as father. What the research space also did was to give Michael a stage on which to play out not so much the events from without but the drama from within.

The group felt that, for any father of a premature infant, his sense of potency and worth as a male is profoundly affected. He may fear that his negative and destructive desires could overcome his positive, creative ones. His idealised role as protector of the mother–infant dyad is distorted, and his challenge to achieve fatherhood may be fraught with guilt and fear, robbing him of the initial joy of attaining parenthood. For any father, there can be confusion, as seen with Michael, between identifying with his baby and with his father, not knowing which of these he is. His relationship with his wife, now a mother, awakens conflicts concerning incest and threats of incest with his own mother. These we see as normal emotions, but against the trauma of prematurity they are distorted and enlarged, as we see with Michael.

We were initially aware of Michael's failure to link emotionally with his baby. We saw his flight to work as a going to a safe place where he knew and was known, and where he had the 'history'. His narrative was the story of how he no longer came to take flight but to make links that were initially precarious and fearful, then falling into a 'reluctant love affair' and finally being able to enjoy Timmy. We saw this as the sensitive unfolding of a story about a father coming alive with his real baby as he came to terms with the birth of his psychic infant within and struggled with old conflicts with his father. We are reminded by Michael that the Oedipal conflict is not a time-limited event but one that is relived continuously for the whole of life. We were awakened as a group to how threatening this external invasion was when an infant was removed prematurely. The lack of continuity, the loss of a timing that was 'right', the upheaval and the vulnerability that was exposed became very real to us as we discussed Michael's narration. Michael's and his wife's preoccupations in those first nights at home were revealing of a normal preoccupation that belongs to the father as well as the mother.

The powerful desire to get it right for Timmy helped Michael to face emotions never before accessible. In the presence of a listener, Michael could express his thoughts and look at the feelings from past conflicts and present trauma in his struggle to achieve fatherhood. The interviewer was, by Michael's choice, the container of Michael's interior battle and fears, a space perhaps, we thought, where he could safely express, experience and look at his feelings. The gathering of information we came to see as a valuable tool in helping him to make links with his past in order to make sense of his present. Michael came to terms with his inner father and hence his external father during the talking-through process. The interviewer was continually surprised at the use made of her presence in what was a research rather than a therapeutic contact; the group wondered whether that had, in fact, facilitated the process.

References

Fonagy P, Steele M, Moran G, Steele H, Higgit A (1992) Measuring the ghost in the nursery: a summary of the main findings of the Anna Freud Centre — University College London Parent–Child Study. Bulletin of the Anna Freud Centre 14: 115–31.

Fraiberg S, Adelson E, Shapiro V (1975) Ghosts in the nursery: a psychoanalytic approach to the problem of impaired infant–mother relationships. Journal of the American Academy of Child Psychiatry 14: 387–422.

Freud S (1950) Beyond the Pleasure Principle. SE 18: Standard Edition of the Complete Psychological Works of Sigmund Freud. London: Hogarth Press/Institute of Psychoanalysis.

Main M, Kaplan N, Cassidy J (1985) Security in infancy, childhood and adulthood: a move to the level of representation. In Bretherton E, Waters E (Eds) Growing Points in Attachment Theory and Research. Monographs of the Society of Social Research and Child Development, Volume 50. New York: Society for Research in Child Development.

Tracey N (1994) Inner world processes during pregnancy. Australian Journal of Psychotherapy 13: 137–53.

Winnicott DW (1956) Primary maternal preoccupation. In Through Paediatrics to Psychoanalysis. London: Hogarth Press/Institute of Psychoanalysis (1977 edition).

Winnicott DW (1965) The Maturational Processes and the Facilitating Environment. London: Hogarth Press.

PART 4
THE FAMILY

Chapter 11
An intergenerational family perspective

Charles Enfield

In this chapter, an attempt will be made to understand a couple with a premature infant through their separate interviews. We will study their reflections on their new baby, the hospital and their own particular culture through my own countertransference and my understanding as a family therapist. Out of their struggle with these intense experiences, a new order was being born, one that would include their new, as yet unknown, infant. Out of the chaos they would write their own future life narrative, including a new baby that would contain renewed hope as well as fear. In this life narrative born out of trauma, they could return to their prior ways of dealing with pain and loss or they could adapt in a new and richer way. This issue is at the core of this chapter.

When I was approached to write about the intergenerational processes that could be observed in the research interviews I had received, it did not seem to be an onerous task. After all, I carried within me many years of experience as a practising family therapist. I could draw on familiar constructs and concepts in order to understand and explore this family's dynamics. Having these ideas gave me a sense of power and of being in charge.

Listening to the audiotapes and analysing the transcripts, however, I began to feel somehow confused, uncertain, even inept. How could I do what was asked of me? I had not faced the experience of having a premature baby, but I could understand prematurity as a doctor well versed in medical and physical processes and procedures. I might also be able to understand – as a man and a husband – why the mother might need to feel supported. I found I had developed intellectual defences against feeling unduly anxious from an event that had within its very process the capacity to confuse and distress me. I did not want to feel too deeply. I was already guarding myself against the pain of 'not knowing' by being detached.

However, it was only when I stood back to reflect on this that I gained insight. I recognised that I was feeling as the parents felt. I was, in an extra-ordinary way, being made to feel and respond as they were. I was being filled with their feelings in facing an event so overwhelming that one would doubt one's being and the meaning of one's life.

I had to begin to think in a new paradigm. I had to try to use this new capacity as a way of getting into the totality of the parents' experience. Although it was clear that the research was not intended to be a therapy, it had a therapeutic effect. It felt to me that the parents had been 'held' respected and valued by the interviewer for sharing their experiences. They had found a 'container' in the immediacy of their trauma, and this immediacy is vital.

Because of the research protocol, the couple were not seen together, nor were the couple seen dealing with their premature infant. Their family system had to be in my mind as a hypothesis. They were in an institutional hospital setting where their baby was delivered. I could feel their incom-prehension of institutional processes, whom to trust or whether to trust at all. It is obvious throughout their narrative that they were angry, frustrated and helpless, not knowing how to turn the institution into a secure base that could hold them helpfully. Out of sync with the institution, they were made to feel observers rather than participants. Their baby had become the institution's baby.

In hospital systems, the doctors and nurses suffer personally when things go wrong with an infant. They defend themselves against their subjective primitive feelings by needing to be powerful and omnipotent. They hide from themselves, and from their patients, their own sense of uncertainty and doubt. They appear distant and authoritarian. For this couple with similarly authoritarian parents, we will see how this aroused their infantile anxiety and guilt. They felt vulnerable and helpless, just like their premature infant.

Ricky's story

I felt I had begun to know Ricky as I listened to his interviews recorded from the birth of his infant to the first few months of life. I responded to his openness, his lack of guile, his feelings for and about others, his capacity to struggle in order to find meaning in what had happened to him.

I heard from him that the couple had been married for two years. They had worked together to provide a secure home where they could take care of their children. Patsy had become pregnant, and they had been very proud of the pregnancy. Suddenly, she had had a bleed at 12 weeks and miscarried:

It broke our hearts to find we'd lost it. It was hell for us, especially her. She swore she would never have more kids.

This pregnancy and birth

Ricky told us that Patsy again became pregnant and early on had had another bleed. For the whole pregnancy, he and Patsy were full of anxiety about once again losing their baby. He tried to support her but 'everything that could go wrong during the pregnancy did'. Ricky very much wanted this baby but kept reassuring Patsy that all that mattered was her being safe. They kept hoping that she would go to full term. However, 'Andrew decided to spoil all that by coming early', and all their preparations for his birth were undone.

'All I kept thinking about premature babies was how sick they always look on telly and you know how they always die', said Ricky. He was full of antici-patory dread, as was Patsy. They were both in tears, clinging to and supporting one another. 'It upsets me that she's upset.' He thought the worst: 'It wasn't going to live anyway ... I was waiting for it to die any second'.

Following the birth of the baby, a nurse had for a moment reassured him that it might survive, 'But the baby was all wired up'. It seemed to me that Ricky was holding Patsy, being there for her, keeping his fears from her and therefore having to manage his feelings on his own. There was nobody there to take care of him. 'I can't do a damn thing about her being upset', he says in the interview. His anxiety is persistent; he cannot sleep, yet when he does, he dreams about the baby, how little he is – worry dreams. His dreams are about thoughts that he cannot face when awake.

Ricky's feelings about the hospital

Ricky comments:

> We didn't know what the hell to think, with different ones telling us different things ... So once again, you don't know what to do. They make it feel as though the impression I'm getting there, it's sort of their patient.

I wondered at this point where his baby was.

> I reckon what I would have liked was facts and figures on premature babies ... I don't know how premature he was or what was wrong with him. It gave me more relief seeing those figures [on premature babies surviving] than anything anybody had told me ... But you just don't find anything and no bastard will tell you. You've gotta find out for yourself.

I also thought that Ricky needed someone to help him to feel better in order to protect himself from his fear of falling apart. The institution was failing him: it was not mindful of him and his baby. Ricky is constantly feeling left out, let down and useless.

Ricky's family

At this time, Ricky looks to his family for support: 'Families are just so important it upsets me how people don't take them seriously'.

Ricky tells us that Patsy's parents live out of Sydney and are not available. He is, however, very attached to his own mother, who remarried having separated from his father, who has himself been remarried for five years. Ricky's mother and grandmother are always available for him: 'I'm very close with my mother and I feel I get all the attention from her'.

However, when he seeks out his father, this reveals his painful family story. Ricky has a need to find his father, and his father is not available. Ricky's father is a senior company manager who has no time away from his work; he never has had, and his father, Ricky's grandfather, was the same. Ricky is determined not to let his relationship with his son turn out the same way but to ensure that history does not repeat itself. In Ricky's family story, men do not father and are not available to their sons. Many deep feelings have been reactivated by the current situation. Ricky had hoped that his father would be there for him now that he has presented him with a grandson, but this is an unrealistic expectation:

> All through the pregnancy I thought he'll be proud to be a grandfather. Now I can't even get him to come and see Andrew – he'll have to make time he said.

Furthermore, it would appear that Ricky has found a wife who cannot be close to her mother.

Andrew's prematurity

In reflecting on his baby's prematurity, Ricky contemplates how it might have been had he had a normal baby:

> that's the sort of feeling I didn't get, that proud look you see on men's faces when they have had a baby. I didn't get that feeling. Whatever that feeling is, I don't know about it. All I could feel was, is he going to live? – just fear. Fear of the not knowing what's going to happen more than anything.

In accepting that his baby is going to survive, Ricky has found a family:

> it's gonna be all right and there is a 'we' like we as in he and I, 'we' as in Patsy and Andrew and 'we' as a family ... He's still in the hospital, started breast-feeding and putting on weight.

Now Ricky could long for Andrew to be at home, but 'you can't get your hopes up too high'. He is anxiously attached:

> I just want to get him home so that we can get to see him. I don't really want to go to work at all, just be home with him.

In Ricky's family script, he needs to be a good father. 'It's starting to sink home that I'm a father – it's such a good feeling.' Ricky's paternal preoccupation remains in his ongoing concern for Andrew and in his recollections of his tiny premature baby and of giving birth to the fantasy adult that this tiny baby will become, as well as in how Andrew will one day be the father of a son and carry on Ricky's good fathering of him. Ricky is in this way finding a generative future.

Ricky's relationship with Patsy

At this point, Ricky exposes a major difficulty in his relationship with Patsy:

> Patsy is not very close with her only brother; she's not close with her mum, she reckons she doesn't want to talk to her mum at all. She just doesn't seem to place the same emphasis on families that I do.

Patsy cannot be close to her family however much Ricky would like this. Because of his anxiety, he and Patsy fight. When they are together, aspects of their relationship as it was prior to the premature birth emerge. Then, they had constantly fought and argued. Their fighting continues, but now it is about Andrew, whom Ricky desperately wants to take care of, Patsy feeling that he cannot be trusted to do so. The baby has become the focus of their rivalrous difficulties. Ricky fights with Patsy as she is in the way of his finding reassurance in being the sort of father that he wants to be to Andrew. 'I've just hit a brick wall at the moment'. I wondered whether he had found in Patsy an unavailable and rejecting object like his father. 'We're at each other's throats. We fight like cat and dog', but neither knows who is right. Ricky is angry at Patsy, whom he feels controls him, 'tells me the way to do it'.

Ricky was saying that nobody is there for him, to support the hurt child in him who is not coping.

Andrew comes home

About three sessions into the interview schedule, Andrew is due to come home. Ricky shows his excitement and relief when Andrew is finally at home, but his good feelings are once again tempered by uncertainty:

> We were two nervous parents who basically did not know what to do. But the settling in and getting to know and takeover phase is not too bad.

Their uncertainty remains over who is the major care-taker, who is going to feed the baby, respond to him when he wakes. Ricky wants to do as much as he can but is apprehensive; Patsy wants both to be in charge and to get away. She very quickly decides to return to work. This creates a problem for Ricky, with his fantasies of the perfect family he is creating:

> I will be the one that gets up when we're both working. That sounds very good in theory, but how will it work in practice. Hopefully, mum's instinct will take over and she'll be the one who wants to get up all the time.

Sadly, we will see later that this does not happen. The conflict now is about Patsy's eagerness to return to work. Ricky says, 'I just don't care about work and I've told them so'.

During the interview, the pain and the memories of how bad this period was keep flooding back: they had had 'seven weeks of Hell'. Now, after all that, Patsy is not wanting to be at home to take care of Andrew and at the same time distrusts Ricky's capacity to look after him. Ricky is aware that if they fight, they will not be able to take appropriate care of Andrew: 'If she tells me something, I have to accept it in Andrew's best interests and not let it affect me'. This is in keeping with Ricky's family script. He is reminded that he was not taken care of because of the fighting between his parents and wants to ensure that the same thing does not happen to Andrew.

Having a normal baby

Andrew has achieved a milestone: he is now at the important anniversary of the expected, full-term, date of his delivery. 'So now we've just got a normal baby', Ricky cries once again with joy. 'It's just good to have him home. So now the fun starts with him, whereas previously it was just like visiting someone in hospital'.

Future children

Ricky now begins to wonder about having other children, concerned once again about the risk to Patsy and whether or not they could deal with another premature birth:

> It is very important that we'll hopefully get a positive answer; if there's any risk to Patsy, well then Andrew's it. I'm prepared to go through this again. I've said to Patsy if we do this four or five times, the odds are that one of them will die; if there's a second then that child will die; could be the second, the third the fourth or the fifth but then it could be none of them. We are prepared to take the risk of one of them dying but how will that affect us if we do.

We can see here that Ricky is vacillating between hopeful feelings and the pain and uncertainty about life and death that still persists.

Passing on a sense of family history

The many losses in Ricky's and Patsy's family background pervade Ricky's thinking and cast their shadow over his view of the future. In this family's past, there have been many losses. All four of Patsy's grandparents are dead, and both Ricky's grandfathers have passed away.

Ricky thinks back to the previous generations and his recollections of his own great-grandparents. In his mind that links with his longing for Andrew to have a history that will exist in his own memory as it does in Ricky's. Ricky is wanting to connect Andrew with the family's past in order to maintain the generative link between a past and a future that seems more likely as Andrew continues to thrive.

Ricky's relationship with Andrew

As Ricky continues to explore his relationship with Andrew, he is now able to acknowledge his ambivalence towards him because of the negative feelings he held about his prematurity. Ricky feels reassured that his anger will not be destructive.

> The way I feel about Andrew, well now, feelings have changed a lot towards Andrew. Now that he's healthy. I know that he's not going to die because he's premature. I don't want to sound mad at him. Why couldn't he have hung on in there a little longer before being born.

However, the actual fact of the baby's presence makes him feel proud to be a dad: 'It makes you feel a bit more worthwhile'.

The family script emerges once again – 'I grew up with parents who used to argue black and blue' – and in his mind, Ricky wonders about his own arguments with Patsy. He recalls that he and his siblings became used to the parents fighting 'so that on the outside it didn't bother us. That's the way all families behave'. Ricky is desperate to give Andrew a better experience.

The rivalry between Ricky and Patsy

For Ricky, Patsy's controlling behaviour:

> just makes me feel as though I'm doing the wrong bloody thing. You don't want to make one person unhappy so you make both unhappy. It's horrible. She makes you feel so bloody guilty about it. Whatever I do is wrong.

Ricky feels burdened by his persecutory anxiety, which Patsy reinforces. Despite this, Ricky feels that he can express his emotions and that this is the major difference between him and Patsy:

> I think she keeps her emotions all bottled up and then takes it out on me. If you can't take it out on the person you're married to, who can you take it out on? I try to make up but Patsy and her emotions, she doesn't want to or can't.

So they do not communicate; they are just 'back to normal'.

Who is going to mother Andrew? – Ricky, because he identifies with his own mother and is confident in his 'mothering', or Patsy, who 'knows best' and, like her mother, appears to be detaching from her own child as her mother did from her. Ricky desperately wants to spend more good time with his son; how miraculous it is that he has survived. He wants to preserve the memory of his smallness and fragility, and to continue to enjoy him and give him a more hopeful, helpful opportunity in life.

Conclusion

Ricky has expressed his narrative in an open and feeling way. We have seen him struggle with his inchoate feelings of fear, loss, danger and death, and with his continuing apprehension that one cannot take anything for granted. He has made known to us his confusion and his need to ensure that his dysfunctional family script is not replicated. This is a script in which parents fight, keep secrets and emotionally detach from their children as Patsy's mother has detached from her and Ricky's father has detached from him.

The nature of Ricky's persecutory anxiety is clear. He wants to change these patterns. He will be the father to Andrew that he had himself wanted when he was a child. Throughout his narrative, Ricky's ambivalence and conflicts about his own parents are omnipresent. Will he be able to alter this script for his new family and for his as yet unborn other children? I respected his openness and his acknowledgement of his pain, struggle and confusion.

Patsy's story

> They tried to stop the labour but they couldn't. When I was in hospital and the baby was taken to King George, I couldn't go over to see him in the first four days 'cause my blood pressure was still too high. ...
>
> He's been there since half an hour after delivery at Hurstville, and I didn't see him till he was four days old [crying, pause], which made it very hard. I didn't even feel as though I'd had a baby. I'd also had a previous miscarriage, which made it feel like it was another miscarriage because I didn't see him after delivery, but all I really saw of him was a hand, and then I was too groggy from the anaesthetic to really see him.

In this first interview, Patsy expresses a complexity of feelings of hurt, confusion and distress. There is a struggle in dealing with her unexpected and overwhelming feelings, which she had not anticipated. She had developed defences against feeling too intensely:

> I had an emergency caesarean. By the time I got to see him, he was already off the life support system and he was just breathing normal air on his own. And

then I'll be able to start feeding him instead of using this pump, so he can be tube fed every hour, which he's just started to tolerate. I find it quite hard when I see him because, being a nurse, I know I can do everything that the nurses are doing for him, but I get the feeling that they don't like us doing much for them, doing much for the baby. I've cuddled him three times [laughs], and he's now oh, how old would he be, about ten days old, and that's only been for about five minutes each time. I still find it extremely hard to take [cries and cries] because if he was home I'd be able to cuddle him a lot more [pause, crying].

Yes, yesterday I had a good day, I didn't cry at all yesterday. I was going to have a caesarean all along because I only have half a uterus and I also have a kidney that's in the wrong position, so I can't have the baby come out naturally because the uterus wouldn't contract properly to push it out.

In the current crisis, Patsy recalls earlier catastrophic events and how she had dealt with them. She struggles with her longing to find her baby, cuddle him and take him home, but it appears that the hospital staff do not understand her feelings or believe that they are acceptable. In the transference, the institution is felt to be the parent who dismisses her and fails to support her. Patsy is herself a competent and qualified nurse, and found her identity and meaning away from her family in her work.

Patsy is filled with her sense of hopelessness, with which she cannot deal. The institution 'didn't understand I was sick'. She's not sure if she or the baby is the patient that needs to be looked after. Her anger at the institution's lack of awareness of how it was for her is intense. She is filled with persecutory anxiety and fear that something has perhaps been kept from her as the baby was hospitalised away from her in another institution: 'Some of the staff were quite good; however, others were telling me he's fine and wouldn't elaborate on anything else'. There was, implicit in what she said, a deep need to be supported by the institution, but it let her down.

Patsy had married Ricky two years previously. He is a very understanding husband. She reflects on how moody she is and feels unworthy of him: 'I don't know how he puts up with me'. She considers how her family are unavailable, whereas, in her view, Ricky's family, especially the women, are supportive. It would appear that Patsy is grateful to Ricky that he can be supportive.

With her nursing knowledge, Patsy knew that she was going to have a premature baby and a caesarean section. She had made rational preparations, ensuring that her baby was born in the right hospital and that it would be well looked after. Unfortunately, the baby was more premature than expected, and there was considerable medical concern about the baby's well-being, so he was separated and placed away from her. Patsy was totally unprepared for this, not anticipating the pain of separation, not knowing or being able to access her baby.

Contact with Andrew

During this first interview, Patsy returns again and again to how difficult it was for her to get together with her baby: 'Not seeing him enough, that was what upsets me'. This initiates her continuing anxiety about losing him. She cannot allow herself to attach in case she does lose him:

> It upsets me more when I do see him. The answers they give me just aren't enough. He doesn't look like a baby ... It just upsets me seeing him in there. He's so skinny, he's got no fat on him. He just looks like a miniature human; he doesn't look like a baby. At first when I saw him I didn't ... well, he still doesn't feel like my baby, it feels like I'm visiting somebody else's baby, and to me it feels like I'm at work; when I change his nappy and do his mouth care and eye care, it feels like I'm at work doing that for someone else's baby. Is this nightmare real?

Patsy is concerned that the intensity of her feelings will interfere with her relationship with Ricky. In this interview, Patsy is clearly making known her distress. She appears to be afraid that she may have difficulty in finding and attaching to her premature baby, who seems not to be there for her. She continues to show her attachment difficulties with the baby, even being uncertain that she wanted to breastfeed: 'It's hard to explain, I prefer to use the pump than to bottle feed'.

Patsy's family

> We have never been a family that's been able to talk; that's why I find it so hard to talk now.

Patsy is not in touch with her married brother; her parents live away but 'anyway they're not the sort of family that you can talk to about anything'. Patsy lets it be known that she has become reconciled to the fact that her family is unavailable. She is concerned that she will cut off from her baby if he makes excessive demands on her: 'I don't know if I would be able to cope'.

Patsy acknowledges that, in following her family script, she too has an inability to relate: 'I just tend to shut people out'. She feels shut out and, similarly, shuts other people out: 'I haven't been brought up to talk to people. You have to work through your own problems'. Like her mother, she is not the sort to express her feelings:

> Perhaps it is easier not to have a baby than to have difficulties like this and not be able to cuddle. I can be very moody at times [laughing] but especially lately. Ricky doesn't understand why I'm crying all the time, and it upsets him and that makes me worse 'cause I see him getting upset. But he comes from a family that are very very supportive: at least one of them rings us up every day to find out how we're going.

Being independent and doing things for herself, Patsy acknowledges the nature of her conflict with Ricky: she feels that he does not do things properly. She finds it difficult to allow him to help her, but in her stress, and being 'dead tired', she knows she needs help.

Patsy's ability to 'mother'

Patsy has doubts about her own capacity to mother. She remains anxious about Andrew's survival but expresses hope that he will be coming home. She is feeling better because the hospital now know that she is a nurse and she is being told more. However, her knowledge exacerbates her irritation with Ricky, whose continuing anxious preoccupation with Andrew raises her own fears concerning her failure to have a normal pregnancy. Patsy cannot allow herself to feel too deeply:

> then I don't really feel anything ... There's not much maternal instinct there at the moment. I don't think there was any maternal instinct to start with, and I don't think having him separated from me for so long helped bring on the maternal instinct.

Patsy sees Ricky as having a greater capacity to mother than she has:

> Ricky's got more maternal instinct than me. Didn't really bother me if we didn't have children. It was Ricky who wanted to have children. All you hear about is the pain and I can't stand pain. I can never have children naturally.

A few weeks later Patsy's ambivalence concerning Andrew and her capacity to be there with him persists. She is even coming to the belief that it is better for Andrew to be in hospital 'so I can recover fully before he comes home'.

Patsy's continuing ambivalence

Patsy is now discovering that she can enjoy breastfeeding, but she still cannot feel that Andrew is her baby. Although Ricky and his family have come to accept Andrew as part of the family, Patsy's ambivalence remains. He might be Ricky's family's baby or he is someone else's baby or:

> I'm just going to work and looking after him, so he's like a patient. I don't know why I feel that but I do.

Patsy once again questions her capacity to be a mother. Are her feelings to do with postnatal depression? Ricky gets upset with her because she is unavailable and unattached to her baby: 'I don't feel as if I'm his mother, but I love to be there when he's upset and needs a cuddle'.

At last, Patsy acknowledges that perhaps one can be allowed to feel pain:

> I'm feeling very sore and sorry for myself. I am more depressed this week. Little
> things just get to me, all of a sudden I just fly off the handle. Ricky gets cranky
> with me but I can't talk about my feelings.

Again and again, Patsy brings to the fore the feeling that she is finding it impossible to attach to her baby. She seems to talk about him as a patient and is feeling guilty and bad, looking to find in herself her own baby. 'A bit more like my baby now because being in the cot, he doesn't seem as distant as what he did in the crib.' She can breastfeed: 'I don't really enjoy it but I don't hate it either'.

Parental rivalry

We will now consider Patsy and Ricky's fight for the control of Andrew's care from Patsy's perspective.

Patsy's ambivalence about Ricky's capacity to mother Andrew irritates her. She gets angry and irritated with him; it is as if Andrew gets in the way, as if he wants to put the baby to his own breast. 'He's become an expert on breastfeeding now', she mocks. Nevertheless, she is in some ways feeling that Ricky is finding a better way to mother her baby. Ricky is needing to compensate and somehow take over the breastfeeding to make up for Patsy's ambivalence and to avoid feeling useless and unwanted by Patsy.

The focus of the conflict between the parents has now become 'Who is going to be the care-taker for the new baby?'. They could share the distress and drama of the premature birth, but now it seems that they are unable to support each other: the needs of this new baby has brought to the fore their own unmet early needs. Patsy deals with this by retreating to work, and Ricky by attaching intensely to Andrew and shutting Patsy out. It now feels as though they are losing each other and returning to their separate ways of dealing with life. Patsy relates to this as being inevitable: her family is separate; they don't make themselves available for her. She struggles with this. Why are they not there for her and her baby?

Andrew's return home

Patsy was unprepared for her baby being suddenly and unexpectedly discharged. It was as if that too concerned having to face the shock of prematurity. The first evening was difficult. With both Ricky and Patsy struggling to adjust to the new situation, Patsy was strained and uncertain, fearing that they would fail. However, Andrew reassured them by progressing satisfactorily.

Patsy is now settling into a more comfortable relationship and can provide a secure base for the new family. She is learning to know her baby and is finding confidence in being able to give. Her baby is also giving back to her by his enjoyment of her breast. However, her uncertainty and ambivalence remain as she is intending to return to work prematurely. She has had difficulty in conceiving, difficulty during the pregnancy, and difficulty in having the baby normally and being there for her baby. She is preparing now to go back to work before she and her baby are settled.

Patsy and Ricky are back to arguing with one another. She feels she has to dictate the way to do things, having to be in control partly because she felt so out of control when her needs were not acknowledged through this very painful period. Because of the baby's fragility, she acknowledges that she and Ricky ought to remain connected to protect him.

Patsy's return to work

One month after Andrew came home, Patsy was back at work full time, having found a secure place in the hospital where she had worked before. In her narrative, this hospital is more of a family than her own family of origin. Patsy is not finding it easy to make a place for the baby as this new pattern evolves. Although she is reassured about Andrew being a healthy baby, a baby who can meet their expectations, it is at work where she feels most validated and competent, and where she can resolve her uncertainties.

Patsy tells the interviewer that she is going blank, appearing to blank out the conflict of having to give up her baby in order to return to work. Because she feels that Ricky is eager to be there for her baby, Patsy can rationalise her need to return to work. She feels that, in an ideal world, it would all have been so much easier for her if she could have had a normal birth in which she would not have needed to suffer so much pain and see her baby being hurt by all the medical procedures.

The conflicts with Ricky and her ambivalence about leaving her baby appear to have been rationalised when she is back at work: 'I love it; I can't find anything to do at home, I get bored stiff'. She can to some extent enjoy breastfeeding, and she can express milk for Ricky to feed the baby: 'that went well, better than I expected'. Patsy fluctuates between her difficulty in attaching to her baby and her simultaneous feeling of detachment. She can find her baby through her breast: 'I don't mind breastfeeding because it's a hell of a lot easier than bottle feeding'. Patsy tries to resolve her guilt about leaving Andrew: 'It sounds like I don't want to be around the baby. But Ricky is available.'

When she gets home, Patsy has difficulty meeting the demands that

Andrew makes on her and adjusting to the new situation of having three of them to care for. 'We're getting used to him being here and not having to worry about unsettling him; we just do it.'

Family issues

Family issues remain disturbing:

> Ricky's really into families. I'm sick of hearing about his family being here all the time, his family wanting to see Andrew when mine doesn't. We're not as close as Ricky is to his family. That's our main bone of contention. I've given up, I don't care.

Patsy does not know how to reconcile their different family cultures other than by going blank and not caring. It appears that Patsy 'does not care' in the same way as her family 'does not care'. Ricky's father does not care, and her father 'is too busy; he's a workaholic'. Perhaps she had been looking to find care from Ricky, but he is less able to care for her now that he is so preoccupied with their baby.

Is Patsy telling the interviewer that she is angry at being displaced by the baby, or is she angry because it appears that Ricky can mother the baby better than she can? There are mothers in Ricky's family who can mother and who want to mother Andrew. In Patsy's family script, mothers are neither available nor trustworthy. She had hoped that her baby would help her to find her mother:

> I thought my relationship with my mother might change a bit after I had Andrew but I don't think it will.

Sadly, she says:

> we've never been close, we're not a mother and daughter that can sit down and talk. When something significant happened, she always sent dad in.

Patsy had to 'work things out for myself'. Her longings for acceptance were revived by her baby, but she is once again giving up. 'I don't really care either.'

There appears to be a myth in both families that daughters are not wanted even though sons are. Even her mother:

> gets on better with Ricky than she does with me. She always wanted boys, she never wanted a girl; she only had boys names picked out when she was having me.

In having a son, Patsy has given the women a boy to love, but the myth is that she and daughters cannot be loved: 'even Ricky's mother is estranged from his two sisters'. Boys get what they want; they get looked after but girls do not.

Returning to 'normal'

Patsy is now settled back at work. In her final interview, she looks back over the recent period of her distress and the fact that she had not had a normal baby. She compares her baby to a normal baby: 'Mark is a little monster compared to Andrew'. But Andrew has settled in and is sleeping and eating, and there are various care-takers who will provide for him while Patsy is at work. She is reassuring herself that she is all right in her independent adjustment. She is more comfortable if Ricky provides the care-taking: 'I'm not keen on having family in all the time, playing pass the parcel. I'm just blank today like every day'.

The past is still present in Patsy's mind, but how difficult it was is being repressed: 'It just seems like such a long time ago that it's virtually forgotten about'. She does not want to continue to talk about babies:

> Which is what happens when you sit at home all day and do nothing but look after the baby. All she [a friend] wants to talk about is babies, babies, babies. I don't know how you can stand it.

The baby reminds her of her depression, which began to resolve when she returned home and she found that she was able to manage Andrew.

It appears as if a new pattern is being set: Patsy can continue to work; Ricky and others can help take care of the baby. In this new situation, they can plan on a future in which she continues to work and find satisfaction as a nurse.

> Ricky and I aren't fighting as much now. Before, we seemed to fight about every little thing. Going back to work helped. We're not together as much, and I'm not stuck in the house all the time.

Patsy is back in a familiar frame and no longer depressed; she is in control of the demands being made on her. She can ensure that Andrew is taken care of and can arrange appointments for him. She is feeling happier, even now trusting Ricky more to take care of the baby. There is a future.

Conclusion

This chapter shows how Ricky's and Patsy's previous experiences in their families of origin helped to shape the way in which they dealt with the crisis of their own premature baby. They revealed to us the overwhelming distress that they had suffered, having to draw on all their strengths and previous ways of functioning.

Patsy and Ricky came from differing family backgrounds and showed clearly what they had longed to find in each other. They moved on from a state of intense distress and fragmentation, clinging to each other and seeking the reassurance they needed. As their baby continued to develop well, they slowly recovered and reverted to dealing with their life and changed circumstances with old and familiar patterns of coping. They were rivalrous and continued to fight with one another, Andrew now being the focus of that fighting.

Ricky showed how much he wished to repair, in this generation with his own son, the lack of fathering that he had received in his own family. His dream of the family he would create in no way matched Patsy's continued pattern of escape from intimacy and attachment, which she saw as a bondage.

Patsy rebelled against mothering, feeling that she lacked the 'mothering instinct', as indeed her own mother had lacked it. She escaped from mothering her baby to the security of her work area. This was her previous pattern now repeated and made extreme by her infant's prematurity and the crisis she had suffered.

There had, however, been opportunities for change in this narrative. Perhaps if help and counselling had been available, the story might not have unfolded in this way, but what did happen is that patterns of family functioning from the past reasserted themselves. Patsy will be to her son the mother her mother was to her. Ricky may well be different, seeking so strongly to change the past with a new present, but this difference may in itself create further problems for the couple.

All too often, trauma does not create a new family script but entrenches an existing one. I propose that in the situation of prematurity, much family counselling is needed if a new script is to be written.

Acknowledgement

To Sylvia Enfield for her invaluable assistance with this chapter.

Chapter 12
A migrant couple with a premature infant

ISLA LONIE

To be a migrant is to be placed at risk of greater distress when life events prove difficult, because there is always an issue of loss in the background. There is, of course, the loss of familiar scenes and places. Often, there is the loss of daily communication with family members who must be left behind. Additionally, there is the problem of differences in religious practice. There is the loss of life-enhancing cultural activities, often made much more difficult by the need to learn an unfamiliar language. The difficulty arises of being ashamed of one's halting speech in a strange country, with the frustration of being, for some time, unable to communicate except in the most rudimentary fashion. There is always the dark shadow of an event or events that led to the migration in the first place as nobody migrates and leaves behind the familiar, the comforting, the known social blanket of their own culture without good reason.

For Alia, leaving Lebanon to come to Australia at the age of 13, the event was, she said, the war.

Norma Tracey, commenting on Alia and Ahmed's interviews, says:

It surprised me how much Alia's original migration experience became confused with her experience of the premature birth of her first child. I have always talked about pregnancy as a migration from womanhood to motherhood. When a woman migrates there is a shock, a rupturing of continuity. There is loss – the loss of the mother country, the harsh introduction to an unfamiliar culture, the loss of identity. Our internal life narrator who holds the past to the present, who carries our history and the continuity of our existence, seems to be cut off with the shock of the change. This shock colours everything.

For some, everything in the new country looks good and the past awful, but mostly the past retains a loving, romantic, unreal hue and the present appears unkind and harsh and unwelcoming by comparison. These difficult beginnings lead to mood swings, to imbalances in dependency between a state of inflated hope, and deep depression with a loss of the neutralising centre.

Alia and Ahmed were a young Lebanese Moslem couple having their first baby. Ahmed had come to Australia when he was five and had few memories of life before that time. On the other hand, Alia recalled her years in Lebanon as a 'very happy time' and her first years in Australia as 'very hard'. This was because she had to learn English and 'everyone was making fun of us because we didn't used to speak that well'. This contrasting of the old and the new in which the old is viewed more favourably is exactly what Tracey is referring to. Certainly, Alia's experience of the trauma of an unexpected premature birth underlined for her a sense of harsh reality in the present.

I first 'met' Alia on the interview tapes when she was interviewed a few days after her baby, Daniel, had been born by caesarean section nine weeks prematurely. The cause of this was Alia's dangerously high blood pressure, which could have been fatal for both mother and baby. Alia and Ahmed were both shocked by the sudden change from a normal pregnancy apparently progressing smoothly to the drama of an emergency caesarean section and all the problems of coping with a premature baby and a totally unexpected event.

The situation was further complicated by the fact that Ahmed was in the midst of the busiest time in his office. He had negotiated to take leave at the expected date of delivery, an arrangement that he was unable to change despite his baby's early birth. Later he was to say, 'I don't think it's fair on a person's family to put in those 60-hour weeks'.

Moreover, Ahmed had an important examination coming up in a few weeks' time, so Alia tried very hard not to be too upset about her baby in case it affected her husband's ability to concentrate on his study. At the third interview she said:

Just these four weeks, I'm just trying to avoid anything – just to hide everything from him so he won't be depressed or anything. I just want him to study, that's all. 'Cause I don't want to feel that I was the cause of him not passing or anything.

Perhaps Alia was also concerned for Ahmed because she had pushed forward their decision to have a baby after only eight months of marriage even though they had originally believed that they would wait for two years. Thinking about this, Ahmed wondered whether Alia's mother had been 'a big force' in Alia's eagerness to become a mother, because parents 'want to be sure their children can have children'.

Over and over again, Alia and Ahmed recalled, in their individual interviews, the trauma of how it was that Alia had gone to the hospital early in
the morning because she had had a bad headache that had stopped her
from sleeping. She was transferred to another specialist hospital and the
next morning was told that they were going to deliver the baby because
there was not enough blood and oxygen reaching the baby as a result of
Alia's dangerously high blood pressure.

When she was telling this story at the first interview a week later, Alia
spoke brightly at first with a frequent nervous laugh, but, remembering
how she had not expected her baby to come so soon and how, as she said,
'I thought he's going to come dead or something', she began to weep and
asked for the tape to be stopped. On continuing, she spoke in a rather flat
voice, still sounding a bit tearful, and the superficial brightness had disappeared. Ahmed, on the other hand, was always determinedly cheerful,
even saying what a cute baby Daniel was, despite all the tubes and
paraphernalia of the intensive care ward. Only later – not until the seventh
interview, when he was finally able to enjoy the sensuality of his baby – did
Ahmed say:

> When he was born I really didn't think he was that cute. I loved him because he
> was my son, and you know I think I had those instincts that normal parents
> have, but as far as looks, I know that parents always – their vision's a little
> blurred because it's their child, and their child is the most beautiful child ever
> born – but I really took a look at him when he was born and I thought he's got
> potential but he's not the best looking child I ever saw. Even when he came out
> of the hospital, six or seven weeks later, I thought he was getting cuter, but I
> still didn't think he was one of the cutest children I've seen.
>
> He wasn't much when he was born. He had a lot of hair and it ran over his
> forehead and shoulders. And naturally his facial features hadn't developed. He
> had a cute little nose – I've always said he's got his mum's nose. That was it.
> What else was there to the child? His skin – his skin was a little withered, was
> saggy, looked a bit too big for him. Sometimes if you touched it, you'd feel it
> was a bit saggy, like it needed flesh underneath it. And perhaps that now,
> because he's got that flesh underneath it you know – it's giving the contours to
> the face and to the body. You wouldn't see this, but now he's got the sexiest
> little thighs! Now he's got baby thighs that've got that little bit of flab on the
> inside.

While Alia spoke of the headache that indicated her raised blood pressure,
it was only later, as she continued to remember with the interviewer what
had happened to her, that she recalled that she had also been 'all swollen
up, and I was really big and I thought, "Oh I don't know if I can go through
with this or not"'. In later tapes, Alia returned to the theme with the

comment, 'I was – god I was ... I don't know, like a Dracula or something, I don't know. I was – my face was all swollen up. I was really like a monster, I show on the video'.

In this process of working through, in which people who have suffered a traumatic event relive aspects of the experience again and again, the opportunity is created to include the events as part of their concept of who they are and what they have experienced. Ahmed's approach was different in that he questioned the process of diagnosis and correctly linked Alia's swollen hands, feet and later face with the problem of raised blood pressure. He avoided direct criticism of the skills of the specialist they had seen ten days earlier but indicated his displeasure with the man's refusal to carry out home visits and his lack of interest in Alia when she was in hospital. This had angered Ahmed sufficiently for him to change his wife's status from private to public patient. On the other hand, Alia did not mention this, probably because she seemed to be very content for Ahmed to deal with the outside world.

The thing that most affected me on first hearing Alia's early tapes was how often she said things like, 'I haven't got him with me', 'He's not here with me', 'He's not here with me at home':

> This is my first baby, and at the moment everybody asks, 'how does it feel, how does it feel?'. And I say I don't know because he's not with me. I don't feel it very much 'cause he's not with me. I don't change his nappy, I don't bathe him, I don't breastfeed him or anything. I haven't got him with me!

While these references were all to her baby, it seemed that Alia was perhaps even more upset by the possibility that her husband would be absent. A week after the event, she recalled with great distress:

> But the next day they came and they told me, 'We're going to deliver it', you know in the evening, and it was like no one knew, no one was over there, I was by myself when they told me. Only I knew!

The next week she told the interviewer, 'When I think of the operation, I'm glad that my husband was in with me, because I needed a lot of support and love, and he was great, and I really love him'. It seemed that she had a tremendous need for her partner to share in her distress, yet she wanted to shield him from it because she also wanted him to pass his exams. 'I try to hide my feelings from him', she said at the third interview, ''Cause I don't want him to think of anything else, because he's got a lot of study to do. I shouldn't be crying. I don't want to cry'. She was possibly more concerned about this than her partner, and was perhaps attributing some of her own distress to Ahmed, for he said with some asperity at the last interview, 'I told you I'd pass. I told you she was panicking for nothing. No one has faith in me'.

It seemed somewhat remarkable that Alia should be experiencing such difficulty about feeling alone and abandoned as her husband, although working long hours, was greatly concerned to be supportive. Also, Alia had a large extended family, with a mother who took her to stay with her while baby Daniel was still in hospital. She did all the work and did not let her daughter do anything. Her mother-in-law, too, offered meals whenever Alia wanted to come.

Ahmed's family was perhaps less involved; his father came to the hospital only once and soon left. Ahmed mentioned this on several occasions, always recognising that his Dad 'didn't like the sight much'. On the early tapes, Ahmed seemed disappointed that his father did not appear to be very interested in the 'first little boy in the family', but he added, 'I know that he's always proud but just that he shows it in different ways'. Later, Ahmed was clearly extremely pleased when his father came visiting after Daniel came home, and was delighted that he wanted to pick him up and hold him.

On the other hand, Ahmed's mother was a frequent visitor, although she went away on an overseas trip intended to last three months when Daniel was just ten weeks old. There were other family members, too, frequently on the scene: brothers, sisters and in-laws of the young couple. In fact, the attentions of the family were so constant that Ahmed instituted restrictions on family visiting for a while as Alia had to spend so much time going to the hospital to visit baby Daniel and was becoming exhausted with the need to entertain.

When Alia was talking to the interviewer and recalling how distressing she had found her birth experience, she moved on at this point to recall an earlier trauma – the painfulness of learning English in her first years in Australia, yet another situation in which she did not feel in control and did not know the language. Not only did she remember how difficult that time had been, but she also seemed to lose her normally good English speech. For example, she repeatedly said things such as, 'I thought I probably would never see that baby you know, probably he'll come die or you know dead or something'.

This regression to an earlier level of functioning was also evident in her loss of fluency later when discussing with the interviewer her concerns about baby Daniel's lack of enthusiasm for breastfeeding.

The inteviewer asks:

Why did a woman praising so highly the satisfaction and the need to breastfeed, and not mentioning any ambivalence in this interview, abruptly wean her baby in the next few days? Why did a woman obviously preoccupied and rapt in her baby give him to her mother, abruptly deciding this in the space of a few days, and choose to return to work well before time, saying, 'She will do a better job with him than me'? It seemed to me there was splitting at a deep unconscious level, some basic dislocation where Alia switched from a state of preoccupation and attachment to no attachment.

For that matter, one may wonder why a woman, breastfed herself for three and a half years, would move on so quickly to the use of the bottle. Could one predict that any of this would happen? It may help to listen to the interviewer saying, 'Trauma brings a terrible loss of the trust in oneself, and the self's capacity to predict and to achieve'.

It may be useful here to look in some detail at how Alia and Ahmed dealt with this issue. In the very first interview, Alia was indicating her impatience to be able to breastfeed her baby, saying, 'I'm just waiting to put him on my breast, you know to feed him and all that, because I haven't tried that yet. So hopefully he'll be OK very soon'.

By the time of the second interview, Alia was saying that Daniel was having a few sucks 'but I think he gets tired very quickly'. At the same time Ahmed was saying:

> The bonding is getting stronger, not only with my son but also with my wife. The expressing and breastfeeding – it's an important part of the attachment. I'm helping out with the breastfeeding – the little things that a father can do. As a male you're very much left out of the whole process. And I mean really, you look at the natural side of it, it is mainly a female process, but you know the more encouragement the fathers are giving, the more the bonding will develop earlier with their wife and their child. It's quite beautiful to see him taking some sucks there. He's having a sleep on the breast actually, which I don't blame him – it's probably nice and warm.

Later, Ahmed told the interviewer that he himself had not been breastfed for as long as his older brothers, his own experience lasting only a couple of months. Certainly, he saw himself as having an important role to play in urging his wife to persist with breastfeeding.

At the third interview, when Daniel was five weeks old, Alia began by excitedly telling the interviewer, 'He's still in the crib, but he's started to breastfeed so I'm breastfeeding twice a day, and he's learning very fast. He's sucking a lot but he's a little bit funny. He's sucking and then resting and then sucking again, and it's so cute'. At this time, Ahmed was saying:

> Bottle feeds – he wants the easy way out, the little cunning devil. He wants the easy way out. He doesn't want to suck the breast sometimes. I didn't think they could be stubborn from this age, but they're pretty clever little buggers. But he just won't take the breast sometimes. On the bottle he sucks so nice and long – one suck, one swallow. He just thrives on it. Although it had breast milk in it.

You can't be expressing and putting in a bottle all the time. Imagine that! For ever. So he's got to get used to it. It gets frustrating at times, especially for my wife. She wants him to take more, and he'll stop sucking and that will really put her on a downer, 'Why isn't he taking it?'. I'll say, 'You've got to give the kid a break he's still only small, and if he doesn't take enough of the breast, you just give him a top-up with the bottle'.

Ahmed was dealing with the anxiety of establishing breastfeeding by becoming the knowledgeable observer, telling his wife how she should do it, just like the lactation nurse.

By the fourth session, the good news was that Daniel was out of the humidicrib. Alia said:

Sometimes he's giving me trouble, trouble to take the breast. He's learning, and the other day he lost some weight and the nurses like, um you know, the um watching him um very closely so he won't lose weight again.

At this point, it seems clear that Alia is having some trouble speaking about this for her speech has become much less fluent and is punctuated by 'ums'. We can think of this as an expression of regression to the time when she was learning English, and we can also recognise what a blow it is to Alia's self-esteem that her baby does not seem to want her breast. She goes on to say:

Every time I go there I stay with him for probably an hour and a half. Sometimes I feel I don't want to give it to him any more – I just want to give him the bottle, because he sucks on the bottle better than the breast. It's easier, and sometimes I think no, I better – I wanna give him the breast just to make sure, because I know the breast milk is better than just formula. So sometimes I get impatient with him.

Ahmed's comment at this time was to wonder whether Daniel was getting milk from the breast. 'Hopefully', he said, 'he'll just get used to the breast. He'll develop more muscles. It's more fun at the breast. I'd really like to see him taking the breast'.

At the fifth interview, Daniel was seven weeks old and had just come home. Alia started the interview by remembering how she had gone to spend the night at the hospital in order to get Daniel used to being breastfed for a whole day. She laughed, as she often did when speaking of painful things, as she reported how she had not slept all night because the baby had fed every five or ten minutes and her breasts were getting very sore. When Alia got Daniel home, every time she tried to feed him he went to sleep but wakened again ten minutes later. Alia was starting to worry that perhaps the baby was not getting enough milk because her breasts were very full. By night-time, she 'just gave him bottles'.

At this stage, Alia sounded more doubtful about her capacity to breastfeed this baby, who had become accustomed to bottle feeds. 'Sometimes', she said:

I think I don't want to give it to him any more. I just want to give him bottles, because I want to see how much he's getting or if he's getting enough. So that's why sometimes I better give him the bottle just to make sure. Sometimes when he cries a lot I get stressed straight away and I get nervous straight away, and I'll just get very angry 'cause he's not taking. I'll have to be patient with him.

She also remarked with a laugh, 'Hopefully when he grows up, he'll appreciate all this. 'Cause we have to tell him what he had done to us, all the pain he caused me and his Dad. Hopefully, he'll appreciate it: "Mummy I'm sorry I caused you all this pain"'.

It was also the case, however, that Alia was discovering the joy of breastfeeding:

Every time I put him on the breast, there's a funny feeling goes inside me and I don't know, it's a wonderful experience. I can't – I don't know – I can't explain it but, every time I put him on the breast I just, just feel very happy, and you can feel something running inside you. It's different if you give him a bottle because you're not close to him, you're not holding him against you and he's not close to your breast. So it's just a wonderful experience and hopefully I'm going to keep going with it. I won't get sick and I'll be patient, but hopefully he'll learn.

At this time, Ahmed was indicating that he felt he should distance himself from the breastfeeding issue:

I don't want to be in there too often while my wife is breastfeeding. I don't know to the extent of a woman what's going on. I felt the night before maybe I was getting a little too involved with the breastfeeding. Fathers have got to know the limit. You don't want to drive your wife to the point of having to tell you. It's still satisfying to see her breastfeeding without getting too involved with doing this and that: 'You're not holding him right'. I wouldn't blame her if she got annoyed. It's really a woman thing.

Ahmed mentioned that he had recently felt that Alia was showing:

a little bit of a lack of motivation, and I've been trying to get her motivated, especially, I said, you know, 'we've done all the hard work, and we've just got to keep it up now. Just let's keep it up'. There was a morning once where she expressed and not much came down from either breast, and she was pretty shocked and got quite depressed about it. That's very difficult and I'm sure must affect a lot of mothers. She's done well – she's been good through it.

At the sixth interview, when Daniel was ten weeks old, Alia proudly showed a smiling baby, saying also that he had kept her awake for four hours during the previous night. He seemed to prefer sleeping with the lights on, maybe because that was how it was in the hospital. She commented that he was really unsettled, perhaps because he had had an injection. Then she said:

> I've stopped – I've stopped breastfeeding because he gave me a really hard time, he didn't take it and I tried and tried and tried, and he didn't take it because he was used to bottles in the hospital so – I'm not breastfeeding him any more and just giving him formula. But he's growing and there's no worries. But I wanted to breastfeed you know – it's his bad luck because he didn't take to the breast at all.

Ahmed began with this topic almost immediately:

> Last time my wife was getting frustrated with the breastfeeding. So we came to a decision – and really it was her decision, and I probably had 5 per cent input into it. I just wanted to encourage her to hang out a little longer with the breast-feeding, which she did, anyhow, but in the end, we wanted the best for him, and so that was, you know, at least he's eating now. And he is, and he's doing well, and he loves the bottle; at least he's eating. So now that's not an issue any more.

Ahmed's voice sounded a bit flat, even though it seemed that he was characteristically trying his best to be cheerful. 'A feed', he said:

> just becomes a pleasure now rather than a struggle with him. It used to get quite depressing sometimes when he didn't take anything in. My wife would always worry about him starving, and there was one period when he actually lost weight over a few days when they next weighed him, and that really concerned us, and I mean it was probably because he wasn't getting much milk out of the breast. He's eating well and we know how much he's eating. We're monitoring everything and so those distractions – destructions – are gone.

Perhaps Ahmed's ambivalence about the decision to bottle feed broke through in his slip of the tongue: his 'distractions/destructions'. Ahmed was in fact quite pleased with the idea that he could now feed Daniel too:

> About the bottle feeding. In some ways it's not so bad. I'm doing a little bit – I wouldn't say I'm doing 50 per cent of it, I mean it's impossible to do 50 per cent being at work. But, where I can, of the evenings, on weekends, I'm putting in my share, and I love it. I'm holding him and I'm feeding him, and previously that was a pleasure only restricted to the mother. She was the only one who was any good at even holding him up to the breast. So there's some joy in that for me, and I knew there would be, even though I used to try and encourage her to keep on breastfeeding. But deep down I've got to admit that I do love holding him there and giving him the bottle. And I think that I'm the master of burps at the moment – he always burps for me.

And I babysat him the other day. She's going to start going to the gym. Now, all there is now is a bottle feeding, whereas the feeding would have been the main problem with doing something like this before. Now there's no problem. I mean I can feed him, I can change him, I can burp him, I can put him to sleep. I can sit up and talk to him, and he loves all of those things, and you know if any of that is what's bothering him he will be quiet.

Alia actually had the possibility of taking quite a long time off work without affecting her employment prospects, yet by the time Daniel was 18 weeks old, she was back at work, and his care was divided between the grandmothers. While the reason given was that the mortgage needed to be paid off, Ahmed's comment was:

We could survive on just my income – we'd get by and we'd keep paying the mortgage, but we won't really make headway and we want to try and make some headway – we've both got the same feelings about that. So, it does mean putting our mothers through a bit. I don't like to burden them but they say they're happy to do it. Until we say we've made enough progress, or another child comes along, and then we say it's worthwhile staying home.

Mum's only been back from overseas for a week and a half or so now. Straight back and basically straight into some child-minding. I feel a little bit guilty about it but they assure me that they're happy to do it. Because you prefer to be looking after your children yourself or you know or, probably in our case, for my wife to be staying home from the start.

Alia did, in fact, begin to think about returning to work as early as the fifth interview, when Daniel was seven weeks old:

I think I'll go back for a while, just until the second baby. Probably I'll stop when I have the second baby. But at the moment I think we need – I need to go back to work – 'cause we've got a mortgage, so we have to just finish it, and then probably I'll think of another baby and I'll stop. But deep inside me, I don't want to go back. Because I don't want to leave him anyway. He will probably be about four months old when I go back.

It often appears to be the case that when the mother is intending to go back to work and find alternative care for her baby, she often turns in her thoughts to the next baby, for whom she has a dream of caring.

Alia was thinking again of returning to work at the time of the seventh interview, when Daniel was eleven weeks old. She spoke of how she really loved to spend time with him, although he was still very wakeful during the night and this tired her. The week before she had mentioned that she felt bored at times, possibly because of Ahmed's long absences, but she could talk to Daniel. Even if he did not understand her yet, it was a kind of companionship. Thinking of his growth, she remarked, laughing, 'He's a grown man'.

During the eighth interview, Alia told the interviewer how exhausted she was because she had not slept for two nights. Daniel had spent nearly the entire night crying and then vomited the next day. He seemed to want to be awake all night and to sleep during the day. Both Alia and Ahmed attributed this to the noise and lights in the intensive care nursery which he had become used to, and they had discovered that he would sleep if they turned the lights on. But then Alia and Ahmed could not sleep. Alia was not only tired, but also had a very bad headache, had lost her appetite and was not eating well.

At the time of the final interview, Alia was sounding extremely uncertain of herself. She talked about how Daniel was becoming naughty, meaning that he liked attention and would not go to sleep by himself. She wondered how she was going to manage to go to work when Daniel was so often awake for much of the night. She had taken him to the doctor, who had said that she did not recommend the 'wind' drops that Alia had obtained from the chemist, which had worked. The doctor had left her with the impression that the drops might cause heart problems when the baby grew up and recommended that she should instead give him Panadol, which did not help. Alia had continued to give Daniel the drops but:

> still I stop and think what she said. I'm just going to get scared you know. That's what she said, and you know everything I tell her what I do for the baby she says no, I don't recommend this, you've got to do this, do that, do that. And the way she tells me to do it, it doesn't work anyway with him.
> ... Just sometimes when he cries I feel like crying with him. I don't know what's wrong with him but I can't do anything with him. I'm trying my best but he doesn't stop crying, and sometimes I feel that I want to cry with him but I hold myself 'cause I don't want Ahmed to see me crying so he feels upset. I think I'm looking forward to going back to work a little bit, just to change my past few months.

Alia and Ahmed often spoke on the tapes about their feelings for each other and about how their love had deepened during this period of adversity. Alia said at the time of the eighth tape, when she was feeling so ill, 'My feelings towards Ahmed – no they haven't changed at all. Probably they're growing a little bit, because when I see him with Daniel I really think, "Oh I'm glad that I've got both of them now"'. She also thought quite often of her choice of Ahmed as a husband. 'I think I made the right choice of getting married to him, so hopefully we'll stay a happy family for ever', she said in the very first interview. Later, when Daniel had come home, she was very appreciative of Ahmed's willingness to help her:

> He's really good with Daniel – like sometimes if he starts crying and he sees me getting upset, and you know probably I'll be a little bit angry if he doesn't stop,

he takes him from me and looks after him for a while, probably feeds him or something, so I can just rest a little bit. He's really wonderful with him.

Ahmed had quite a few thoughts about his marriage:

Because she understands me, that makes me a good husband. Although I try to be – I am – flexible, it does come pretty naturally with her though. We haven't been married all that long – 15 months. We knew each other for about two years. I know she was the right person.

In thinking about the accelerated pace of their lives since Daniel's birth, Ahmed said:

I think that'll keep going for a while. It's hard to get good, er – I don't know how you say it – private time together these days. There's a lot of verbal emotion between us. It's just been difficult with physical emotion, not just sexual even, just showing it in other ways. We went out to dinner – we needed it – we took him with us; the restaurant was good, he slept all the way through it. OK we got out – a change of atmosphere – she really needed it. I just did it as a surprise; I think it went down very well. I think you've got to do these things – we used to do them a lot before we had Daniel. It used to be a lot easier.

Both Alia and Ahmed set a high value on making the best of things. For example, they tried hard to see Daniel's time in hospital as helpful because of Ahmed's need to study. Alia said with exquisite ambivalence:

So it's good in a way, it's so bad in a way, because [Daniel's] far away from – no, he's not far away, but he's not at home – he's down in the hospital. We don't see him much, and it's good in a way because it's a relief for us and for my husband. Probably he'll get some study done or something. I don't know.

At the time of the sixth interview, Ahmed was saying:

I wouldn't want to go through it again but if we had to I think we are strong enough to go through it again, and I wouldn't wish it on anybody. To go through it unscathed. It's one thing to go through it, and another thing at the end of it to have a good relationship between the parents and not to have let any of the depression or anything like that get between you.

And there's probably a lot of areas where conflict could have arisen or where just a lack of support to the other partner could have sparked some conflict. Even if it wasn't direct conflict, maybe just depression or something like that, and I don't think that happened. It didn't happen with me and I don't think it happened with my wife. I think she thinks I stood by her well and gave her the support that I think she required. It was hard sometimes, it was.

Alia was also finding the transition to motherhood difficult in terms of the loss of freedom and the company of other people. She mentioned this herself rather shyly, without emphasis, but Ahmed was characteristically eloquent for her:

> There's one bit of frustration coming through and that's being home all day. And even though she's got the car here, and basically as long as she's providing for him, she can do whatever she wants, go wherever she wants; as long as she's looking after his nappy changes, feeds, sleeps, whatever. But it's not that simple, and if he's asleep you don't want to be disrupting his sleep, putting him in the car. And if he's awake, you don't want to take him, because he's probably going to cry.
>
> So, at first it was hard to work out. I'd come home and she'd say, 'Can't we go somewhere?' And I'd think, 'Well OK, I'm pretty tired, but you haven't been at work all day. Why are you the one wanting to go?'. The only place she's been able to go, really, is her mother's place – and that's because you don't have to care for him the same as if you take him to the shops or anywhere else.

This couple were also thinking through some of the issues to do with the differences between male and female roles, which their culture perhaps delineated more clearly than did Australian culture in general. In talking about Alia's decision to go back to work, Ahmed reported that she wanted to go back to university to undertake some further study and that he was happy for her to do that. 'It could be', he said, 'just part-time, and by the time she's done with it the kids are probably ready to go to school. So it could work out very well for us'.

Alia was not particularly interested in a career, but, Ahmed said:

> It's different with my work, because I see myself as the breadwinner and we both think and see it that way. Not only because I'm earning more money, but also because I'd be hopeless staying home and looking after kids, I really would. I mean I'm fine if I'm looking after them for a day here and there and looking after them when I come home – but I think to stay home for the whole day and night as well, I don't think I've got that knack. Men are hopeless, aren't they? No, we've had this with some friends who've come over – a couple of her friends are the same age as her and they're studying at the university. They're single. And of course they've got the attitude of – that if women could do it, any man could do it. Well I believe, yes, some man could do it, but I don't believe any man could do it.
>
> I think that's something that takes a lot of educating – it's a whole lifestyle that has to change, right? It takes a lifetime of enrichment and of taking in the attitudes – the new attitudes – but to not have had that as a child and a youth, and to not have had it in my family with my parents playing their roles. I think, 'Well I'm doing things that my Dad didn't do for example – OK, so I've come part way there'. Perhaps my son will be able to do that. But from the background that I've come – from the upbringing – from the community attitudes when I was growing up – it's a huge step and it takes more education than – not only education but exposure along the way, because if you've got constant exposure while you're growing up then you don't feel so out of place.

The bond is a three way triangle. My relationship with my wife is not separate from that with my son. It's just difficult if you're going in [to the hospital] in the morning. In the past, I've liked to help my wife express her milk, to help to change nappies. These are usually the mother's roles and the mother's pleasures. They shouldn't be restricted to just the mothers. There was a time when she did get depressed for no apparent reason, maybe because she wanted him home. It seemed to be out of the blue. The tears did flow quite easily – she's quite a softie. I guess the more you see him the more you do wish to have him home.

Ahmed's recognition of Alia's sadness around this time was a response to her saying things such as:

I don't know how I feel sometimes, sometimes I feel happy, sometimes I feel sad, not sad but I don't know, probably I worry too much, because I'm not seeing him in front of me all the time. And I don't know when he cries whether there's something wrong with him or something, 'cause I only see him once a day.

'Pregnancy is like a migration' reports the interviewer:

Identity changes, mapping strange territory; not sure if you are the infant or the mother; a final severing of the ties with the mother, just as migration severs one from the mother country. It is not so different.

Alia, I thought, regressed as one does in crisis to this earlier trauma of migrating, awakened now by the present one, and seemed temporarily to lose the gains she had made in Australia. In the early days of Daniel coming home, she told me, 'Everyone of the women tell me what to do. When I come home, I do as they tell me, but I cry'. This was in contrast to a couple of sessions later, when I arrived and she was in her leotard just back from the gym, and Ahmed was left to mind the baby.

It was surprising that in the beginning she seemed to lose her new language. Her English became 'broken' to say the least, and she seemed to have lost words: 'I was afraid he would come dead'. Later, you get a shock – her English is fluent. You can see it change as she and her infant recover. She sounds simple, almost peasant-like at first; then you later find she is a university student and finished high school in Australia. The memories of her bad school days and awful early beginnings in Australia are now confused with this awful beginning to motherhood.

Chapter 13
A couple with a premature infant from an attachment perspective

BRYANNE BARNETT AND MARIJA RADOJEVIC

In this chapter, we will discuss the experience of one mother, as recounted in her nine interviews, within the framework of attachment theory. Some of the key features of the theory will be outlined, and then the dramatic narrative of Susan, the mother of a premature infant, will be considered. James, Susan's partner, played a significant part in these events.

The constructs used as a foundation for this chapter derive from the attachment theory of John Bowlby (Bowlby 1969/1982, 1973, 1980), developed on the basis of evolutionary and ethological principles. This new theory proposed that infants arrive in the world 'pre-wired' to participate in a social relationship with a care-giver because that relationship, through protection from predators and so on, will ensure their survival. As Ainsworth (1967) was later to describe it, the care-giver provides 'a secure base', where the infant feels safe and from which the child can later venture forth to explore the world.

Bowlby considered that the capacity to form strong emotional bonds with particular people, sometimes giving care and sometimes seeking it, was an important aspect of effective personal functioning. The pattern of these attachment bonds is a significant determinant not only of resilience or vulnerability throughout our life's journey, but also of our capacity to enjoy life.

For the purposes of the present chapter, the major features of attachment theory are listed below:

1. Attachment is a highly specific type of social bond, a complementary, asymmetrical relationship in which one participant seeks comfort and safety from the other. The one who is deemed stronger and wiser, that

is, capable of providing the security, is known as the attachment figure, while the one in need or distress is said to show attachment behaviour. Thus care-giving is complementary to care-seeking.

2. The availability and responsiveness of the attachment figure promotes an experience of felt security.

3. Although attachment behaviour is manifested from birth onwards, evidence of a coherent, integrated pattern, constructed on the basis of repeated interactions with the particular care-giver, is not seen until late in the first year of life. These mental representations, which include both sides of the dyadic relationship, are called internal working models (IWMs), and they become part of the personality structure. Working models form the prototype for subsequent relationships and, over time, become increasingly resistant to change. Nevertheless, as care-giving circumstances change (for better or worse), some revision of working models is possible.

4. Different patterns of attachment organisation (IWMs) develop. The *secure* attachment pattern maximises the subjective experience of security. In *insecure* patterns, felt security is compromised to varying degrees.

5. The formation of attachment bonds is an ubiquitous human phenomenon that serves the biological function of protection. Only in cases of the most extreme infantile deprivation does an attachment bond fail to form. The bond may be very strong without necessarily being 'secure' (see below).

6. Attachment behaviour characterises human beings throughout the lifespan.

A corollary of attachment is separation. What happens when the bond is threatened or actually severed, either temporarily or permanently? Although the attachment pattern has formed by around 12 months of age, the IWM remains fragile. Three-year-olds find it hard to cope with unaccustomed separation from their main attachment figures. By around the age of four or five years, the child has usually developed sufficiently to keep the bond in mind long enough to be separated from attachment figures for some hours without disintegrating. Nevertheless, if the child is stressed in any way, attachment behaviour is elicited and an attachment figure will be sought. The more distressed the child, the greater the need for the comforter to be the actual parent, especially the mother. Adults too usually find loss of significant attachment figures, such as spouse, parents or siblings, hard to endure.

Separation elicits attachment behaviour and reveals the attachment pattern or IWM. Ainsworth and her colleagues devised a reliable procedure called the Strange Situation Procedure (Ainsworth et al 1978) to assess the infant–parent attachment relationship. A secure pattern and two insecure patterns were found by carefully observing the infant's attachment behaviour towards the parent when stressed by two brief separations from the parent in a laboratory situation. Mother–infant and father–infant attachment security patterns may be (and often are) independent of one another (Main 1981).

Secure infants are unambivalent in seeking proximity, interaction or contact with their parent on reunion. The parent is emotionally available and contingently responsive.

Insecure/avoidant infants avoid the parent on reunion and show few, if any, signs of having missed the parent during separation, even though they were distressed. In the developing relationship with the baby, this parent has shown reduced sensitivity to the baby's cues, not responding, or responding negatively, to bids for comfort. The infant learns that it is better 'not to ask'.

Insecure/resistant infants display ambivalence towards the parent. They cry and signal that they want contact, but also clearly show anger. They are not easily soothed by the parent and find it hard to separate and return to play activity. This pattern is associated with a degree of parental insensitivity to infant signals, including inconsistency and therefore unpredictability.

More recently, a third insecure category, *insecure/disorganised/disorientated*, has been identified by Main and colleagues (Main and Solomon 1990). The behaviour of these infants on reunion is characterised by approach-avoidance. They may, for example, approach backwards or with their heads turned away. They appear frightened, confused or dazed. The parent has usually suffered considerable trauma in childhood, such as the loss of a parent (either physically or because the parent was affected by mental illness) or abuse.

An adult's 'state of mind with respect to attachment' can be assessed using a semi-structured interview (Main and Goldwyn 1999). The Adult Attachment Interview (AAI; George et al 1985) identifies four patterns corresponding to infant attachment status. During the AAI, adults are asked to speak about their perceptions of the parenting they received in childhood and how they consider that this is influencing their lives, especially the parenting of their own children.

Secure adults, termed *autonomous* or *free*, have a relatively easy and free-flowing recollection of their childhood attachment experiences. They neither idealise nor disavow these experiences. Most importantly, they are able to integrate both positive and negative aspects into a coherent and compassionate narrative. Insecure children may also become autonomous adults. This is termed *earned secure*. Thus, an individual who experienced adverse childhood circumstances may nevertheless have reflected appropriately upon the past and modified his or her IWM. The difficult experiences have been integrated adaptively into their personal narrative, thus freeing the individual from the burden of repeating the traumatic pattern. Autonomous adults tend to have securely attached infants.

Insecure/dismissing adults have difficulty remembering attachment-relevant childhood experiences or profess to regard them as being irrelevant to their current lives. The parenting they received tends to be idealised, and personal distress (either past or current) is dismissed. There is a marked discrepancy between the generalised and idealised recollections of parenting and specific recollections, the latter actually indicating varying levels of rejection of the child's attachment behaviour. Insecure/dismissing adults tend to have insecure/avoidant infants.

Insecure/preoccupied adults are still angrily preoccupied with the actual or perceived shortcomings of their parents. Negative experiences are related at length with little evidence that they have been reflectively integrated. The care-giving histories of these adults reveal considerable parental overinvolvement with, or role reversal of, the child. Insecure/preoccupied adults tend to have insecure/resistant infants.

Finally, *insecure/unresolved* adults relate a history of either unresolved abusive trauma or unresolved mourning for the loss of a significant attachment figure during childhood – often a parent or sibling. Their infants tend to be insecure/disorganised/disorientated.

As we have noted, attachment is an important determinant throughout life of self-esteem and resilience. New or substitute attachment relationships form readily when the individual is in a vulnerable situation, for example through illness or in circumstances of potential physical or psychological danger. A pregnant woman, especially if there are concerns about her own welfare or that of the fetus, will quickly establish such bonds with medical and nursing attendants.

In his last major work, Bowlby (1988) wrote:

> Whilst attachment behaviour is at its most obvious in early childhood, it can be observed throughout the life cycle, especially in emergencies. .... To remain within easy access of a familiar individual known to be ready and willing to come to our aid in an emergency is clearly a good insurance policy – whatever our age.

This passage will come dramatically to life as Susan journeys through her highly risky pregnancy, struggles to cope with the crises of the birth and survival of her daughter, falteringly assumes the role of first-time mother, and courageously works to maintain a close relationship with her husband, James, as well as trying to hold their large family together.

Interview 1

Susan, aged 36 years, is still in hospital following an emergency caesarean section. Her first baby, Lucy, is nine days old, having arrived some ten weeks prematurely.

In this first interview, we learn that the new husband whom Susan has chosen is significantly older, and that he has in her eyes amply demonstrated his capacity to be an adequate attachment figure. James has had to be both mother and father to his three children since his first wife died when their twins (now 19 years old) were aged three. James clearly also had to cope with the loss of his wife. Susan feels that he will be a competent attachment figure (secure base) not only for her, but also for her child. For his part, James considers that he is at a different developmental stage. He is unsure whether he wishes to repeat the earlier parenting experience, which for him included the burdens of being a sole parent and attachment figure in addition to coping with a significant bereavement.

Susan has experienced several losses of her own, including her mother, two miscarriages and a divorce from her first husband. However, her relationship with James makes her feel sufficiently secure to try again to create a new partnership and a family. In spite of James's reservations, Susan pursues her plan and conceives very quickly. Problems begin to arise almost immediately. The problems – bleeding, abnormal test results and termination having to be considered – were sufficiently grave for Susan to postpone attaching too strongly to the fetus. She says:

> I think I was postponing you know going out and looking at baby things and setting up a room ... just because of all these stalling events.

Perhaps partly for the same reason and also because they anticipated a mixed response, James and Susan did not tell his children about the pregnancy until around five months' gestation.

At this stage, Susan starts to be physically very unwell, with early signs of pre-eclampsia. Her obstetrician is overseas so her attachment behaviours are directed to a medically qualified woman friend. She obtains good advice and acts on it. In fact, Susan has taken the precaution of collecting several attachment figures. For example, we learn that she is attending a hypnotherapist. She is also maintaining her usual practice of attending the gym and keeping fit, all very sensible activities for keeping her anxiety level down.

Then things really start to go wrong. Susan's concern for the welfare of the child is evident in her reluctance to take the medication prescribed for her high blood pressure. She is admitted to hospital but has to be referred urgently to a specialist in a teaching hospital. Her blood pressure is apparently uncontrollable, and both mother and baby are at risk.

Susan telephones her husband and arranges for him to go directly to the hospital where the emergency caesarean is to take place. Like a good attachment figure, her husband drops everything and proceeds to the hospital immediately. She tells us:

> I rang him and said ... meet me over at [the hospital] because I think I'm going to have the baby really quickly, so you know he acted very fast and got over there, so he was there when I was there, which was nice ... and comforting that he got there so quickly. And he was really calm.

The baby, a girl, arrives ten or eleven weeks prematurely, and her survival is initially in doubt. Susan is also in acute care. Nevertheless, she makes a point of seeing and touching the baby as soon as possible. She says, 'I touched her little hand and her little foot, very tentatively of course, and James didn't, but that's OK'. Like most fathers, James is more reluctant to commit himself to this baby while her survival is uncertain. Susan would undoubtedly have been too ill to acknowledge it, but James must have been very frightened that he might lose another wife.

Susan believes that some of these events, such as receiving a general anaesthetic and not having the baby placed on her tummy immediately after birth, may have jeopardised the bonding process, and she is delighted to be able to express breast milk for the baby. To the nurses' surprise, she is fit enough (and determined enough) to make early and frequent visits to the nursery, taking every opportunity to perform as many tasks for the baby as possible. She notes that her husband is still avoiding holding the baby and she rationalises this:

> James hasn't cuddled her yet, but I'm sure he'll work himself up to it [laughing]. I think he thinks that he doesn't want to hurt her.

It would not be surprising that he should be hesitant given that this infant nearly cost him his wife.

Susan lets us know that she has a supportive social network. To her delight, members of this have visited not only her, but also the baby in the nursery, some of them illicitly taking the opportunity of touching Lucy. Susan believes this to mean that they will also bond well with her infant. She presumably she wishes to create an extended family for Lucy – a good safety net.

Various items of information, including a document on postnatal depression, are given to Susan. This topic is of some concern to her as her mother apparently suffered from the condition. One might conclude that Susan's attachment to her own mother was thereby jeopardised. Susan does not offer any further details at this point apart from saying that her mother is now dead. She realises that she may have inherited a tendency to similar problems but is too busy to worry about it at the moment. She is concentrating on the positive role models offered in the nursery, including a young mother who comes a very long distance every day to visit her baby.

Towards the end of the interview, we learn that Susan is beginning to think about her own discharge from hospital. We also discover that the household to which she will return now includes seven adults: James and Susan, Susan's father, James's three children and a student (as well as two dogs and a cat).

Interview 2

Susan was discharged the day after the first interview and has now been at home for a week. She spends a large part of each day in the neonatal intensive care unit (NICU).

The nurses are now being used as attachment figures. Susan is learning as much as possible and coping as best she can with her not inconsiderable anxiety. We also notice evidence of attachment behaviours directed towards others, such as her work colleagues, who respond positively, as she had anticipated.

Susan relates with amusement how James has been 'roped ... into changing his first nappy' by the nurses. She then immediately changes the subject to discuss her alarm when she is told that the baby is well enough to be moved to another ward, and goes on to acknowledge her apprehension regarding how she will manage when the baby is finally discharged from hospital altogether. Although she is now able to take the baby out of the humidicrib and hold her, Susan discusses with the nursing staff the 'cotton wool syndrome' – a tendency to overprotection. James is also making progress in his relationship with the baby, but he is not at the same stage in this process as is Susan.

We are now told that James is a perfectionist ('a neatnik') while Susan is a hoarder. She is unsure of how compatible everyone in the household will be. It seems that their house, which is very large and old, requires extensive renovations, which are even now underway. In spite of all this, and only partly because Lucy arrived too soon, Susan says, 'we haven't got a room to put her in'. She adds, 'there's really four households that are blended'. Many of the established attachment relationships are being subjected to considerable strain in this process.

In the meantime, Susan is progressing nicely in her relationship with the baby: 'running around and doing all this expresso type stuff but you know ... general baby equipment, little carry things and prams and nappy supplies and all that sort of stuff'. She remains anxious about separating from the attachment figures in the NICU. When talking about the baby being discharged, she says laughingly, 'better give me some warning or I'll die'. She has joined the Nursing Mothers Association of Australia and has received help from them regarding breastfeeding.

Susan now offers some details regarding her previous marriage and academic involvement. Her life has now changed emphasis, but she is nevertheless not sure that she will be able to take care of her daughter 'like regular mothers'. She is afraid that the baby will not be 'regular', that is normal – a common worry for the parents of very premature infants. She has been told that breastfeeding will raise the baby's IQ, this being one of the reasons she perseveres with it.

Susan comments that she has not seen James hold the baby yet, but he has said: 'I'm going to become really attached to this little girl'. She then talks about his hesitation regarding the pregnancy, contrasting that with his present statements. He now feels that he must keep himself healthy and stable because he wants to see Lucy grow up.

Susan proceeds to talk about her mother. It becomes clear that her current state of mind with respect to attachment is, in the terms described above, 'unresolved'. For example, she says, 'I'm motherless at the moment'. She has noticed that other women in maternity shops and similar places have their mothers with them; 'Where's my mother?'. We learn that Susan's mother suffered from manic-depressive disorder and committed suicide some six years before Lucy's birth. Susan was actually pregnant at the time and miscarried a few weeks later. She still feels as if the death of her mother were recent. Susan is aware that she may have inherited a vulnerability to manic-depressive illness but is undaunted. She misses her mother and is conscious of acquiring other women to fill the gap. James's mother is definitely seen as a potential attachment figure ('she's a real sweetheart and she's a very strong lady as well'), although his very large family is both attractive and intimidating.

Next we learn that Susan actually has a half sister, about whom she is positive: 'she really likes little babies and she's been around and very helpful ... I think I've got a pretty extensive support network'. One is inclined to agree with her, and it needs to be emphasised that a good support network is unlikely to be a matter of chance – it is something the individual creates for him- or herself. Susan is extremely insightful and has reflected extensively regarding her 'dysfunctional family'. This augurs well for her potential to move into a more secure attachment mode.

Interview 3

It is now a week later. The baby is doing well, but the family has been hit by yet another bombshell.

Susan initially comments that James has 'really bonded well' with the baby. She dates this from the occasion when the nurse encouraged him to change a nappy: 'I think once he got hands on you know, he hasn't looked back'. Susan also heard him saying to his mother, 'I saw them [that is, Susan and Lucy] feeding together and it was nice to watch'. Although Susan has so far minimised his problems, and he has undoubtedly tried to protect her from these, Susan is aware of some of them. For example, she is sensitive to the possibility that a husband might not be entirely happy about sharing his wife with a baby. Indeed, James must be feeling very insecure as he at this point becomes unexpectedly unemployed. Susan tries to be very positive about this, saying, 'secretly it's nice to have him around'. Because her place of employment is 'in the business of finding people work', Susan sends James there for help.

Although she offers practical advice, Susan is not able to offer much emotional support for James because she is, appropriately, preoccupied at this stage with creating an emotional relationship with Lucy. This she tries to enhance by 'writing little messages and putting them on the humidicrib' and by buying some crystals. She says:

> I don't have much contact with Lucy and a lot of that sort of softer type interaction I don't think is really there ... there's a lot of medical blips and squeaks and this sort of thing, and I just wanted something to soften that when I'm not around.

Susan is aware of the need to leave something of herself in the ward to maintain the connection with the baby when she is not around.

Paediatricians on the ward become instant attachment figures for the mothers. In Susan's case, one of them offers her comfort, reassurance and validation when he comments that it requires great dedication and persistence to continue with expressing breast milk. He adds that over 50 per cent of women who have premature babies are not breastfeeding when the baby leaves hospital.

Staff often do not realise that they become attachment figures and that this makes all of their comments, both positive and negative, highly significant to parents. Such comments (from other parents as well as staff) tend to tap into any 'unfinished business' that the mother may have. For example, one ward assistant says that Susan, because she has had a caesarean section, has avoided the pain of 'a regular birth'. Instead of refuting this statement by pointing out all the trauma that she has suffered, Susan immediately feels that she has 'gotten away with something and it's just like I've got the reward ... but I haven't gone through the pain and the anguish in the process of earning that reward'. She has 'feelings of unworthiness' because 'other women have done it the hard way'. How easy it is to make women feel guilty.

After some further musing on the subject, Susan reaches the conclusion that, on the contrary, she has as usual done it the hard way; she actually feels that 'something has been taken away' rather than that she has 'got something for nothing', a loss that will somehow need to be 'replenished' in the future. Is Susan thinking of another pregnancy where everything goes according to plan for a change?

Increasing physical contact with Lucy is also proving reinforcing for Susan. She is now able to bath the baby and put her to the breast. Nevertheless, she continues to be apprehensive about assuming full responsibility.

James is very supportive about the enormous efforts required to produce the small amount of breast milk. Her father, however, makes a less supportive comment: 'there's a lot of equipment for such a small amount of milk'. Susan replies, 'that's not a small amount of milk, it's all I've got; it's all relative', and laughs. She goes on to talk about 'issues about one's own upbringing and whether we felt deprived or nurtured'. She now feels very fortunate to have a partner who is so understanding: 'there's not a day that goes by that I don't you know I don't acknowledge that'. She proceeds to talk about herself as a critical perfectionist, asserting that James is 'totally non-judgemental' and that he is helping her to 'soften the edges', meaning that because of him she is less anxious and, therefore, has less need for defences such as perfectionism. She contrasts this with her previous relationship, which clearly did not provide her with a secure base and an opportunity to grow and mature.

Interview 4

This interview took place a week later. James is looking for a job, and Susan is doing her best to support his endeavours. His previous work was of late proving extremely stressful, and Susan feels his health is now actually improving. Susan discusses the positive and negative aspects of her interactions with the baby and with various members of the NICU staff.

Although Susan considers that James is becoming more relaxed, he has in fact had a third attack of 'flu. In her usual fashion, Susan sees this positively, talking of it as a 'cleansing' and 'shedding' process rather than something that happens when a person's resistance is reduced by stress. James has been seeing more of his friends and his mother, which is good according to Susan, who feels that his mother needs support in her efforts to 'contend with a husband who has Alzheimer's disease'.

Because of his illness, James has been unable to visit Lucy, and Susan is maintaining the continuity by reporting details of Lucy's progress to James. Susan herself is more involved in physical care of the baby and notes that, 'it's not really a bonding experience, it's a bit anxiety producing'. In fact, it is, of course, both.

Susan expresses concern that she may have upset one of the nurses by asking 'an inappropriate question'. Susan thinks that she may have hurt the feelings of this nurse, who 'can't have babies', and also worries that she may not be forgiven. With another nurse, Susan apologises for getting in the way, but this nurse comes back later to tell her that an apology was not necessary. This allows the two of them to become involved in a useful discussion of their individual strengths and the importance of a good relationship for meeting life's challenges. Susan concludes that 'it's really really important ... to have that really solid foundation and then you can always weather any storm'. It seems that, like many new mothers, Susan has an intuitive understanding of attachment theory.

The relationship between Susan and Lucy is going well. Susan is breast-feeding, and the baby 'seems to want to feed and she doesn't get all stressed'. The baby's enthusiasm and aptitude for feeding are a powerful reinforcer of the mother's feelings of competence in her new role.

Susan has formed a bond with many of the other mothers. She is looking forward to maintaining contact with some through a reunion that one of the younger women, described by Susan as the 'wonder mother', is organising, and will be sad to lose contact with others.

Susan also continues to idealise her husband, who is actively looking for work. Although she considers that she would not do as well in his situation, it seems to an outsider that she has clearly demonstrated her competence in meeting a variety of challenges. From Susan's point of view, however, she is not attending to day-to-day routine tasks of paying bills, contacting her employer and so on. In fact, she remains appropriately preoccupied with the baby. She is, as she notes, very self-critical: 'The responsibilities that I feel as a new mother ... really daunting and ah ... I guess I'm really hard on myself'. Susan thinks that her own unfinished business may contaminate the beginning of the baby's life, but, like most parents, she is determined to make sure that her child has 'something better' than she herself has experienced.

Early attachment relationships are a powerful determinant of how one manages negative emotions such as anxiety and anger. Susan believes that these issues are better managed in James's family than they were in her own. As we learn in the next session, her 'passionate feelings of rage' in childhood were dealt with by mother locking her in the bathroom – a painful experience. Nevertheless, Susan was a resourceful child who fantasised that she had the capacity to fly out the bathroom window and was not trapped at all. She has learned not to express her anger, but, as so often happens in such circumstances, this simply ends up in an explosion.

Interview 5

The weekly sessions are changing to fortnightly ones. James has two casual jobs, but his son has now just become unexpectedly unemployed. Two teenage students from Japan have joined the already crowded household. Susan is concerned that James is finding it hard to tolerate his son being around, whereas we might feel that the discomfort lies in the reminder for James of his own situation and how some of it came about.

Susan mentions the baby 'being in the driver's seat', but she actually continues to be very empathic, accommodating and attuned to the baby. Although there have been some very mixed experiences in her attempts to breastfeed Lucy directly, Susan has reached a stage at which the baby does not get cold quite so quickly and can fall asleep briefly at the end of a feed while still attached to the nipple. This is touchingly described as:

> she's really tired and she just had her little arms around and a singlet ... I just sort of held her and ... she fell asleep in an upright position, like a little koala that hangs onto a gum tree ... this is really nice, it sort of all fell into place.

Not only is Susan still concerned about the baby's fragility and the need for medical expertise to be close at hand, but she is also afraid about James's survival, 'if he wasn't around any more, oh what a disaster'. He has been arranging an insurance policy to cover the mortgage – an appropriate part of paternal responsibility, but it arouses extreme anxiety in Susan, who thinks, 'God, can I cope with this baby on my own?'.

This leads her to consider who else is an important support for her. Her father is a major support person, but they have 'quite a few clashes ... big ones, big cerebral things', and again it seems that she and her father are alike. An acknowledgement of this potential problem allows her to plan how it might be managed. Without such insight, the pattern would almost certainly be repeated. This feeds into her anxiety about the possible loss of James, which would leave a triad of herself, her father and the little girl, uncomfortably reminiscent of her own childhood. In contrast, James is idealised and seen as providing both emotional (motherly) and instrumental (fatherly) support. In her turn, she is doing her best to support him through the ordeal of continued employment uncertainty.

As noted in the previous session, Susan's family has difficulty expressing negative emotions. Like her father, she says nothing for a long time and then explodes like a volcano. Susan goes on to describe how her mother could not handle Susan's anger, speculating that this may have meant that her mother could not handle her *own* feelings of anger. Susan is clearly wondering how she will handle similar situations with Lucy.

Interview 6

It has been two weeks since the previous interview. James has still not found full-time employment, and Susan is unwell. Lucy will soon be coming home, and Susan has to plan her own return to work.

Susan is briefly separated from the baby because she contracts 'flu. This is a setback for her: 'all of a sudden I wasn't the primary care-giver'. James delivered the milk and brought her daily news from the front. She is anxious about the discharge date, and it seems the nurses are also concerned about her ability to handle the baby. Nevertheless, there is some reluctance on their part to allow her to spend a night or two in the hospital, gradually taking over the care of her baby.

At home, meanwhile, the problems include the impending renovations, the lack of a dedicated area for the baby, the fact that the whole household only possesses one car (Susan's, and unreliable) and the question of whether the young people should have their lovers to stay over night. Susan is already pondering the possibility of taking the baby to work with her when she resumes part-time employment at the end of maternity leave. She compares herself with her car and suggests that she needs 'a make-over'. She is aware of losing confidence about returning to work, a common problem for mothers.

James has had several unsuccessful job interviews, but Susan is now more able to include him in her thoughts and understand his probable feelings. She is relieved that he is remaining positive about both work and the new baby, trying hard to make room for the baby in the life of his family. In his turn, he acknowledges the inequality inherent in caring for a baby, that is, that the mother does most of the care-giving.

Susan notes the strong bond developing between her father and Lucy – his first and only grandchild. He has been visiting the baby in the ward, singing, talking and touching her, to the surprise and pleasure of the staff. He is clearly going to be very involved, and Susan, although delighted, wonders whether he will criticise her own efforts.

Interview 7

Since the last interview, Lucy has come home. An important component of this session is Susan's extreme anxiety on the subject of the very real danger of lead poisoning from the paint that is being stripped from the old house. As is so often the case, she receives conflicting advice from the experts, which compounds her anxiety.

Like most mothers in her position, Susan is filled with dismay and engages in 'stalling tactics' when a discharge date for the baby is announced: 'I thought I had an extra week'. With her husband's support, she agrees to the discharge date but insists on an overnight stay in the hospital, "cause if something really went wrong then they're there'. Despite their reluctance, the staff agree and also allow her a few hours sleep on the first night when the baby is unsettled. On the second night, she determinedly manages on her own. During her inpatient stay, Susan learns several useful things, for example how to discern that the baby is tired and needs help with settling. At this stage, a temporary space has been made available at home for the baby. This happens to be in their bedroom, so Susan at times insists that James must sleep in another room to ensure that he is rested in preparation for his job interviews.

Susan admires Lucy's capacity to be 'totally oblivious to all of this'. Meantime, the baby is making good progress, including in the relationship with James. When the baby is hard to settle, Susan gets angry and James helps by reflecting this to her. She then works out strategies such as breathing techniques and meditation to calm herself. The 24-hour emergency hotline is important. Although it is not clear whether she has used it, Susan is tempted to telephone and check 'are you really there?'.

Susan is beginning to be aware of how close she, like all mothers, is at times to being overwhelmed. Part of this relates to a feeling of being trapped while other members of the household have much more freedom.

Interview 8

Susan is preoccupied throughout this session with Lucy, who is in her arms. The baby has now been home for three weeks.

James is still described as 'wonderful' and 'patient', although Susan is cross when he is not sufficiently attentive to the baby and herself. She concedes that his life is very difficult and would have been easier without this new infant. Mother and baby are attending a group at the hospital. Susan also visits her chiropractor, and the baby has had a neck manipulation. She is taking the baby for daily walks around the area and getting to know the neighbours. She is clearly reconnecting with the outside world. Susan can at times separate from the baby, trusting her father to look after Lucy while she visits a friend.

Susan has developed a positive relationship with ward staff and the nurses who visited at home. She is also confident about establishing a good relationship with the next attachment figure, who will be the early childhood nurse. Susan's return to work is on her mind, and she is aware that her fantasy of taking the baby with her may not eventuate in practice. It is also obvious that she is (appropriately) looking forward to some baby-free days.

Interview 9

This is the last interview. Susan is now addressing the tasks that have to date been avoided, and is now clearly moving out of the primary maternal preoccupation phase. Since the previous session, she has been involved in a serious motor vehicle accident (not her fault), which resulted in a whiplash injury. Fortunately, Lucy was not in the car at the time. The household now has no car at all, but Susan takes this in her stride ... .

There is some pressure from Susan's colleagues for her not to return to work; it seems that others have taken over at least part of her role. Susan also has some concerns about expecting such a lot from her father (who will be minding the baby), wondering how feasible her work plans are. Nevertheless, she would like to return to work and expand her life again, feeling that this will add to her relationship with Lucy; 'on the good side you know I'll be all replenished, have more perspective on things'. Her conclusion for the time being is that if things do not work out at the office, she will resign. She is doing her best to give the baby the highest priority.

Susan is very aware of the importance of her relationship with James and that it represents the key to the success or failure of this complex household. She also gives indications that she has grown through the vicis-situdes of her experience. Reading through the transcripts makes it clear that this is indeed the case. It is also likely that the interviews offered her the opportunity to reflect upon and integrate her past experiences with current events, a prerequisite for offering her infant a secure base.

Conclusion

Both James and Susan experienced much personal anguish before and after Lucy's conception and birth. During her childhood, Susan had to deal with harsh, critical parenting practices and the recurrent serious mental illness of her mother, who was in all probability very sick in the early months of Susan's life. Susan later suffered the death of her mother by suicide and further loss through miscarriages and then divorce. Although her parents loved her and did the best they could, Susan's early attachment and loss experiences left her insecurely attached and thus vulnerable in the face of subsequent adversity.

Over the course of the interviews, we learn about her personal strengths, including her evident intelligence, self-discipline and considerable reflective capacity. These protective factors have allowed her not only to face the challenges, but also ultimately to set, both consciously and unconsciously, various goals towards which she has struggled unswervingly. These goals include physical fitness, job satisfaction, establishing a satisfactory social support network, and, last but not least, finding an appropriate partner and creating a happy family, with herself at the centre as a competent mother.

Susan's coping skills include tackling her problems head on if necessary: 'fly straight to the heart of danger for therein lies safety', she says in an early interview. Past experience has taught her that pregnancy may be hazardous, but she does not avoid it: she very deliberately conceives and then does everything in her power to anticipate and manage problems. Susan keeps fit, attends for medical guidance, undergoes all the screening tests, obtains other advice and support when required, involves herself in Lucy's care as soon as she can, takes an interest in everything that is being done to and for Lucy, even when it is unpleasant, and works to maintain good relationships with the staff. She struggles through discomfort and exhaustion to provide breast milk, even when at times she is 'only a tablespoon ahead' of the baby's requirements.

James too has suffered a disruption of attachments, through the loss of his first wife and more recently the serious illness of his father. His family have no doubt supported him and may have provided positive attachment experiences in early childhood that gave him a more secure internal working model than Susan's. Nevertheless, the imperative of being sole parent to three small children after his wife's death would have made the resolution of mourning for her a complex experience. From Susan's description of James's children, it is evident that he has been remarkably successful in providing a secure base for them. Despite his doubts and the additional burden of becoming suddenly unemployed, James is able to maintain the traditional masculine role of 'keeping a stiff upper lip' with regard to his own problems, doubts and fears, while supporting his wife.

Although they each have a history of loss and deprivation of their attachment figures, James and Susan are at different developmental stages in their lifespan when they meet. James has essentially completed the most pressing period of active parenting while Susan has not yet begun. Her determination and his empathy allow his reluctance to repeat a difficult experience to be overcome. Together, they form a strong bond that helps them to weather the appalling stresses befalling them in this new venture. James offers Susan unconditional support and, in his turn, is supported by her practical approach and clearly expressed appreciation of him.

Susan's perseverance and single-mindedness are rewarded, but not without cost. It is clear, for example, that not only James, but also his children have doubts, that the household is noisily chaotic, that Susan feels at times isolated and trapped, that the smooth return to part-time work that she planned is not going to be possible.

The literature suggests that the crisis of a very premature birth tests any marital relationship to the limit. The inherent physical and emotional stresses are managed in different ways and at different rates by each partner. If they cannot tolerate this situation, separation is sooner or later inevitable. If they can tolerate it and empathise with one another's method of coping, the relationship is much strengthened and will stand them in good stead for the future. Fortunately, the latter description seems to fit with Susan and James's partnership. They certainly make a formidable team.

References

Ainsworth MDS (1967) Infancy in Uganda: Infant Care and the Growth of Love. Baltimore: Johns Hopkins University Press.

Ainsworth MDS, Blehar MC, Waters E, Wall S (1978) Patterns of Attachment: A Psychological Study of the Strange Situation. Hillsdale, NJ: Erlbaum.

Bowlby J (1969/1982 revised Edn) Attachment and Loss. Volume 1: Attachment. New York: Basic Books.

Bowlby J (1973) Attachment and Loss. Volume 2: Separation. New York: Basic Books.

Bowlby J (1980) Attachment and Loss. Volume 3: Loss, Sadness and Depression. New York: Basic Books.

Bowlby J (1988) Developmental psychiatry comes of age. American Journal of Psychiatry 145: 27.

George C, Kaplan N, Main M (1985) The Berkeley Adult Attachment Interview. Unpublished protocol, Department of Psychology, University of California, Berkeley.

Main M (1981) Avoidance in the service of attachment: a working paper. In Immelmann K, Barlow G, Petrinovich L, Main M (Eds) Behavioral Development: The Bielefeld Interdisciplinary Project. New York: Cambridge University Press.

Main M, Solomon J (1990) Procedure for identifying infants as disorganized/disoriented during the Ainsworth Strange Situation. In Greenberg M, Cicchetti D, Cummings EM (Eds) Attachment in the Preschool Years: Theory, Research and Intervention. Chicago: University of Chicago Press.

Main M, Goldwyn R (1999) Interview-based adult attachment classifications: related to infant–mother and infant–father attachment. Developmental Psychology (in press).

PART 5
THE BABY

Chapter 14
The experience of early infancy for the preterm infant

HELEN HARDY

The poignant sight of a fragile immature infant lying isolated and exposed in a humidicrib, under the constant surveillance of electronic monitors and deprived of human intimacy, touches the most vulnerable part of any observer. There is a sense of abandonment, even though the baby is being carefully watched and attended to medically, and even though the parents visit. In closely observing the baby's behaviour, some insight can be gained into the efforts that the baby makes to deal with the multiple challenges of immaturity and an alien environment. What this experience may mean to the baby while in hospital, how it might influence development and how it might be improved are the topics of this chapter.

The paradoxical and stressful circumstances of the preterm baby

The very survival of a preterm baby means that the baby must forego the normal continuum of intrauterine nurturing, flowing on to mothering care and a secure holding in the arms at birth, and the loving scrutiny by the parents of every small detail of the newborn baby's appearance and behaviour. In contrast to a full-term baby, the newborn preterm baby, biologically unprepared for extrauterine life, suddenly becomes reliant on technology and specialist medical and nursing care in a neonatal intensive care unit (NICU) in order to sustain the most basic functions of temperature control, respiration and nutrition. Instead of building on the threads of familiarity of tastes, odours and sounds known in prenatal life, the transition to extrauterine life is a jarring disruption and an introduction to a clinical world. Instead of encountering the welcoming human environment that the term baby is psychobiologically ready to meet and interact with, the immature baby is essentially alone in the midst of a busy and, from the baby's perspective, impersonal NICU. The whole situation is a product of cultural rather than biological evolution (Als 1986), for which there can be no biological preparedness. The difficulties and stresses encountered in breathing, taking in nourishment and dealing with incongruous, unco-ordinated and uncomfortable sensory experience can be overwhelming for even a healthy preterm infant, whose capacity to manage stress is also immature (Kuhn et al 1991). For many infants, illness, congenital abnormalities, surgery and pain are additional stressors.

Among the recognised stressors affecting babies in a NICU are excessive levels of environmental noise and light (see, for example, Lawson et al 1977, Gottfried and Gaiter 1985), resulting in both unnecessary stress and possible damage to hearing (American Academy of Pediatrics 1997) and vision (Glass et al 1985). These effects are compounded by stressful, ill-timed handling (see, for example, Long et al 1980, Gorski et al 1983), and the stress of painful or uncomfortable procedures such as heel-pricks (Harpin and Rutter 1983, Owens and Todt 1984, Franck 1986), handling that is part of neurobehavioural testing (Gunnar et al 1987, Morrow et al 1990), chest physiotherapy (Gajdosik 1985, Greisen et al 1985) and routine procedures (see, for example, Norris et al 1982, Lagercrantz et al 1986, Mok et al 1991, Bernert et al 1997, Quinn et al 1998).

The behaviours that equip a full-term baby to respond specifically and preferentially to people, especially to his or her mother, and to elicit nurturing and comforting responses from care-givers, are undeveloped or distorted in the preterm infant. Even though all the baby's sensory systems are structurally complete, physiological instability, an inability to sustain periods of calm alertness, immature movement patterns and poor self-regulation all adversely affect the baby's responses and communication. The kinds of cues that the baby gives may not be as readily understood as the signals of a more mature and robust baby. In particular, facial expressions indicative of pain may be less obvious (Johnston et al 1993).

The baby is likely to be too fragile to be held, and too weak to snuggle in if able to be nursed, and touch may be experienced as aversive instead of comforting, especially if painful medical or nursing procedures are involved. The baby cannot initially feed orally, and thus misses out on the continuity of experience that normally occurs when the containing uterus is exchanged for being wrapped and gently held, and amniotic fluid is replaced by breast milk, with a taste and odour profile similar to that of amniotic fluid (Hepper 1996, Marlier et al 1998).

The subjective experience of preterm babies

Parents often express concern about the possible effects of pain and isolation on their babies and wonder whether the baby will remember what he or she has been through. Although conscious memories are not retained, evidence from several sources seems to suggest that there can be enduring effects on the baby's emerging sense of self and ultimate behavioural competency and learning ability. In looking for links between experience in the perinatal period and later mental health and educational outcomes, I would like to consider the following areas:

1. the neurophysiological effects of stress;
2. the behavioural language of preterm infants;
3. the nature of earliest memories;
4. states of mind inferred from observed infant behaviour.

Neurophysiological effects of stress

Exposure to stress, and the accompanying release of cortisol, may be damaging to preterm infants. In infancy, the hippocampus is particularly vulnerable, and its development can be impaired by high levels of cortisol (Lewis 1995). Animal research (Sapolsky and Meaney 1986) indicates that a stress non-responsive period (SNRP) occurs in newborn rats, which is thought to be protective of the developing brain, especially the hippocampus. High glucocorticoid levels at this time lead to a permanently diminished number of glucocorticoid receptors in the hippocampus, and consequently to a permanently reduced capacity to manage stress.

The least mature of preterm infants are described as hyporesponsive (Minde et al 1978, Tronick et al 1990). This behaviour may indicate that there is a SNRP for preterm infants, coinciding with the time when habituation is unavailable. Once established, habituation can be protective against the impact of too much stimulation. In human fetuses, habituation emerges gradually, being discernible in healthy fetuses by 30 weeks (Leader et al 1982). Consequently, excessive stress in very preterm babies, or in any infant lacking habituation, might have permanently detrimental effects on the capacity to cope with stress. There may also be adverse effects on long-term memory, for which the hippocampus is thought to be important (Lewis 1995).

This could account for some of the subsequent learning problems of children who were preterm, as rats subjected to stress during the SNRP have later been shown to have impaired learning ability. In rats, the stressful effects of maternal deprivation are reversed specifically by stroking, which simulates maternal licking (Schanberg and Field 1987). In stable preterm infants, too, stress behaviours are reduced, and habituation improved, by touch (Field et al 1986, Scafidii et al 1990), and stress hormone concentrations are reduced (Acolet et al 1993, McIntosh 1994). This suggests that infant massage might be beneficial both in comforting a preterm baby and in improving the potential for later learning, as has been seen in a group of children, assessed at seven years of age, who received specific tactile stimulation as preterm infants (Adamson-Macedo et al 1993).

It is known that even the preterm newborn is aware of pain (Anand and McGrath 1993), but there is continuing concern among NICU clinicians about achieving optimal pain management (Porter et al 1997). The particular stress associated with pain appears to be different for preterm compared with full-term infants. Their responses to noxious stimuli are more unpredictable, and more easily elicited, than those of term babies (Fitzgerald 1998), and soothing techniques may be only superficially effective, the underlying stress persisting (Porter et al 1997). In addition, persisting tactile hypersensitivity can result from tissue damage (Fitzgerald 1998), and it is often the case that the feet of babies who have had many heel-pricks while in the NICU remain hypersensitive to touch for a long time after they go home. Tactile defensiveness, more common in preterm than term infants (see, for example, Case-Smith et al 1998), is possibly a consequence of these experiences, and a further factor influencing behavioural outcome.

The endogenous opiate system is also responsive to stress signals, and with extended exposure to inescapable stress, stress-induced analgesia (SIA) has been demonstrated in animal studies (Grau et al 1981). A component of learned helplessness behaviour, this hypersensitivity of the endogenous opiate system persists so that, on subsequent occasions, small shocks induce analgesia. The same adaptation appears to occur in some preterm babies. Pain sensitivity is significantly lower among low birthweight toddlers, compared with those who were full term (Grunau et al 1994), following the repeated painful experiences of neonatal intensive care. In contrast, a single painful episode in a term neonate can have a sensitising effect. Circumcised newborns are reported to react more to the pain associated with subsequent immunisation at 4–6 months of age, achieving higher scores on objective measures of pain (Taddio et al 1997).

The behavioural language of preterm infants

'However gratifying it is in later life to express thoughts and feelings to a congenial person, there remains an unsatisfied longing for an understanding without words' (Klein 1963). This quotation crystallises for me the position of an immature infant who needs our understanding. Behaviour is like speech for the preverbal infant, and everything even the youngest baby does can be thought of as a spontaneous communication, hinting at how the baby is feeling and suggesting what the baby might be needing.

It is presumed that how a baby looks is generally how that baby feels, although there may be exceptions. For example, a baby may suck on a dummy and appear to be soothed while an uncomfortable procedure is taking place, yet still have high levels of cortisol circulating (Gunnar et al 1984). Similarly, when stimulation is overwhelming, a baby may sleep defensively. In the case of healthy term babies, it appears that novel stimuli, whether of a positive, noxious or neutral nature, precipitate both behavioural changes and a rise in cortisol level. When the non-noxious stimuli are repeated, there can be the same behavioural distress or arousal as before but without the elevation of cortisol level (Gunnar 1990). This habituation of the cortisol response does not occur in compromised newborns (Gunnar et al 1991), so the preterm baby's behavioural responses to any stimulation, including pain, might be a closer reflection of accompanying physiological stress than it would be for a more mature baby.

The baby's behavioural communication consists of observable autonomic reactions, body movement, varying states of arousal and a range of facial expressions and gestures. Autonomic signals include changes in skin colour, heart rate and respiration, as well as gastrointenstinal signs. Motor indicators include muscle tone and the use of flexion and extension. The level of arousal ranges from deep sleep to an awake, alert state, to robust crying. In the preterm infant, these states will be less clearly defined than in a full-term infant, diffuse light sleep states initially predominating. Facial expressions include grimaces, gaze aversion, sucking and smiling, while gestures include grasping and bringing the hand to the mouth.

A synactive model of development has been proposed by Als (Als 1982, Als et al 1979, 1982), based on the observed behavioural responses of the preterm neonate, to provide a framework for determining optimal care. Five hierarchical, sequentially maturing and interdependent areas of function are described:

- the autonomic system;
- the motor system;
- the state organisational system;
- the attention and interaction system within the state system;
- a self-regulatory and balancing system.

Autonomic homeostasis is seen as forming the core, in terms of being the earliest system to achieve some stability and because of being required, not only in the newborn period, but also in an ongoing way, as the foundation of other behaviour. A similar hierarchy of neuromaturation is observed in fetal development (DiPietro et al 1996).

Within each subsystem, a repertoire of behaviours, indicating either approach to or withdrawal from stimulation, can be identified. These range from mild and subtle indications to dramatic and global expressions. With increasing maturity and stability, fluctuations between avoidance and engaging behaviours become more discrete, and responses more smoothly modulated. The preterm infant, because of the immaturity of all physiological functioning, is significantly challenged in striving to achieve and maintain a secure base for more sophisticated activities.

Homeostasis – harmony in internal functioning, and balance in interactions with the world – is also conceived of as the first phase in emotional development (Greenspan 1991). The achievement of this stage of development is dependent on a predictable and comforting milieu for the infant, which a NICU does not typically provide. This places the infant at risk of establishing poorly regulated patterns of behaviour, of either hyperexcitability or withdrawal, of hyperarousal or dissociation (Perry et al 1995), that could be the basis of later attention and behaviour problems in ex-preterm babies (see, for example, Wolke 1998).

The nature of earliest memories

The brain is sufficiently developed for long-term memory traces to be laid down before 40 weeks' gestation even though the cortex is still immature (Prechtl 1984). However, myelinisation of the hippocampus remains incomplete, leaving episodic memories without sufficient context cues of time and space for retrieval, although something of their sensory quality may be retained (Reviere 1996). Earliest memories are more procedural, sensorimotor, non-verbal, implicit ones rather than declarative, conceptual, verbal and explicit (Squire 1987, Nelson 1994).

Memories of this kind are processed in the phylogenetically older areas of the brain within the limbic system, which is also involved in emotional experience. They cannot be accessed voluntarily. Examples of implicit memory include sensitisation, habituation and simple conditioning, behaviours that are acquired automatically with repeated stimulation. These habitual ways of responding are then reactivated in circumstances like the ones in which the learning took place, without recall of the original situation. Conditioned emotional responses of this kind, independent of cortical input, appear to be relatively fixed (Post and Weiss 1997) and may have a profound effect on subsequent behaviour, as well as on setting basic emotional tone.

In the case of traumatic perinatal experiences, these also appear to be retained, as specific bodily memories, with a predisposition for the events to be re-enacted. Jacobson et al (1987) compared birth data relating to 412 forensic victims, comprising suicide cases, alcoholics and drug addicts, with the data for 2901 controls, all born since 1940. This showed that suicide by asphyxiation was associated with birth asphyxia, suicide by violent mechanical means, such as strangulation, with mechanical birth trauma, and drug addiction with opiate and/or barbiturate obstetric medication. Winnicott (1949) also mentions a desire for suffocation as a common legacy of traumatic birth. Suicide is not, of course, necessarily an outcome of adverse birth experiences, given that protective factors may operate as well, but an individual may be primed by the early experience and in unfavourable circumstances feel compelled to repeat the trauma.

Evidence from psychoanalysis (Winnicott 1949, Rose 1992) and hypnosis (Chamberlain 1988) suggests that explicit memories from the perinatal period are also recoverable during psychotherapy. These recollections, although fragmentary, can extend back to intrauterine experience (Winnicott 1949). It appears quite likely that preterm babies will carry lasting impressions of their early experience, and these could be a factor in shaping their later behaviour.

States of mind inferred from observed infant behaviour

While it is useful to have theoretical frameworks within which to organise observations of a baby's behaviour, and to act as a source of ideas for interacting more appropriately with the preterm infant, I have also found it necessary to allow intuition to guide and inform more formal thinking about a baby. The infant's presentation can legitimately be taken at face value, even though observers' perceptions are naturally shaped by their own experiences of having been an infant. The process of being attentive to the baby's signals makes it possible to share something of the baby's feelings.

What I often sense when watching a preterm baby are feelings of panic and terror, of being isolated and fragmented, helpless and vulnerable, misunderstood and ignored, and exposed to experiences that are intrusive and disjointed. Such feelings must be sensed most keenly by a baby's parents. Then there are times of more reassuring feelings, when the baby seems to be 'heard' and embraced; and in states of reverie with an infant, or perhaps with the deep sigh that sometimes follows the successful comforting of a baby, one is perhaps close to feeling how the baby feels, at his or her best, while in hospital. The main issue is not so much precisely understanding the meaning of the baby's cues as the active process of thinking with and for the baby. As Schore (1998) has said, 'self-organization of the developing brain occurs in the context of a relationship with another self, another brain'.

The holding environment, necessary while the infant is in an absolutely dependent state psychologically, is based on reliable and empathetic, rather than mechanical, care-giving. This care enables the infant to maintain an ongoing sense of being, unaware of the adaptations being made for them by the care-giving environment. Failure of the holding environment means that the very sense of existing is under threat (Winnicott 1960). Given the frequently precarious circumstances of the newborn preterm infant, it seems that intensely painful experiences of this kind are unavoidable. Recurrent life-threatening episodes are often in fact a reality for a preterm infant.

Personality development, based on the repeated need to react to and recover from environmental impingements, to adapt to the environment instead of the environment meeting the baby's needs, leads to the formation of a false self (Winnicott 1960, Bick 1968). Without some containment of the baby's unintegrated personality parts, the baby struggles in terror to achieve this alone. It is not uncommon to see premature babies striving to assume a more curled up posture, or moving around until they can find firm surfaces against which to brace their feet, often squirming about inside a humidicrib until curled up in a corner with their feet resting against the wall of the crib, in an attempt to hold themselves together.

> Mary, born at 33 weeks, is now just one week old. She is lying unclothed in an open crib under phototherapy lights. Mary is on her back, with a nappy placed underneath her, on a shallow sheepskin covered 'nest'. This provides some support on either side but leaves her feet free. Her head is turned to the left-hand side, and her eyes are covered by an eye mask to shield her from the phototherapy lights directly overhead. There is a large arm-board taped to her right forearm, a nasal endotracheal tube taped to her nose, an orogastric tube taped to her face adjacent to her mouth, and leads attached to her body and her right foot. Mary seems to be awake, but it is difficult to be sure as her eyes are covered and she seems to be uncomfortable. She is restless, moving much of the time and repeatedly trying to tuck her limbs in closer to her body. She is able to keep her arms tucked in, and she then brings her left hand close to her mouth. Each time she flexes her legs, she holds the posture briefly, and then her legs collapse back onto the bed, the knees still flexed. There are twitching movements of both feet and tremors of her left foot, and then she manages momentarily to brace her left foot against her right knee.

Mary is 'asking' to be held. For Mary, and for all immature infants, physical holding is the beginning of a basic sense of security. Without this, uncontained terror and pain are retained in insulated autistic spaces (Tustin 1994). True containment requires both reassuring physical handling and emotional contact through the reverie of a mother (Likierman 1988). In the NICU, this closeness to the baby may be more equally shared between the parents than it would be in some other settings, as it is often the father who has the earliest contact with the baby.

Behavioural outcome of preterm birth

Throughout the period of late gestation and early infancy, the brain is undergoing rapid development and is particularly vulnerable. Small neurological insults and subtle distortions in brain development may be reflected in the high incidence of behaviour and learning disorders, negative temperament characteristics and lower levels of social competence (Chapieski and Evankovich 1997) among surviving preterm infants.

In children with a birthweight of less than 1500 g, the estimated prevalence of learning difficulties is 40 per cent, and that of attention deficit disorder 30 per cent (Paneth et al 1994), and early trends towards depression are reported in a follow-up study of seven-year-old low birthweight children (Hoy et al 1992). Compared with normal birthweight controls, and independently of social class or cognitive level, the children's scores on measures of sadness and unhappiness were significantly higher, and they were withdrawn and lacking in social skills. Even at four months' post-term, preterm infants smile and laugh less than term infants in playful interactions with their mothers, and continue to show poorer self-regulation, first evident in the neonatal period (Field 1982).

Factors such as stress and the inappropriate stimulation of immature, slowly responding sensory systems during the neonatal period may contribute to these outcomes through the effects of early experience in shaping the maturation of experience-dependent areas of the brain. Lasting effects on cognitive and emotional development are probable. The specific basis of behavioural difficulties in a child born preterm may be unclear, since they can occur in the absence of gross neurological lesions and there may be more than one possible cause. However, the potential for care-giving after discharge to counteract any maladjustment that is present will be limited if some aspects of brain functioning are already determined by the experiences of neonatal intensive care, or if subtle damage has occurred in later maturing areas of the brain (Moore 1986).

Intervention

The earliest possible intervention is required if the most favourable outcomes are to be achieved. This essentially consists of nurturing the baby's place within the family and providing the infant with a mothering environment that is constantly adjusting itself to his or her specific and changing needs for comfort and support, as an integral part of total patient care.

In comparison with infants receiving routine care, a number of studies have shown that the medical, developmental and behavioural outcome for preterm infants can be improved by individualised, family-centred developmental care (Als et al 1986, 1994, Becker et al 1991, 1993, Buehler et al 1995, Fleisher et al 1995). Significant changes demonstrated by this type of care include a reduced dependence on mechanical ventilation and supplemental oxygen, earlier oral feeding and better weight gain, improved neurobehavioural organisation and self-regulation in the first month post-term, a shorter duration of hospitalisation and being younger at the time of discharge from hospital. Developmental and behavioural gains have so far been shown to persist to a corrected age of nine months (Als et al 1986, 1994). It has also been demonstrated that brain function is enhanced in preterm infants receiving individualised supportive care. In the study by Buehler et al (1995), neurobehavioural and electrophysiological measures at two weeks' post-term showed that attention and frontal lobe functioning in preterm infants free of medical complications were comparable to those of full-term infants. This suggests that the later learning and behavioural problems frequently found among preterm infants in later childhood might be averted by lessening the stress of neonatal intensive care.

In planning care-giving to reduce stress, intrusive environmental noise and light should be minimised. Positioning and supports that facilitate flexion and provide boundaries and soft surfaces, such as sheepskin to lie on, are required. Handling and routines should be modified to be more in keeping with the baby's cues. It is recognised that an infant is capable of organising their own behaviour and seeking out beneficial stimulation (see, for example, Thoman et al, 1991), and is able to give signals that are meaningful. By following the baby's cues, defensive behaviours are less likely to be dramatic. If stimulation is reduced in response to an early, subtle message such as a yawn or gaze aversion, for example, there is less likelihood of the baby being totally overwhelmed and of disorganisation progressing to physiological instability. At the same time, contingent support will be offered to the baby, building on the baby's efforts to achieve self-regulation and to explore their social and sensory environment. The introduction of any social or supplementary sensory stimulation needs to be gradual, gentle and in keeping with the baby's readiness, as indicated by the state of arousal and engaging cues. The following scenario illustrates how this approach can work in practice.

Jane was born at 31 weeks and is now three weeks old. She is in a humidicrib, with a cover over the crib to protect her from bright light. The surroundings are noisy – alarms are sounding, several conversations are in progress nearby, there are rattling and rustling sounds as equipment and charts are manipulated, and audible footsteps can be heard as numerous people walk through the unit. Jane is lying on her back, comfortably cradled in a soft 'nest' and loosely covered with a sheet. She has an arm-board strapped to her right forearm, a cannula in her scalp on the left and an orogastric tube taped to her face. Her face is turned to the right, and there is a tiny dummy beside her. She is in light sleep, her breathing and heart rate being steady.

As some of the activity of the unit moves close to her crib, involuntary twitching movements and active movements of her arms and legs are seen, and she makes makes grasping movements with her free hand. There is a loud noise as something is dropped not far away, and Jane startles briefly. Her nurse opens the crib door quietly, uncovers her slowly and changes her nappy. Jane becomes very active, intermittently tucking up her legs, then arching her back, squirming and extending both legs in the air. Her nurse pauses, supporting Jane's legs in gentle flexion and talking to her softly. Umbilical cord care follows, and is clearly painful as she cries, her face reddens and she again arches and extends, as if trying to get away. Her nurse resumes cradled holding and some gentle patting, Jane then actively flexes her limbs and holds on to the edge of the sheet, becoming calm again. Her nurse attends to the leads, which need to be repositioned, and strokes Jane's hand, giving her a finger to hold and talking reassuringly. Jane has some difficulty retaining her composure and seems disturbed by the noise around her.

Her mouth is cleaned with cotton buds and cleansing solution, and she bites on the cotton buds as this is done. Her nurse is surprised when this happens and laughs gently. Jane now appears flaccid and exhausted, but she recovers slowly once settled, by being repositioned, turned now towards the left side, curled up with the nurse's hands supporting her and sucking her dummy. She is lying quietly awake, alert and visually attentive looking out through her crib wall, and the ward is a little quieter now.

For Jane, slowly paced interventions, with pauses for regaining stability, together with supportive holding, enable her actively to participate in becoming settled by grasping, sucking, curling up and having something to look at. She is trying to keep herself together by maintaining a flexed posture and by holding on with her hand, her eyes and her mouth. Jane demonstrates that she can communicate with, and respond to, a sensitive care-giver. She epitomises vulnerability, evokes tenderness in her nurse and is soothed by the nurse's calm approach and touch.

For other babies, similar strategies may be applicable, based on the particular way in which each one will respond to handling and to the environment in which they are being cared for. Both parents and staff can learn to read the baby's behaviour. The interplay between what the baby 'says' and how we respond is like a conversation, unique to the individuals involved. Thus, for each person involved in caring for a baby, there can be different, but equally appropriate, ways of responding to a particular cue from the baby. The baby's reaction to what is done, and felt, by the care-giver will tell us how well we have understood what they are saying and what they need.

Maximising continuity and consistency in the way in which the baby is cared for requires the hospital to be 'family friendly', ensuring that parents are supported and unpressured by the hospital system and ambience, well informed about their baby's condition and involved in decision-making concerning care. They need opportunities to participate in the care of their baby and to have some privacy in their contact with the baby. Mothers need to be supported in keeping up their breast milk supply, knowing that this is their unique link with the baby while other ways of parenting may, for the time being, be limited. In addition, fathers, given their early involvement with their babies, are more likely to remain available as care-givers than the fathers of full-term babies might be (Minde 1990).

Parents who would like to help with the baby's treatment, and who might need to learn special techniques for looking after their baby if there are going to be continuing medical problems to manage at home, are often concerned about being in a position in which they would be required to carry out a procedure that is painful for the baby. They are worried about hurting the baby and about becoming associated, in the baby's mind, with inflicting pain. The more unwell the baby is, the more probable it may be that parents will be hesitant, or perhaps less encouraged by staff, to interact with their baby (Minde et al 1983). They may need to move slowly but, once skilful, often perform procedures with great sensitivity because they know their own baby so much better than anyone else does.

There are also opportunities for rewarding activities with the baby while in hospital. When the baby's medical condition allows it, skin-to-skin holding (see, for example, Charpak et al 1997) and infant massage by the parents (for example, Harrison et al 1996) may be options, as may feeding and play time later on. Audiotapes of the parents' voices may also reinforce the positive bond between the baby and parents.

Besides having the parents involved in as much of the baby's care as they are ready for, ideally other care-givers will also know the baby well, as an individual person, and have similar approaches to handling. Explaining the differences between preterm and full-term behaviour, in order to allay some of the concerns that parents are likely to have, and providing antici-patory developmental guidance during hospitalisation and on discharge, may also assist parents in gaining some sense of mastery (Affleck et al 1991) in uncertain circumstances. Improved developmental outcomes for their babies may also be gained since positive social and environmental factors are known to be the best predictors of good developmental and behavioural outcomes in low-risk preterm infants (Wolke 1998). Assisting mothers to become more attuned to the behaviour of their preterm babies during the neonatal period has been shown to have lasting beneficial effects on development up to at least the age of seven years (Achenbach et al, 1990). Having shared the NICU experience with their baby also places parents in a position to later help their child to understand the circumstances of their earliest infancy, and to know that their parents were with them.

In working intuitively with parents and infants while both are in a distressed state, it is necessary to just be with them, without an agenda. Listening, but not knowing in advance what a baby will 'say' or need, and being sensitive to the trauma and grief that parents are negotiating, helps to create a space in which parents are able to think more about their baby. Differences in parenting styles, psychosocial circumstances and cultural backgrounds also need to be taken into account, but an accepting and supportive presence is a buffer against some of the extreme anxiety and thus enhances ongoing relationships between the preterm infant and the parents.

Conclusion

The experience of neonatal intensive care itself, independently of the effects of prematurity *per se* or of specific medical conditions, has both immediate and long-term impacts on a preterm baby. There is the potential for acute distress to go unrecognised and unrelieved, and for this adversely to influence the organisation of stress responses, the tactile system, experience-dependent brain maturation and self-regulation, all of which could have effects on later behaviour.

Optimal care aims to make the experience more gentle in the present, and less harmful in terms of outcome, by fostering contact between the baby and family, acknowledging the baby's cues and fragility, and responding empathetically. The baby is handled in ways that enable the baby to feel contained and safe, to experience stimulation that is appropriate in type, complexity, intensity and timing, so that self-regulation can grow. The care received is both life-saving and enriched by the warmth of human touch and understanding, and the baby's protective envelope of parental dedication is safeguarded.

References

Achenbach TM, Phares V, Howell CT, Rauh VA, Nurcombe B (1990) Seven-year outcome of the Vermont Intervention Program for low-birthweight infants. Child

Development 61: 1672–81.

Acolet D, Modi N, Giannakoulopoulos X, Bond C, Weg W, Clow A, Glover V (1993) Changes in plasma cortisol and catecholamine concentrations in response to massage in preterm infants. Archives of Disease in Childhood 68: 29–31.

Adamson-Macedo EN, Dattani I, Wilson A, DeCarvalho FA (1993) A small sample follow-up study of children who received tactile stimulation after pre-term birth: intelligence and achievements. Journal of Reproductive and Infant Psychology 11: 165–8.

Affleck G, Tennen H, Rowe J (1991) Infants in Crisis: How Parents Cope with Newborn Intensive Care and its Aftermath. New York: Springer-Verlag.

Als H (1982) Towards a synactive theory of development: promise for the assessment of infant individuality. Infant Mental Health Journal 3: 229–43.

Als H (1986) A synactive model of neonatal behavioral organization: framework for the assessment of neurobehavioral development in the premature infant and for support of infants and parents in the neonatal intensive care environment. In Sweeney JK (Ed.) The High-risk Neonate: Developmental Therapy Perspectives. New York: Haworth Press.

Als H, Lester BM, Brazelton TB (1979) Dynamics of the behavioral organization of the premature infant: a theoretical perspective. In Field T, Sostek A, Goldberg S, Shulman HH (Eds) Infants Born at Risk: Behavior and Development. New York: Spectrum.

Als H, Lester BM, Tronick EZ, Brazelton TB (1982) Towards a research instrument for the measurement of preterm infants' behavior (APIB). In Fitzgerald HE, Lester BM, Yogman MW (Eds) Theory and Research in Behavioral Pediatrics, Volume 1. New York: Plenum Press.

Als H, Lawhon G, Brown E et al (1986) Individualized behavioral and environmental care for the very low birth weight preterm infant at high risk for bronchopulmonary dysplasia: neonatal intensive care unit and developmental outcome. Pediatrics 78: 1123–32.

Als H, Lawhon G, Duffy FH, McAnulty GB, Gibes-Grossman R, Blickman JG (1994) Individualized developmental care for the very low-birth-weight preterm infant. Journal of the American Medical Association 272: 853–8.

American Academy of Pediatrics (1997) Noise: a hazard for the fetus and newborn. Pediatrics 100: 724–7.

Anand KJS, McGrath PJ (Eds) (1993) Pain in Neonates. Amsterdam: Elsevier.

Becker PT, Grunwald PC, Moorman J, Stuhr S (1991) Outcomes of developmentally supportive nursing care for very low birth weight infants. Nursing Research 40: 150–5.

Becker PT, Grunwald PC, Moorman J, Stuhr S (1993) Effects of developmental care on behavioral organization in very-low-birth-weight infants. Nursing Research 42: 214–20.

Bernert G, Siebenthal KV, Seidl R, Vanhole Ch., Devlieger H, Casaer P (1997) The effect of behavioural states on cerebral oxygenation during endotracheal suctioning of preterm babies. Neuropediatrics 28: 111–15.

Bick E (1968) The experience of the skin in early object-relations. International Journal of Psychoanalysis 49: 484–6.

Buehler DM, Als H, Duffy FH, McAnulty GB, Liederman J (1995) Effectiveness of individualized developmental care for low-risk preterm infants: behavioral and electrophysiological evidence. Pediatrics 96: 923–32.

Case-Smith J, Butcher L, Reed D (1998) Parents report of sensory responsiveness and temperament in preterm infants. American Journal of Occupational Therapy 52: 547–55.

Chamberlain D (1988) Babies Remember Birth. Los Angeles: Jeremy P. Tarcher.

Chapieski ML, Evankovich KD (1997) Behavioral effects of prematurity. Seminars in Perinatology 21: 221–39.

Charpak N, Ruiz-Peláez JG, Figueroa CZ de, Charpak Y (1997) Kangaroo mother versus traditional care for newborn infants ≤ 2000 grams: a randomized, controlled trial. Pediatrics 100: 682–8.

DiPietro JA, Hodgson DM, Costigan KA, Johnson TRB (1996) Fetal antecedents of infant temperament. Child Development 67: 2568–83.

Field T (1982) Affective displays of high-risk infants during early interactions. In Field T, Fogel A (Eds) Emotion and Early Interaction. Hillsdale, NJ: Lawrence Erlbaum Associates.

Field TM, Schanberg SM, Scafidi F et al (1986) Tactile/kinesthetic stimulation effects on preterm neonates. Pediatrics 77: 654–8.

Fitzgerald M (1998) The birth of pain. MRC News (Summer): 20–3.

Fleisher BE, VandenBerg K, Constantinou J et al (1995) Individualized developmental care for very-low-birth-weight premature infants. Clinical Pediatrics 34: 523–9.

Franck LS (1986) A new method to quantitatively describe pain behavior in infants. Nursing Research 35: 28–31.

Gajdosik CG (1985) Transcutaneous monitoring of PO2 during chest physical therapy in a premature infant. Physical and Occupational Therapy in Pediatrics 5(4): 69–75.

Glass P, Avery G, Subramanian K (1985) Effect of bright light in the hospital nursery on the incidence of retinopathy of prematurity. New England Journal of Medicine 313: 401–4.

Gorski PA, Hole WT, Leonard CH, Martin JA (1983) Direct computer recording of premature infants and nursery care: distress following two interventions. Pediatrics 72: 198–202.

Gottfried AW, Gaiter JL (Eds) (1985) Infant Stress Under Intensive Care. Baltimore: University Park Press.

Grau JW, Hyson RL, Maier SF, Madden J, Barchas JD (1981) Long-term stress-induced analgesia activation of the opiate system. Science 213: 1409–11.

Greenspan SI (1991) Clinical assessment of emotional milestones in infancy and early childhood. Pediatric Clinics of North America 38: 1371–85.

Greisen G, Frederiksen PS, Hertel J, Christensen NJ (1985) Catecholamine response to chest physiotherapy and endotracheal suctioning in preterm infants. Acta Paediatrica Scandinavica 74: 525–9.

Grunau RV, Whitfield MF, Petrie JH (1994) Pain sensitivity and temperament in extremely low-birth-weight premature toddlers and preterm and full-term controls. Pain 58: 341–6.

Gunnar MR (1990) The psychobiology of infant temperament. In Colombo J, Fagen J (Eds) Individual Differences in Infancy: Reliability, Stability, Prediction. Hillsdale, NJ: Lawrence Erlbaum Associates.

Gunnar MR, Fisch RO, Malone S (1984) The effects of a pacifying stimulus on behavioral and adrenocortical responses to circumcision in the newborn. Journal of the American Academy of Child Psychiatry 23: 34–8.

Gunnar MR, Isenee J, Fust LS (1987) Adrenocortical activity and the Brazelton Neonatal Assessment Scale: moderating effects of the newborn's biomedical status. Child Development 58: 1448–58.

Gunnar MR, Hertsgaard L, Larson M, Rigatuso J (1991) Cortisol and behavioral responses to repeated stressors in the human newborn. Developmental Psychobiology 24: 487–505.

Harpin VA, Rutter N (1983) Making heel pricks less painful. Archives of Disease in Childhood 58: 226–8.

Harrison L, Olivet L, Cunningham K, Bodin MB, Hicks C (1996) Effects of gentle human touch on preterm infants: pilot study results. Neonatal Network 15(2): 35–42.

Hepper PG (1996) Fetal memory: does it exist? What does it do? Acta Paediatrica Supplement 416: 16–20.

Hoy EA, Sykes DH, Bill JM, Halliday HL, McClure BG, Reid MMcC (1992) The social competence of very-low-birthweight children: teacher, peer and self-perceptions. Journal of Abnormal Child Psychology 20: 123–50.

Jacobson B, Eklund G, Hamberger L, Linnarsson D, Sedvall G, Valverius M (1987) Perinatal origin of adult self-destructive behavior. Acta Psychiatrica Scandinavica 76: 364–71.

Johnston CC, Stevens B, Craig KD, Grunau RV (1993) Developmental changes in pain expression in premature, full-term, two- and four-month-old infants. Pain 52: 201–8.

Klein M (1963) Our Adult World and Other Essays. London: Heinemann. Quoted in Thoman EB, Browder S (1987) Born Dancing. New York: Harper & Row.

Kuhn CM, Schanberg SM, Field T et al (1991) Tactile-kinesthetic stimulation effects on sympathetic and adrenocortical function in preterm infants. Journal of Pediatrics 119: 434–40.

Lagercrantz H, Nilsson E, Redham I, Hjemdahl P (1986) Plasma catecholamines following nursing procedures in a neonatal ward. Early Human Development 14: 61–5.

Lawson K, Daum C, Turkewitz G (1977) Environmental characteristics of a neonatal intensive-care unit. Child Development 48: 1633–9.

Leader LR, Baille P, Martin B, Vermeulen E (1982) The assessment and significance of habituation to a repeated stimulus by the human foetus. Early Human Development 7: 211–19.

Lewis M (1995) Memory and psychoanalysis: a new look at infantile amnesia and transference. Journal of the American Academy of Child and Adolescent Psychiatry 34: 405–17.

Likierman M (1988) Maternal love and positive projective identification. Journal of Child Psychotherapy 14(2): 29–46.

Long JG, Philip AGS, Lucey JF (1980) Excessive handling as a cause of hypoxemia. Pediatrics 65: 203–7.

McIntosh N (1994) Massage in preterm infants. Archives of Disease in Childhood Fetal and Neonatal Edition 70: F80.

Marlier L, Schaal B, Soussignan R (1998) Neonatal responsiveness to the odor of amniotic and lacteal fluid: a test of perinatal chemosensory continuity. Child Development 69: 611–23.

Minde K (1990) The long-term impact of prematurity on the family. Ab Initio 2(2): 1–3.

Minde K, Trehub S, Corter C, Celhoffer L, Marton P (1978) Mother–child relationships in the premature nursery: an observational study. Pediatrics 6: 373–77.

Minde K, Whitelaw A, Brown J, Fitzhardinge P (1983) Effects of neonatal complications in premature infants on early parent–infant interactions. Developmental Medicine and Child Neurology 25: 763–77.

Mok Q, Bass CA, Ducker DA, McIntosh N (1991) Temperature instability during nursing procedures. Archives of Disease in Childhood 66(7 Special Number): 783–6.

Moore JC (1986) Neonatal neuropathology. In Sweeney JK (Ed.) The High-risk Neonate: Developmental Therapy Perspectives. New York: Haworth Press.

Morrow CJ, Field TM, Scafidi FA et al (1990) Transcutaneous oxygen tension in preterm neonates during neonatal behavioral assessments and heelsticks. Journal of Developmental and Behavioral Pediatrics 11: 312–16.

Nelson K (1994) Long-term retention of memory for preverbal experience: evidence and implications. Memory 2: 467–75.

Norris S, Campbell LA, Brenkert S (1982) Nursing procedures and alterations in transcutaneous oxygen tension in premature infants. Nursing Research 31: 330–6.

Owens ME, Todt EH (1984) Pain in infancy: neonatal reaction to a heel lance. Pain 20: 77–86.

Paneth N, Rudelli R, Kazam E, Monte W (1994) Brain Damage in the Preterm Infant. Clinics in Developmental Medicine No. 131. London: MacKeith Press/Cambridge University Press.

Perry BD, Pollard RA, Blakley TL, Baker WL, Vigilante D (1995) Childhood trauma, the neurobiology of adaptation, and 'use-dependent' development of the brain: how 'states' become 'traits'. Infant Mental Health Journal 16: 271–91.

Porter FL, Wolf CM, Gold J, Lotsoff D, Miller JP (1997) Pain and pain management in newborn infants: a survey of physicians and nurses. Pediatrics 100: 626–32.

Post RM, Weiss SRB (1997) Emergent properties of neural systems: how focal molecular neurobiological alterations can affect behavior. Development and Psychopathology 9: 907–29.

Prechtl HFR (Ed.) (1984) Continuity of Neural Functions from Prenatal to Postnatal Life. Clinics in Developmental Medicine No. 94. Oxford: SIMP/Blackwell Scientific Publications.

Quinn MW, de Boer RC, Ansari N, Baumer JH (1998) Stress response and mode of ventilation in preterm infants. Archives of Disease in Childhood Fetal and Neonatal Edition 78: F195–F198.

Reviere SL (1996) Memory of Childhood Trauma: A Clinician's Guide to the Literature. New York: Guilford Press.

Rose L (1992) A stream of sensation. . . . Australian Journal of Psychotherapy 11: 35–46.

Sapolsky RM, Meaney MJ (1986) Maturation of the adrenocortical stress response: neuroendocrine control mechanisms and the stress hyporesponsive period. Brain Research Reviews 11: 65–76.

Scafidi FA, Field TM, Schanberg SM et al (1990) Massage stimulates growth in preterm infants: a replication. Infant Behavior and Development 13: 167–88.

Schanberg SM, Field TM (1987) Sensory deprivation stress and supplemental stimulation in the rat pup and preterm human neonate. Child Development 58: 1431–47.

Schore AN (1998) The experience-dependent maturation of an evaluative system in the cortex. In Pribram KH (Ed.) Brain and Values: Is a Biological Science of Values Possible? Proceedings of the Fifth Appalachian Conference on Behavioral Neurodynamics. Mahwah, NJ: Lawrence Erlbaum Associates.

Squire LR (1987) Memory and Brain. New York: Oxford University Press.

Taddio A, Katz J, Ilersich AL, Koren G (1997) Effect of neonatal circumcision on pain response during subsequent routine vaccination. Lancet 349: 599–603.

Thoman EB, Ingersoll EW, Acebo C (1991) Premature infants seek rhythmic stimulation, and the experience facilitates neurobehavioural development. Journal of Developmental and Behavioral Paediatrics 12: 11–18.

Tronick EZ, Scanlon KB, Scanlon JW (1990) Protective apathy, a hypothesis about the behavioral organization and its relation to clinical and physiologic status of the preterm infant during the newborn period. Clinics in Perinatology 17: 125–54.

Tustin F (1994) The perpetuation of an error. Journal of Child Psychotherapy 20: 3–23.

Winnicott DW (1949) Birth memories, birth trauma, and anxiety. In Through Paediatrics to Psychoanalysis (1978 edition). London: Hogarth Press.

Winnicott DW (1960) The theory of the parent–infant relationship. In The Maturational Processes and the Facilitating Environment (1979 edition). London: Hogarth Press.

Wolke D (1998) Psychological development of prematurely born children. Archives of Disease in Childhood 78: 567–70.

PART 6
THE WARD

Chapter 15
'Whose baby is it?'

BRYANNE BARNETT

This chapter discusses the behaviours, attitudes and relationships that occur among staff and family members when a baby spends the first months of his life in a neonatal intensive care unit (NICU) instead of in a uterus.

The birth of a wanted, healthy baby, born on the due date, without prior struggles with infertility or pregnancy, or delivery complications, to healthy, well-supported parents, is a very positive milestone in a family's life. The emotional development of all concerned may be expected to continue smoothly. The parents feel competent, confident of their capacity to exert some control and mastery in their lives, and optimistic about the future. Similarly, brothers and sisters, although temporarily disconcerted by the new (ar)rival in the household, look to their parents and extended family for support and, receiving it, decide that the gains outweigh the losses and life can proceed positively.

The birth of a premature or unwell infant, often after a worrying or complicated pregnancy and to a seriously ill mother, disrupts the smooth developmental process for everyone in the immediate and extended family. This is a crisis (Redshaw and Harris 1995), a major acute stress or trauma – war veterans are not the only ones who can suffer traumatic stress and post-traumatic stress disorder. It may also prove to be a matter of chronic stress, since the infant may hover between life and death for many weeks or months, experience many traumatic medical or surgical complications and interventions, and even then remain unwell. The parents cannot relax and get on with the task, actually begun long before, in their own childhood, of bonding to their baby. Indeed, they frequently wonder whether to stop or undo the process of attaching to this baby since they cannot be confident that the child will survive and not be hopelessly damaged. There are times when they wish or fantasise that they did not own this baby.

Meanwhile, the grandparents (the 'forgotten grievers' according to Blackburn and Lowen 1986) are intensely stressed, and the other children in the family experience a poorly understood disturbance in their daily routine. The mother and father are at the centre of this emotional chaos: all communication is channelled through them; everyone is looking to them for information, explanations and reassurance. All involved are in limbo until life settles down again, which may take quite some time. Indeed, it may never do so. In these circumstances, we should not be surprised if powerful emotions, both positive and negative, are evoked in all concerned.

Such feelings, thoughts and wishes may not be recognised or acknowledged by those experiencing them, especially when some of them might be deemed socially unacceptable. Thus, defences have to be mounted against these feelings and thoughts, and it is the results of these defensive activities that we note in behaviour, attitudes and conversation. If we are reluctant to interpret puzzling or difficult behaviour in a child as implying distress rather than their 'being bad', we will be even less tolerant of such behaviour in an adult – and stressed or distressed adults, be they family or staff, are capable of such behaviour. They may, for example, drive recklessly, drink too much, take their feelings out on partners and children, or complain about and berate other people. They may also distance themselves, finding excuses (such as a crisis elsewhere requiring their attention) to avoid facing the problem.

Not everyone reacts in the same way; much depends on the state of mind and context prevailing when the trauma occurs. Issues of gender, socialisation, age, mental and physical health, available social support, psychological resilience, previous experiences of loss and other trauma, financial circumstances and so on are important. If we do not understand the underlying issues, it is hard to understand and accept the behaviour and, conversely, only too easy to judge and criticise (parents and staff) rather than offer them support.

Ownership

To an observer, one striking feature of the situation of admitting an infant to neonatal intensive care is the way in which the biological parents are extruded and marginalised, the mother and her uterus being supplanted by an incubator and a plethora of tubes, instruments and other people. Nursing staff tend to take possession of individual infants, viewing one or several of the infants as their 'baby', while medical staff may see the unit as a whole as their 'baby', taking particular pride and proprietorial interest in its size and technology.

In fact, the parents lost exclusive ownership much earlier. The midwife or obstetrician became a part-owner, indeed was invited to do so, as soon as antenatal care was sought. This is a joint venture; and appropriately so. The pregnancy may proceed as a joint effort, but all too often the health professional takes control, with or without the mother's acquiescence (and sometimes to the almost complete exclusion of the father). It is as if the obstetrician or midwife assumes total accountability for the outcome when this responsibility actually needs to be shared throughout. Very little of this is overtly negotiated. It is not a problem if all goes well, but it can certainly become one if significant problems arise. If one takes the credit for a good outcome, one might be expected to shoulder the blame for a poor outcome. Not surprisingly, such a situation sometimes ends in litigation.

When things start to go wrong, there may be little time to discuss options; decisions may be urgent and parental consent given despite poor understanding. This is a matter of trust, but the unspoken contract usually implies that the situation should return to one of power-sharing (joint ownership) as soon as possible. The intervening step, in which the events of the crisis are reviewed and feelings are shared, often does not take place, or may occur only in a somewhat perfunctory fashion. This is not merely because of avoidance on the part of staff or parents, although this is part of the explanation; it is simply that everyone is now concentrating on the infant's physical survival, often placing a great deal of emphasis on the miraculous powers of the technology, so other aspects tend to seem less critical. If, however, the parents are not helped to work through the double grief, that is, the loss of the full-term healthy infant they were expecting and the anticipatory grief as they realise that they may lose the baby who has arrived, it is hard for them to resume the relationship with this baby and avoid depression.

Elkan (1981) describes how important it can be for someone who was present at the delivery to set aside time for a discussion with the parents. A dialogue regarding the sequence of causes and effects will facilitate their understanding and mitigate the guilt and anger that can lead to their unnecessarily blaming themselves or staff. There is also an opportunity to validate the parents' own feelings about the life and death crisis that they and their infant have experienced. It is important to stress that such discussions should be a dialogue. In these circumstances, the doctor or nurse often tends to be anxious and resort to a monologue, which prevents the parents from participating actively and therefore achieves little.

If no debriefing occurs, there is a gap or block in the narrative sequence. Prugh (1953) describes this as an 'emotional lag' or alienation, which the woman experiences in the first few days. The mother is emotionally stuck at the time the impending disaster was identified and she went into crisis coping mode, which often means partial dissociation. This may be exacerbated by the general anaesthetic or other medication that she received. Somehow she was separated from her baby and strangers took the infant away; sometimes disappearing down the corridor but sometimes leaving for a different hospital – an unknown destination. The baby is out of sight and cannot be pictured accurately in the new surroundings, and so may drop out of mind.

Thus, the question, 'Whose baby is it?' has another dimension. If, as is often the case, the infant has been delivered under general anaesthesia, the mother is extremely unwell or the two have been separated immediately after the delivery, the mother may have a feeling of unreality about the events. Has the baby been born? Where is the baby? Is this baby they are showing me really my baby? How do I know? Although common, these feelings may not be transient or may come and go over many months.

In such circumstances, the woman concludes that she has not been able to do what a mother should naturally be able to do – be a safe and efficient incubator – so someone else has taken both the baby and her place as mother. She is both dismayed and relieved. If the woman herself is recovering from major surgery and is physically very ill, the nurse must indeed take over the maternal role and provide 'an intermediary attachment, and a thread of continuity to sustain the baby through the time of waiting' (Szur 1981). This *locum parentis* situation will always be the case initially, and will continue to be a vital ingredient if the infant is in a distant hospital as well as during those many day- and night-time hours when neither parent is available.

Thus, when the infant is first installed in the NICU, the parents, especially the mother, are overwhelmed by shock, numbness, bewilderment, denial, feelings of abject failure, loss and grief, and submit readily, even eagerly, to the ministrations and direction of those whom they perceive as stronger, wiser and more competent to help the infant to survive. Sooner or later, however, the human urge to master trauma and not feel helpless, in this case to survive and acquire the skills necessary to be a competent mother to her infant, motivates a move for most (but not all) mothers towards contact and repossession. Nevertheless, parents struggling to stay close to their infants are aware of being in the way, and apologise. When a procedure has to be undertaken, they know to make themselves scarce. It is a rare mother who insists on staying to see what is being done to her baby. If the procedure were unpleasant, she might regret having stayed, although it is important that someone besides the infant has a memory of the events that the infant experiences. The nurse and the parents have to talk to one another to maintain a continuous narrative. An undervaluing of this *in loco parentis* aspect of the nurse's role is detrimental not only to the mother and infant, but also to the nurse herself.

Anger, so often viewed in a purely negative light despite its importance in many other struggles in human existence, provides much of the necessary energy, the fuel, for this struggle too. If all goes well, the relationship between staff and parent moves quickly from 'no contest' to active competition to collaboration, and then the staff gradually relinquish responsibility to the parents. This process can be something of a roller-coaster ride even at best, and it may also take a surprisingly long time to complete.

According to Caplan et al (1965), signs of appropriate coping on the part of the parents include:

- an active gathering of appropriate information and attempts to retain or regain some control and sharing of decision-making;
- a lack of, or minimal, distortion of the facts;
- an acknowledgement of ambivalent feelings towards the baby, with a verbal and non-verbal expression of these feelings, and an active seeking of help to express the feelings and find out about the special needs of the infant.

There are certainly times when staff 'forget' that the parents are the joint owners of the infant, for example when a decision is made regarding an intervention for the infant, such as a blood transfusion, without anyone thinking to consult the parents. The parents might have found it difficult to make this decision and would perhaps have deferred to the staff anyway, but, after the event, they may feel safe to complain about it! Conversely, staff often question the parents' motives in decisions regarding life-and-death interventions. Each wonders whether the other is thinking more of sparing, or even putting an end to, their own pain, alleviating their own distress rather than considering what is best for the baby. Of course, they may at times be correct in this assumption, but the long-term outcome for most infants cannot be reliably predicted, and, unless we have somehow gained considerable insight, we are all making decisions based on a mixture of motives, some conscious, others unconscious; some rational and others emotional. All important decisions are significantly influenced by emotional factors; to forget or deny this can be hazardous.

The mother

First, let us look at the mother's situation. The mother of a frail, very premature baby will experience most if not all of the following emotions:

anxiety; sadness; loneliness; disbelief; fear; a loss of confidence in herself as a mother and as a woman; guilt over the prematurity or illness of the infant (Is it because of something I did? Is it because of something I should have done? Am I being punished for 'misdeeds' in the past?); resentment and revulsion towards the strange-looking creature that purports to be her baby; resentment, anger, envy (of staff's skills and competence as care-takers for the baby) and jealousy (of their relationship with the baby) (cf. Prugh 1953).

At first, the mother is too grateful to the staff and too needful of their best efforts to express any anger about the staff's possessiveness. She feels ashamed of harbouring such thoughts – if she recognises them at all. As she regains confidence, the mother's anger with the staff may be expressed in a variety of ways. A legitimate 'peg' on which to hang some of these angry feelings is available if decisions are made regarding the infant without prior consultation with the parents. If staff react defensively rather than adopting a conciliatory stance, a battle of quite disproportionate dimensions may ensue. This seems at times to be exacerbated if the circumstances of the prior traumatic birth have not been adequately discussed with the parents. The feelings of loss of control, powerlessness and being excluded from decision-making build up and finally are expressed.

The mother's wish to re-establish her importance to the baby's survival results in positive as well as negative behaviour on her part. She may, for example, if she lives within a reasonable distance of the hospital, struggle valiantly to express breast milk and bring it for the baby; she may spend a lot of time on the ward despite the alien feel of the environment, and stay near the baby, talking, singing, touching, even learning to undertake some of the nursing procedures. Thus, the mother actively works to establish her relationship with the baby.

An atmosphere of goodwill is essential for success in this. If the mother is able to enlist the co-operation rather than the hostility of staff in her endeavours, so much the better. Some people are better at doing this than others, knowing from past experience how to get people on-side rather than off-side. Mothers often act as the nurse's aide in the ward and take an interest in the nurse's personal life, asking about her time off, her family and so on; they may also offer gifts. These activities, which are all valid ingredients of interpersonal negotiation, have sometimes been described as 'bargaining for' or 'buying back' the baby.

While the competition for ownership of the infant proceeds, other parent–child relationships are in evidence. An important aspect of the relationship with staff is their assumption in the mother's eyes of a parental role *vis-à-vis* herself. Nurses and doctors instantly become attachment figures (that is, they are viewed as being stronger, wiser and able to provide comfort and safety), while the mother manifests attachment behaviours towards staff and hopes that they will offer competent care – a secure base – for her as well as the baby.

Whether the mother actively seeks this care or does not ask for help, and whether she is confident or not about receiving it, depends on her previous experiences in care-eliciting situations, especially in infancy and early childhood. Thus, the relationships with the mother's own parents, both in the past and currently, influence her attitudes and behaviour. If she enjoyed a secure, affectionate relationship with her own mother or father, she will probably behave in ways which elicit a similar positive response from at least some of the staff. Unfortunately, the reverse is also true. The mother may long for staff, especially the ones who resemble her parents in some other ways, to behave differently from them, to care for her unconditionally, to approve, to praise, to be emotionally available and supportive, and not to criticise or punish. If she is fortunate, some or all of this may happen, and if such positive input is a new experience for her, she will benefit enormously in terms of personal growth.

Szur (1981) has commented that the emphasis placed on maximising the family's presence on the ward for infant inpatients might actually exacerbate the stress for parents, perhaps also increasing the burden of guilt and resentment. The parents may be distantly located or there may be maternal illness that keeps the mother and her partner away from the NICU, especially if there are other children or relatives to be cared for. If the mother spends every spare moment visiting the NICU and when at home is preoccupied (with the sick infant or with expressing breast milk, for example), her partner and their other children may resent as well as worry about the new infant. Szur suggests that such distortions in relationships may be long-lasting and detrimental to all, including the newcomer.

When the time comes for the discharge of the infant into exclusively parental care, we again see behaviours that are puzzling if we do not remember the workings of the unconscious mind and the need for defensive activity. For example, it is common for mothers who have eagerly awaited the moment when they can at last take the baby home and celebrate full possession – exclusive ownership – to try to postpone this moment when they are finally given a specific day: they are too busy, there is no transport available, the baby's room is not ready (why not?). Depending on their own reluctance to let the infant go, on their need for him/her to go quickly without prolonging the pain of parting or on their doubts about the mother's competence, staff may agree to or refuse this request without addressing the underlying issue.

Parental anxiety about taking on total responsibility without the back-up of the unit's expertise and equipment is understandable, but this is to be expected so anticipatory plans to address this issue can be implemented. A sensitive handling of this well-known crisis of confidence on the mother's part can smooth the transition, but, if the staff are also doubtful about the parental capacity to care for the infant, or one staff member is not ready to relinquish the baby, the mother's requests to delay discharge may be granted for the wrong reasons.

Some units offer the mother a day or two in the hospital, usually outside the NICU. This validates the concerns felt by all and allows a more gradual assumption of the total care of the infant on the part of the mother. This graduated discharge process, although 'officially' available, is sometimes not offered at all or is offered in a reluctant, half-hearted, even discouraging fashion, which the mother senses. She may rationalise that the staff are overworked and that their reluctance is understandable on that basis. Depending on her personality, she may then either insist on her right to stay overnight within reach of staff or accept her dismissal with or without openly expressing her dismay. If the parent's appropriate anxieties are accepted and verbally reflected in an empathic fashion by staff, the appropriate solution to the dilemma will be found. This solution may or may not include a maternal stay in the hospital.

The nursing staff

Meanwhile, what is happening from the staff's point of view? Since staff rarely have any training in understanding these interactions, a positive experience for the parents is by no means the rule. In addition, the staff themselves have needs and wishes for the very same items as the mother – for care, approval, praise and so on. Their work is constantly and extremely stressful. Even if they were resilient to start with, this may become attenuated through constant strain. Who is available to provide for them? Who actually does so? The NICU is a very unusual place, although for those who work there on a long-term basis, their perspective alters and it becomes familiar, even comfortable. Do they understand why they have chosen to work in this stressful and often depressing environment, so full of loss and grief? Very rarely. The stress of working in such an intense environment, where life and death are everyday matters, needs to be balanced by an equally significant life lived outside the NICU. An appropriate system of checks and balances to ensure good health for staff, and thus for the tiny patients and their anxious families, is not in place as routinely as one might wish.

Morale in difficult workplaces is often maintained by developing close, even intimate, relationships within the unit – the team – and excluding outsiders. In the case of the NICU, even staff working in related areas, such as the maternity unit and other paediatric units, may be regarded as outsiders – potential intruders – as may the families of the infants. The mother's obstetrician or midwife may not feel welcome to visit the unit, and the parents, though ostensibly welcome, may find that the room set aside for them to rest, have a cup of coffee or support one another, is actually full of surplus ward furniture.

Staff may compete rather than collaborate with the mother to prove to themselves that they are competent care-givers (better even than the baby's mother?), to expunge guilt, to promote their own self-esteem, to receive affection and approval. Doctors and nurses may be engaged in this work for a variety of reasons, not simply to defeat or compete with nature, to defeat death so to speak. Their reasons may include an altruistic desire to save lives and help families, a wish to offer others the care that they would like to have received themselves, and a desire for omnipotence to overcome their human feelings of powerlessness.

In their efforts to save, protect and care for the babies, staff inevitably become involved in a relationship with them. Because of the inherent inequality of the individuals involved, this will be a very unequal relation-ship between a very powerful parent substitute (the staff member) and a particularly helpless infant. Anyone who has been involved in saving a life, or has observed this event, knows that the rescuer is often more strongly bonded to the person saved than the other way round. The issue is, however, more complex than this. Helpless infants are, of course, powerful in their own right, that is, in eliciting care from attendant adults. In the past, it was common for NICUs to discourage nursing staff from 'becoming involved' with particular infants and their parents. It was thought that this would protect the nurses from the grief resulting from the inevitable separation from and loss of every infant in their care, whether through death or simply discharge into the care of the parents. Complex attachment issues are involved here, but suffice it to say that unless the nurse brings an avoidant, dismissive stance or model to all her close relationships, she cannot avoid becoming involved. She will assume a parental role towards the infant and will be in a similar role, or sometimes a sibling one, with regard to the parents. These repeated, brief, intense relationships require very considerable skill in managing appro-priate degrees of engagement and detachment, more skills perhaps than most of us possess.

Even when the infant is discharged home with mother, the nurse may be anxious to keep in touch or undertake home visits to ensure that 'her' baby is being properly cared for. Many nurses will say exactly that: 'It's our baby too, we have to make sure they're OK'. As was the case when the infant was initially admitted to intensive care, the parents are so anxious when the baby is first discharged home that they gratefully accept the nurse's ongoing involvement. A gradual weaning process may be necessary on all sides, but, as with weaning proper, some people can only manage this difficult separation by doing it abruptly – 'cold turkey', as it were.

Some mothers have an effect on the staff that is called 'splitting', dividing them into 'wonderful' and 'horrible', with nothing in between. In their turn, some staff will be very concerned for the mother, sympathetic and positive, willing to go out of their way to support and assist her. Others may take a dislike to her, considering her 'difficult' or 'manipulative' and being critical of her as a mother: 'She shouldn't be having children', 'She doesn't deserve this child' (often with the unspoken corollary 'I would do a better job' or 'This should be my baby').

To some extent, this criticism will occur for every mother. Whatever her behaviour, some will find positive reasons for it, others negative ones. For example, if, after her own discharge from hospital, she returns every day and spends long hours in the unit, some will praise her, while others will imply that she is neglecting her partner and other children. If she does not visit frequently, some staff will be concerned for her (the distance, the cost, her poor health, other commitments must be preventing her; how terrible she must feel, not being able to stay with the baby), while others will conclude that she is not trying hard enough. If she weeps a lot, this may be viewed sympathetically – or it may not : 'She should pull her socks up'.

Both medical and nursing staff, like parents, tend to expect 'children' to express gratitude, verbally and through gifts, and may be angry if this is not forthcoming. Such expressions also help the staff to cope with the repeated 'loss' of infants to whom they have become attached while caring for them so intimately and whom they have to return to the parents at the time of discharge. It is noticeable that staff actively maintain contact with 'favourite' infants or families, visiting and becoming literally part of the extended family, especially at times such as the child's birthday. For parents with no extended family available, this can be very positive. This staff member will hear from the family if another baby arrives safely, the father receives a promotion and so on. Sometimes the nurse remains in a parental role, sometimes she moves to that of a sibling or close friend, possibly depending on the relative ages of the individuals involved, although this is not always the case.

After the baby's discharge, the parents are likely to wish at some point to revisit the ward and to keep in touch for various lengths of time with particular staff members. This is appropriate and need not be discouraged: it is part of the psychological work for all concerned of processing the traumatic experience. Staff vary in their capacity to tolerate this. Many are aware that they too need to know that the baby is surviving; others cannot acknowledge their feelings, either positive or negative.

While most staff assume that the contacts will be infrequent and taper off in due course (which usually happens), some fear that the mother will become 'too demanding', an interesting concept perhaps acknowledging that the staff are already stretched to their emotional limits. If contacts are very frequent and do not subside, this should indicate to staff that all is not well with 'their baby', so action must be taken to enlist further assistance for the family. It is rarely either necessary or appropriate for the nurse to offer such additional assistance herself. If the nurse experiences requests for further contact as intolerable, he or she needs to seek increased sources of personal support, either within or outside the work context. A well-run unit keeps all these aspects in mind and under constant review in order to ensure neither staff nor parents become overwhelmed.

Discussion

Freud (1981) comments that although the mother and the hospital staff 'manifestly have the same aims: 1. that while the baby is in neonatal intensive care the mother should be helped to become confident in looking after him herself, and 2. that mother and infant should thrive so that they can be at home together as soon as possible', some of the behaviours and attitudes that we observe do not fit this paradigm. He states that these 'puzzling manifestations' only make sense when 'we acknowledge the double-edged nature of the conscious and unconscious functioning in both staff and parents'.

Although all the protagonists know, at least at some level, what they are supposed to be doing, actually doing it is obviously more easily said than done. To cope with anxiety, impending or recurrent loss, and conflicts of ownership (of expertise and competence, never mind the baby), authority and control, staff may have to distance themselves emotionally (and even physically at times – leaving the ward for a cup of tea, to collect pathology results or on sick leave) from both infant and parents. Similarly, the parents, although desperate to regain contact with the infant prematurely separated from them, do not want to face reminders of the trauma, the failure, the guilt, the painfully obvious frailty of the baby. At times, staff and parents clearly collude. Defences such as denial, avoidance, rationalisation, displacement and procrastination are all in evidence in any NICU and are well illustrated in the transcripts of the interviews with the parents in this volume.

It must be emphasised that these comments do not imply that the use of such defences is pathological; on the contrary, both staff and parents have to survive, so it is not surprising that these behaviours occur and are tolerated. Problems arise only when the defences are used excessively, that is, emotional contact between staff and infant, parent and infant, or parent and staff is not occurring sufficiently or positively enough to sustain a mutually supportive relationship.

Norma Tracey's research in this book illustrates how well some parents can use an empathic listener. Nevertheless, when individuals are traumatised, it is not clear how important an ingredient is provided by someone taking a specific interest in them, be it someone allocated to them or someone selected by the mother herself for a discussion of her concerns. Patteson and Barnard (1990) report that the relationship of the parents with their health professional might be more important than the actual content of any specific intervention targetted towards the infant or parents.

Debriefing interviews have been advocated for both partners following all deliveries, but this seldom occurs in busy obstetric units. There is also a tendency among professionals in the field to suggest that discussion should be avoided because the parents will be upset if they are encouraged to talk about their stressful experience. It is tempting to dismiss this attitude as self-defensive, but it requires more careful consideration. For example, does any discussion require a particular person (for example, a staff member who was present at the birth) or particular skills (a trained psychotherapist, a midwife) if harm is not to ensue?

It is not unreasonable to hypothesise that some parents will manage well without additional help, whereas others, perhaps less resilient through prior trauma and/or a lack of intra- and interpersonal resources, will benefit, while still others might need offers of both practical and emotional support. Although it is obvious that painful issues were raised in some of the research interviews that could not have been resolved over this short period of contact, the fact that the parents themselves were unanimously very positive about the interviews seems to suggest that, if those issues did require further work in the future, the parents would feel more comfortable and be active and hopeful about obtaining appropriate help.

Our health system does, in fact, make someone available to new parents — initially the hospital staff, and then the community nurse who sees the mother and baby to check on their progress after the discharge from hospital, and the family's general practitioner. Should hospital staff be more emotionally available to new parents? Should the community nurse be involved with the family before discharge, especially where the baby is in neonatal intensive care; should the family doctor be encouraged to play a more active role even before the mother and infant are discharged to their care? These professionals might well agree that this would be beneficial, but it does not seem to happen very often, partly because of the way in which our health services are structured – indicating a pressing need for change – and partly because of the unrealistically heavy workload shouldered by most nurses and doctors in this situation. They may be well aware that they are already working close to their emotional limits, which perhaps also indicates a need for change in work practices and our work ethic.

In addition, the training of these health professionals rarely includes the very particular skills of counselling (especially of the non-directive type), although they all offer a degree of support and advice. If all is going well, the routine visits to the baby health centre or doctor's office are adequate for the task of supporting the changes in the family system. Nevertheless, we know, for example from research on postnatal depression, that many women who are significantly distressed or depressed are not recognised as such, and that skills beyond those provided by the usual training are required if health professionals are to intervene effectively.

In our efforts to achieve the best outcome for the infants and their families, it is essential to maintain a balanced perspective. Szur (1981) wonders, for example, whether too much emphasis on parents undertaking care for the patient might 'tend to undervalue and undermine the essential nurturing aspects of nursing care and ward structure'. Similarly, too much emphasis on technology undervalues the importance of the reciprocal human interactions in the unit. It is hard to disagree with Szur when she stresses the need for 'a respectful partnership between parents and professionals, which includes a shared commitment to the present needs of these often very fragile patients, and also to their future development as people'.

Conclusion

Behaviour that seems irrational or uncaring may simply be a way of coping with a painful situation and surviving. Every crisis is stressful, but it also affords the opportunity to grow and mature. The NICU offers such an opportunity, not only for the infants in its care, but also for the parents and the staff, although we do not always make the most of this.

References

Astbury J (1996) Consumers' Perspective on Preterm Birth. Unpublished consultant's report to the Care Around Preterm Birth working party. Cited in Care Around Preterm Birth. A Guide for Parents (1997) NHMRC.

Blackburn S, Lowen L (1986) Impact of an infant's premature birth on the grandparents and parents. Journal of Obstetric, Gynecological and Neonatal Nursing 14: 173–8.

Caplan G, Mason E, Kaplan D (1965) Four studies of crisis in parents of prematures. Community Mental Health Journal 1: 149–61.

Elkan J (1981) Talking about the birth. Journal of Child Psychotherapy 7: 11–15.

Freud W E (1981) To be in touch. Journal of Child Psychotherapy 7: 7–9.

Patteson DM, Barnard KE (1990) Parenting of low birth weight infants: a review of issues and interventions. Infant Mental Health Journal 11: 37–56.

Prugh D (1953) Emotional problems of the premature infant's parents. Nursing Outlook 1: 461–4.

Redshaw ME, Harris A (1995) Maternal perceptions of neonatal intensive care. Acta Paediatrica 84: 593–8.

Szur R (1981) Infants in hospital. Journal of Child Psychotherapy 7: 3–6.

Chapter 16
The experience of staff who work in neonatal intensive care

CAMPBELL PAUL

Survival

The neonatal intensive care unit (NICU) is one of the few places in the field of paediatrics where the clear primary task is that of survival – the physical or emotional survival of the babies, parents and the staff. The unit consists of a community of souls engaged in the same mission but coming from different beginnings and orientations. There is an inevitable feeling that all demands cannot be met by each person. To cope with and meet the real and urgent needs of the sick premature baby, we all need a range of defences, from detachment and objectivication to humour and tears. Fostering a capacity for thought and reflective supervision in the unit seems crucial for the ultimate optimal care of the baby and their family. In the past 10 years, there have been vast improvements in the care and ultimate survival of the very low birthweight and sick baby. This is an astonishing phenomenon that stands as a major testament to those nurses and doctors who devote so much of themselves to the most vulnerable children. But how do they manage to pursue such an enormous task for so long?

In this chapter, we will look at some aspects of the experience of medical and nursing staff in this complex situation. The NICU is relatively unusual within the scope of paediatric medicine since prolonged complex hospital admission and death are the constant companions of those living and working there. I have had the privilege of being able to play a small role alongside the staff of one particular NICU. Each unit is very different. Some provide service to those infants with very rare, complicated or grave illnesses and disorders, who require a superspecialised multidisciplinary team of neonatologists, surgeons, anaesthetists and nursing staff. Other units are able to provide more routine care for very premature infants who require time to grow and develop before they can leave hospital. We might use the processes, issues and dilemmas that arise in the specialised NICU to highlight and illustrate some of the problems that might be applicable to all special care baby nurseries.

The bulk of this book describes and analyses parents' own accounts of their babies' experiences in the neonatal unit. In this section, I propose to look at some of the experiences of the staff, especially of the nurses and doctors who work with babies and their families. It seems important to try to understand how staff cope, how they survive and how they arrive at the remarkable outcomes that can be achieved with infants so tiny and so young.

It is a very difficult job to grasp just how vulnerable a very low birthweight baby is, lying there under the constant gaze of the staff. We tend to be struck by the babies who do not survive and by those who have a prolonged and painful course, but it is important to be aware that there are many infants who graduate, leave the unit and do well. This can be seen vividly and concretely by looking at the photographs on the walls of the units, the 'rogues' gallery' of those who have done well and made it into the community.

It is not always easy for the staff working in the unit to keep in mind the successes to which they have contributed. Many parents find it difficult and traumatic to return to the unit, even to pass on thanks. For many others, who have come from remote and distant places, it is, in practical terms, very difficult. Thus, the unit staff must develop a range of mechanisms for dealing with the high-level stress and uncertainty that is inevitable. Sometimes the direct rewards, such as christenings, birthday parties and school graduations, can compensate for the sadness of the funerals of those not so lucky.

The basic task of the unit seems clear enough: to provide urgent and acute treatment and care for very low birthweight and sick young babies. Attendant on this task, however, are many profound anxieties. Isabel Menzies-Lyth (1970) has talked about the social systems that have developed as a defence against anxiety in institutions such as hospitals. She sees these defences as quite ordinary but not always helpful in undertaking the basic task. Menzies-Lyth focused particularly on the way in which nursing activities were structured in an apparent attempt to keep the nurse at some distance from the patient in order that the relationship would not be too close. In some units, there was strong pressure to diffuse responsibility, obscure it and diminish the autonomous role of each individual in the workplace. Part of the process was to deny feelings and encourage detachment and eliminate decisions by falling back onto ritual. In the modern NICU, it may seem difficult to avoid some of these unhelpful defensive processes.

The relationship between nursing and medical staff is also of major importance when life-and-death decisions are frequent. Strong, sometimes charismatic leadership is essential since governance by democracy would most probably lead to chaos rather than order. There is, however, always the risk that such a leadership style can lead to the disruption of teamwork, and units are always looking for ways to facilitate lively and imaginative, collaborative teamwork.

There are many reasons why staff are under extreme stress when working in NICUs. When dealing with so many very sick and fragile infants, the margin for error in their care is narrow, but the level of scrutiny in the unit is very high. Computerised readings of the infant's physiological progress throughout the day are recorded and available for others to see. It must sometimes feel as if someone is looking over the nurse's shoulder all the time and someone is constantly watching over the doctor. The nurse must continuously monitor and adjust sophisticated and sensitive equipment attached to the baby. She must do this in addition to her nursing care of the infant – bathing, feeding, changing dressings – as well as being at every moment responsible for the baby's state and well-being. The nurse must also try to support the baby's parents, often feeling unprepared and at times unsupported him/herself.

Knowledge concerning the medical and physiological needs of the very premature baby has increased dramatically in recent years, and nursing and medical staff are increasingly called upon to be totally vigilant with complex and sensitive machinery while still being responsible for the care of the body and soul of the infant. There can be a sense of feeling observed and persecuted by the machinery, much of which records, from moment to moment, the baby's progress for others to see. The neonatal unit has become a workplace where everybody's actions are monitored, closely linked and interrelated with the work and role of every other person in the unit. This is further complicated by the fact that parents are often present for prolonged periods in the unit, learning much about the equipment and how it works. Parents can monitor the activities of staff with anxious vigilance. It is not only the baby who is observed as if in a fishbowl: each person observes the other.

The staff group in the unit in which I worked proposed regular meetings of nursing staff to discuss their experiences both with the families and with each other during the course of their work. These regular fortnightly meetings initiated by nursing staff proved to be powerful and intense sessions. Many critical issues were raised, and these were particularly highlighted when considering the experience of working with those infants who stayed a long time in the unit and had an uncertain outlook in terms of actual survival or disability.

The carers' role

The nature of the work demanded of the nursing staff in NICU follows some of the traditional nurturing aspects of the nursing role. There is a powerful and poignant tension in being able to meet both the constant and extensive technical aspects of the nursing role while at the same time being able to find the emotional space to provide for the broad range of the infant's and family's own psychological needs. The formation of dedicated small teams around each infant is an attempt to address the problem that each person alone might not be able to meet all the diverse needs of the patient. Aspects of the complete role can be shared within a small group of three or four staff, ensuring that critical aspects of total care are not missing.

Specific models of neonatal nursing care have been developed to address the needs of the infant and family. Als and Gilkerson (1995) have described the evolution of developmentally supportive care and family centre care, which involve detailed behavioural observations of the baby's own behaviour. Nursing interventions are tailored to this understanding of the infant's own early psyche and soma development. The nursing team is able to develop a care-giving plan that is consistent and relates to the structure of each infant's daily routine. The plan provides for extra support in times of stress for the baby and focusing on such aspects as the positioning of the infant, support for feeding, important opportunities for skin-to-skin contact and holding, and adjustments to the infant's external environment: sound, lighting and temperature. Similarly, a sensitive understanding of the family leads to the development of supportive integrated strategies for each infant's family.

Als and Gilkerson stress the need for NICU staff to have regular opportunities for reflective supervision since the technical and emotional demands of the task are so great and the moment-to-moment opportunities for stepping aside from the immediate task while with the baby so rare. In the process of reflective supervision, a space is developed in which one is able to think about the overall milieu of the unit and to consider some of the defensive processes that interfere with optimal care and practices. It is an extremely difficult task for all staff to be able to hold all aspects of the patient's care in mind. In fact, with modern medicine and nursing, it may be impossible when working at such a constant and intensive level for each individual to hold both the baby's mind and body in mind at once.

Splitting responsibilities between people in the care team may be quite appropriate, but along with this runs the danger of developing an unhealthy split by overvaluing the urgent and constant technical aspects of care above the emotional aspects of the baby's care. To accept that some staff are as good with technical aspects of patient care as others are equally good in a different way with the emotional aspects is to see them as complementary parts of the team approach, meeting the overall needs of the infant.

This splitting process can be driven by a sense of inadequacy as each person may expect that he or she too should be able to provide everything for the baby all the time. Such self-doubt can then be projected onto others, who then feel that they are not competent.

These splits can also be conceptualised as labelling some staff as being too emotionally involved and enmeshed with the baby or the family, and others as, in contrast, too cold, too distant and unsupportive. The unit should provide means for making these processes explicit and ensuring that all staff members are valued and supported in what they do, and that the overall needs of the baby and family are actually met. A failure to understand these issues can lead to the development of an unsettled and sometimes paranoid setting in which mutual trust is one of the first casualties.

Staff who are reflective and trusting of each other are able to provide the containment that is necessary for the families and babies in this prolonged traumatic situation. Bion (1962) has talked about the container–contained model for the mother with her young infant. A mother capable of the experience of reverie with her baby is able to receive her infant's projected rages and frustrations, despairs and excitements, and hold these in such a way that the infant is not overwhelmed by her own intense and potentially disorganising affects. In carrying out their ordinary care, the nursing staff also provide something of a therapeutic container for the young baby's emerging self. As with ordinary maternal care, the way in which the nurse talks to, strokes, holds and comforts the infant provides structure and containment for the baby's developing psyche–soma organisation.

In a parallel way, the unit provides containment for the powerful feelings experienced by all the staff who work within it. Within the unit, this containment can be embodied in its general ethos or identity and enacted through the leadership of the senior and longstanding staff. The group as a whole provides a role that somewhat mirrors the role of a mother in the care of her developing infant. If all goes well and the 'work group' develops (Bion 1961), the focus is on the basic task in a healthy sustained way.

There is, however, a real predicament for the NICU. The staff, particularly the medical staff, have a dual role. They must constantly strive to ensure the baby's survival with a healthy outcome, yet a major part of their role is to know when to allow the baby to die, to know when the baby has had enough treatment and that to do anything further would be unfair and futile. When lodged in the one individual, the neonatologist, this dual role can seem intrinsically contradictory. In order to carry out necessary, painful and intrusive procedures, the neonatologist must identify with the baby as the courageous infant who is struggling on and who cannot and will not give up. It seems very important to have this investment in the baby's own striving for life.

Without the projection of the doctor's own self into the baby, and without the idealisation of the baby and their tenacity, it can be hard to do what is intrusive yet necessary for good treatment. Equally, when it is clear that further treatment is no longer appropriate, it can be extremely hard to contemplate the end of a life that has only just begun to begin, a life for which it seems that there is nothing to look back on except the parents' hopes, dreams and expectations for their child. Perhaps, paradoxically, by seeing the person in the baby, such decisions as when to cease vigorous treatment can be made more clearly. Identifying the real person inside the infant, the baby who responds to pain, to comfort, to the soft voice or the touch of their carer, can make it easier to make the hardest decisions about the baby's care. As time goes by, it perhaps becomes a bit easier to identify with the baby's present and future suffering as well as the baby's developmental potential.

Whose baby is it anyway?

Attachment is a universal human phenomenon (Bowlby 1982). The small infant elicits quite powerful feelings of attachment across many different circumstances and settings. The primary attachment is clearly with the baby's parents, who have experienced their own thoughts and fantasies, hopes and desires through the preconceptive phase, the pregnancy and the birth. With the premature baby, however, much of this process is fractured or disrupted, and parents can even experience a conscious attempt to avoid coming too close to their own baby. This is often the focus of intervention by the infant mental health worker in the NICU.

Some similar processes are inevitably at work, however, with the nursing and medical staff in the unit. The process of providing frequent daily physical and emotional care for a baby over a long period of time inevitably leads to the development of a powerful emotional attachment. This might be in spite of conscious attempts not to become too close to the infant for whom the care is being provided. Doctors and nurses on the unit get to know their tiny patients very well – their sensitivities, their responsiveness, the way they look, the way their tiny bodies respond to touch when they are held, the way in which they respond to painful and disruptive procedures. Indeed, the NICU staff often have more intimate and prolonged contact with the baby than the parents have been able to have during the first months out of the womb. This is an area that is not often addressed or discussed.

'Overinvolvement' or too close a relationship with the patient has often been seen as an impediment to good care. Avoiding 'overinvolvement' has, however, neither stopped nor prevented the development of a close attachment between carers and their infant patients: it may simply become covert.

In the unit, parents can describe feeling that their baby no longer belongs to them, and this can lead to quite intense and troubling relationships between parents and staff. Both parents and staff are in an invidious position. Parents want the staff to provide their baby with the best care possible; they want the staff to know their baby as well as they can and to care tenderly for the baby as well as they can, but they do not want to relinquish the love of their baby to someone else. Staff, on the other hand, want to be able to provide the best level of physical and technical care that the baby can receive and fear that developing too close a relationship might obscure their judgement and professional objectivity.

Nurses talking about one infant who had been in the unit a long time, having been very sick and through many crises, vividly described the real person that they had come to know: 'We were really upset; we could see how she pulled out her central venous line. She tears at her own skin as if she is distressed and wants to get out'. The staff have entered the world of this baby. Their identification with her and her experience is deep and profound, and they were themselves traumatised by her distress. A doctor described another infant, seeing him as having become sad and distressed: 'You look into his eyes and he looks straight back at you. The look he gives is like he has just given up'. Of course, staff more often describe the tenacious and courageous qualities of the babies for whom they are caring: 'She is a real fighter; she is not going to give up. She's got real guts and determination'. Many of these positive things are recorded in the communication books that are shared with parents about their babies.

These are overwhelmingly encouraging comments, but at times parents feel angry that someone else should know their child better than they do and could love their child more than they do. Equally, the unit staff can feel angry or distressed that parents who have been unable to visit or stay for lengthy periods with their baby do not seem very attached or connected to their child. The feeling may be that they will not be able to provide the appropriate emotional and physical care for their baby when he/she is ready to go home.

These processes are very powerful, Bynghall (1997) describes how a doctor's personal experience can be a major influence on why they enter medicine to care for people. Within families, Bynghall reports, there is a classical relationship dilemma: to get close or to keep a suitable distance. This dilemma applies in the health care-giving system as well. Those working in hospitals bring with them a diverse range of emotional and relationship histories. Consequently, there are many different ways of relating to infants and their parents in the neonatal unit, and different attachment relationships. It seems important to acknowledge this diversity rather than expect each staff member or each professional group to follow one stereotypic line. This underscores the value of small working teams in which different tasks and different relationships can be developed over time to suit the real needs of each baby, family and staff group. It seems wrong and arrogant to expect each staff member to be all things to all patients at all times.

Trauma for the staff

Given that close relationships are formed with families and babies, and that the identification of staff with their patients is deep and profound, the trauma experienced by the baby and the parents can be also painfully experienced by the staff. They can be traumatised by this process. After months of working intensively to keep a baby alive, to give them the best chance in life, staff often report symptoms of their own such as sleeplessness, profound anxiety, tearfulness, nightmares, dreams and difficulty in leaving their work behind at the end of a shift. When talking in groups about this process, the impact on their own relationships is discussed. The families with whom we work can sometimes provide an unwelcome echo of our own family narratives, and it can be hard to deal with these experiences when they remain out of consciousness.

A more concrete manifestation of the phenomenon of work intruding into staff's personal lives is when the babies' families lean so much on the nurses that they seem to become part of their own home life. Out-of-hours contact, telephone calls, meeting for coffee or meals can creep across and break the boundaries of emotional safety. It can be very difficult to talk about this process of being engulfed by the babies' families and their dramas, leaving nurses painfully alienated from their peers. The reflective listening space of the staff group can enable the nurse to share and defuse the strain of feeling that they have to hold the family on their own .

Useful defences

We all have some ways of bringing such issues to the light of day to be dealt with.

Humour

'You have to get used to our weird sense of humour ... we need it.' Humour provides a major outlet for pent-up tension, anxiety and despair. Medical staff especially are adept at the use of appropriately called 'sick humour'. This is part of a tradition going back in time to medical student training: to exaggerate, to make bizarre and shocking some of the awesome, frightening and sad experiences when dealing with disease, despair and death.

Christie (1994) reviews the place of humour, stressing its creative and playful aspects, which can be used to provide timely transient relief. It also can provide a transformation of otherwise warded-off fears, anxieties and impulses to something more manageable. He suggests that humour is especially good at providing a means for us to creatively tolerate intolerable or irreconcilable ideas and feelings. At times, humour between colleagues can diffuse the shock of working with a tiny human being: 'no heavier than a pound of butter ...'. Simultaneously, we are seemingly disrespectful yet making light of the situation to cope with the awesome nature of the premature infant's supreme vulnerability. When I joined a ward round within one neonatal unit, one of the medical staff said, 'he's coming on the ward round; people think we are all crazy here – and he's here to prove it!'.

Tears

In the tea room and other settings away from the ward itself, tears often flow as staff unburden their accumulated tensions from the long shift of the day. The tea room often provides a safe debriefing environment where emotions can be expressed with colleagues who are experiencing similar trauma. Some of the tensely ambivalent and at times angry feelings about the babies, their families and colleagues can be given an airing and have the poison removed from the sting. These defences are not always successful: splits in the staff group can be quite distressing as unwanted feelings can be lodged on to others whether or not they belong there. When the issue of the baby's survival and whether to continue vigorous treatment is in the air, confusing, intensely ambivalent feelings are common. Exhausted parents can wish for a peaceful end to their child's struggle yet at the same time desperately hope for a miracle, a reprieve. The doctors and nurses can share the same apparently irreconcilable feelings. It is equally hard, however, for the staff to talk about the sometimes macabre experiences surounding a wished-for death.

Who decides?

Reaching the decision to discontinue intensive or active treatment is an agonising process in itself and, despite a cohesive team, can be a very lonely one for the consultant. Newspapers often report on a 'miracle baby' who has defied death over and over, and the public are encouraged to believe that the hospital is capable of snatching any child from the jaws of death. Ultimately, it is the doctor who feels responsible. Such decisions generate intense feelings in the unit and the community, but as one neonatologist affirmed, 'A doctor must have insights into the limitations of medicine and thus be able to recognize the unthinking preservation of life is not always in the patient's best interests'. Different staff arrive at the conclusion that the baby's situation is hopeless at different times, which can lead to tension between the nursing and medical staff. As one consultant observed, it occasionally emerges, during the process of resolving these tensions, that 'the nursing staff feel that we went on too long and the medical staff feel that it wasn't long enough'. Can it be that they are both right, each coming from their own legitimate perspective?

The NICU is a very complex microsociety. Leadership is provided by a group of senior neonatologists and nursing staff. They are in an extremely rewarding but at times lonely position. Maintaining the apparently contradictory dual role of striving to keep the baby alive and knowing when to cease active treatment is a heavy load. The senior staff have a very difficult task in generating and sustaining hope in the unit. Hope has its two faces: optimism and pain. There is the joyful expectation that we will come through the trial and tribulation that faces us, but the other face of hope is that of pain, the pain of hanging on, of knowing that hope is not a certainty but only a possibility for the wished-for outcome. The neonatologist is responsible for nurturing hope as well as despatching it at the appropriate time. Being able to follow up the successful graduates of the unit over time to see them develop into lively, responsive children must be one of the main engines that drives this dissemination of hope.

The responsibility put on the staff, the parents and the hospital by the media can be enormous. The medical and nursing staff are placed high on a pedestal with huge responsibility, as great as any in medicine. But in the NICU 'the miracle' is achieved only with constant vigilant work. Rarely do single acts effect a prolonged cure. It is from this position on the high pedestal that the staff have judiciously to manage hope. It can be as intensely difficult a task to allow an infant to die with dignity as it is exciting and exhilarating to see those survivors go into the world, leaving behind their life in perspex boxes, gladwrap and watchful monitors. It can be exhilarating to experience the joy of helping parents to get to know a new person and to go home with that person. It is equally important to help those parents whose children do not go home to get to know their child as well as they can while they can.

What is helpful for staff

The milieu of NICU caring for the very sick baby can be an unforgiving and frightening one for those who work within it, despite the marvellous joy of the babies who do so well. Some systems appear to be quite helpful in supporting the workers in their role of caring for babies and families.

The social worker clearly has a critical role, especially in the life of the parents. It is a privileged position being both 'inside' and 'outside' the unit. Parents can share much with the available social worker. It can feel safer to tell the social worker about one's ambivalence towards one's baby or to tell him/her about one's resentment of the unit staff seeming to take over the baby. The social worker can then hear and contain the parents' fears and despair, which might otherwise perturb the direct care staff in their work with the baby.

A constant challenge confronting the NICU is how creatively to incorporate the social workers' experiences with families into the care of the baby and the overall running of the unit. Gorski (1984) argues for 'structured systems for sharing or communicating personal feelings among peers' in order to benefit both infants and families. A person who is somewhat outside the ward can be a useful facilitator in these sharing processes. However, recognition must be given to the fact that each person has his/her own style and way of coping, which need real consideration and respect. There may need to be a variety of settings available, both homogeneous and mixed. Some things can only be said in front of one's professional peers, and some dilemmas must be explored together by the range of all professionals in the unit. These systems should lead to the capacity for a free and regular therapeutic conversation to exist between the staff.

Each neonatal unit has its own peculiar properties, so the form of communication between parent groups and staff will also vary. Nonetheless, consideration should be given to the judicious engagement of these parent groups. Families visiting for long hours over many weeks become an integral part of the ward community. Although often reluctant to talk to other parents, they usually strike up their own connections in the cafeteria or sitting room. Taking the opportunity for some structured, if low key, input from staff into the shared parent network can by very successful. Issues that are important to the parents can be shared in staff meeting, which can relieve staff of the onerous burden of supporting anxious mothers and fathers.

The nurse is in a seemingly impossible position: being on the one hand the primary carer – the substitute 'mother' and comforter — and on the other the person responsible for inflicting so many painful and distressing procedures upon the baby. Sharing this dilemma with colleagues and, when appropriate, parents can release the nurse to be even more emotionally available to the baby. There must always be ways of ensuring that staff do not lose sight of the importance of their own feelings about and interaction with the baby as the baby depends on these emotionally invested behaviours for their own development

The establishment of a small primary care team around each infant, especially those who are likely to be very sick or stay in hospital a long time, is also to be encouraged. As with the larger staff group, there will be within each team different perspectives of and identifications with the baby, the parents and again the nurses' own personal past. The teams should be open and flexible enough to allow for these differences as well as meeting the urgent technical care needs of the sick infant.

In this unique type of human setting is played out an extravagant ocean of human emotions – hope, despair, joy, hatred, confusion and love – in the midst of this being the families, staff and babies. The pressures on the nurses and doctors are profound, but the pleasure can be great when seeing a child graduate and later return to tell of their successes in life. Working in neonatal intensive care involves great strain and trauma for the staff, but human systems have evolved useful ways of containing such stress in order to survive for the sake of the infant.

References

Als H, Gilkerson L (1995) Developmentally supportive care in the neonatal intensive care unit. Zero to Three 15(6).

Bion WR (1961) Experiences in Groups. London: Tavistock Publications.

Bion WR (1962) Learning from Experience. London: Heinemann.

Bowlby J (1982) Attachment and Loss, Volume 1, 2nd edn (revised). London: Hogarth Press.

Bynghall J (1997) Towards a coherent story about illness and loss. In Papadopoulos RK, Bynghall J (Eds) Multiple Voices: Narrative in Systemic Family Psychotherapy. London: Duckworth.

Christie GL (1994) Some psychoanalytic aspects of humour. International Journal of Psychoanalysis 75: 479.

Gorski PA (1984) Experience following premature birth: stresses and opportunities for infants, parents and professionals. In Call JD, Galenson E, Tyson RL (Eds) Frontiers of Infant Psychiatry, Volume II. New York: Basic Books.

Menzies-Lyth I (1970) The Functioning of Social Systems as a Defence against Anxiety. London: Tavistock Institute.

Chapter 17
Social work in the neonatal intensive care environment

NORMA TRACEY, LISIANNE LA TOUCHE, LORRAINE ROSE,
BEULAH WARREN, HELEN HARDY, MEGAN GOSBEE,
DEIDRE CHIU, JILL DITTON, TERESE SHERIDAN,
LOUISE POLES, ANNE MAYO AND LYNNE TRIPET

> For this chapter, we invited some of the professionals who had written
> chapters for *Parents of Premature Infants* to join with social workers from
> the major Sydney hospitals' neonatal intensive care units (NICUs) for a day's
> audiotaped workshop. The workshop was entitled 'Care of Parents and
> Staff in NICU Wards'. This chapter is the edited transcription of that day.
> We have purposely left the format of the chapter in the group discussion
> mode, but individual speakers are not identified.

Two issues are discussed: how can we as social workers and therapists
help the parents of infants in NICU, with special reference to their
emotional care, and how does working in a NICU affect us as professionals?

Worker A: Mothers with a baby in neonatal intensive care are actually
suffering the loss of their baby in the sense of not being able to be close
and with them. My primary task is to help these mothers to be with their
babies, not just in a physical sense but emotionally. I do this by acting in a
non-judgemental, protective capacity while the mother is actually with the
baby in the unit.

Worker B: I wonder whether the mothers are not only mourning not
having this baby by their side, but also not having a healthy full-term baby?

Worker A: I'm sure they are, but I think the struggle for me as a professional is to help them to be able to find their own supports with my encouragement, rather than me becoming their support, which I can't do because of the limited time and the large number of mothers we have in the unit.

Worker C: I have had experiences of mourning an infant myself, and I used to struggle with the dichotomy between bringing my personal experiences to a therapeutic setting and being the objective neutral social worker. As I have gained more experience over the years, I feel a synchrony between allowing myself to be guided by my personal awareness and at the same time providing a safe therapeutic setting for the families I work with. I look to them to guide me in what they need from me and balance this with what I am able to give.

Worker D: The thing I find hardest is the incredible effect it has on me after I leave each interview. The mothers are so open and sensitive to what is going on at a very deep level, and so then am I. Other staff can close off, but as the professional who takes emotional care of them I cannot. I'm the one who straddles between the hospital and the presence of the real mother of the baby on the ward.

Private Worker: Because the mother is in an autistic-like, traumatised state, she's not in a position to mobilise her own resources. There is a place for the worker to mobilise the family. Is there a place for you, as facilitator, to do what she herself is unable to do at this time? What about Dad?

Worker D: Well, I try to see both the parents together. Sometimes I don't get a chance to, sometimes Dad's had to go back to work. The fathers often miss out on our services, and I think that is a real issue our unit hasn't yet addressed.

Worker E: Before I look for supports, I acknowledge what is going on for them. Many of our mothers on the ward feel disenfranchised; they can't break down on the ward. They think, 'I shouldn't be feeling this way; I should be a lot stronger, I should be coping!'. The biggest hurdle is letting them know it's OK to feel the way they do. My biggest problem is that there isn't enough space and time to do this work on the ward with them.

Worker A: We all have this problem. We all try to do what is called blanket cover. I become really overwhelmed at the level of illness of the babies who are there, but I still try to see all parents who come into the unit. We are not always successful in that, and it gives me the feeling of not keeping up, of not doing enough. In that initial interview, I assess, 'How much is this woman, this family, going to need us?', I see people just two or three times and that will be it. It's even more complicated for us because we have the NICU on level 3 and our special care nursery is on level 6. I feel as if I run up and down all day. This researcher had 18 one-hour interviews. We could never have that kind of time. Yet we feel as if the traumatised parents need every bit of it.

Worker F: One of the ways that we get around our lack of hours to cover parents adequately is to try to create a support group in the unit. The parents' group meets once a week, and I find that group works really well, in fact in some ways it's better than me just working with individuals. They hear other mothers saying, 'This is how I feel' or 'This is where I am and I've had these feelings'. And they say, 'Thank goodness she said that because I was feeling that!'.

Worker B: I find that the support they get from each other is more meaningful to them than that of their families because their families are often anxious too and therefore not able to support them or really understand what they're feeling and going through. For example, if the baby has a good day, the family might expect the mother to suddenly feel better, but the mother gets tossed up and down because the next day the baby might be worse again. I think the group is something for them in a ward that is not for them.

Worker G: One of the groups of parents that miss out in the high-tech nurseries are 30-weeks plus. These are seen by the medical staff with a cursory look, but the trauma for these parents is amazing. A ward parent group picks up and validates their feelings. The medical model is a problem-orientated approach, whereas we should assume that every parent on that ward is in a state of grieving. Often when they go home, they do all their crying, and it's because we haven't the resources really to deal with their issues while they are in hospital.

Worker C: Professional mothers also get left out, yet most mothers who come into a postnatal care unit are totally disorientated, irrespective of their professional background, and totally vulnerable. I think maybe I could be a coathanger for a little while, so that they could hang their coat (that is, their pain and grief) but then take it back, regardless of who they are and what their background is. Why do we equate being professional with being a good mother? Sometimes it makes it harder.

Worker D: Recently, two of the mothers had their babies moved without being told that the babies had been moved to another ward, and one mother used the entire interview to talk about her shock at walking in and not finding her baby on that ward. She thought the worst. They are so impotent it must be so painful.

Private Worker: How much power do you think you've got on a ward, in a sense of professional-centred power? For example, to be able to say to staff on the ward that no infant should be moved without some sort of notification to the mother.

Worker G: Well, it's even in the name, isn't it? You've got 'neonatal intensive care unit'. You need a name like 'mother and newborn unit' or 'family neonatal intensive care unit'.

Worker A: When the new hospital was being built, we as professionals researched what the parents wanted in the unit, and on the basis of that we asked for 30 beds for mothers. We said it could be the best in the world having 'living-in' facilities actually integrated into the unit (there are such models overseas). We designed a floor plan of this new unit too, with all the rooms off the neonatal unit, and the babies only had to be in the neonatal unit when they were desperately ill. At other times, they could be wheeled into the mother's room. Of course, it didn't happen. There are three rooms where parents can 'live in' adjacent to the unit. It's to do with a way of thinking – thinking about a mother, a family and a baby instead of just a baby.

Worker B: The singular complaint of every mother is to do with being unable to access her baby. Babies who are in level 3 are in a life-and-death struggle, and parents put their feelings very much on hold because they're concentrating on the day-to-day survival of their infant. When they get into the less intensive parts of the unit, particularly level 1, this is where the parents start to fall apart. They feel so frightened as they become more aware of what they have been through, about the prospect of being on their own and going out with the baby in their arms. Yet most of the nursing staff don't like working there because it means that they have to interact more with parents, and it lacks the high-tech status of working in level 3 nursery. It is level 1 that is most important!

Worker H: It's so hard having to take the baby home after the baby has been attached to monitors and respirators to make sure the baby's breathing. They go home without any of these supports. As well their anxiety is, 'Am I going to be able to be a mother to this baby after all that we've been through?' and also, 'Is my baby going to be all right? What am I going to do if my baby stops breathing? How will I know?'. I think they're really big concerns.

Worker F: There have been half a dozen professional people looking after this baby, and parents are told glibly, 'Now just take your baby home, it's all right!', and you know they are thinking, 'I can't do the work of half a dozen'. Even having the assurance of knowing it is normal to be scared and not be told, 'Look you shouldn't be anxious!' would help them. New mothers, especially the traumatised mothers of premature babies, *are* anxious.

Worker C: We have two rooms where parents can room-in for the last 24 hours before they take their baby home. That acknowledges their feeling of 'It's hard to go cold turkey straight out of an intensive care unit', but in our hospital there would be an absolute jam-packed routine of what they had to be taught, like bathing and sometimes quite difficult medical procedures that they were going to take responsibility for. Add to this trying to sleep in a room with the bleeps just outside the door and having your baby with you in this strange environment for the first time in its two or three months of life. Even if you took everything in, which you couldn't, you still don't even know your baby.

Worker A: Many mothers have a genuine fear, 'Have I actually bonded enough with this baby to take it home?'. That issue comes up over and over and over with the women I see. It is not just emotional barriers but distinct physical barriers that women in our hospital face. The postnatal ward is three floors down, and they have to very carefully waddle down, very sore, to see their baby. Then they have to go through glass barriers to even touch their baby. All these bonding and attachment fears are really present for them, and they need to be addressed before a mother can take her baby home.

Worker D: It is the lack of privacy in the NICU that parents find hardest – this makes the ward so intimidating to them. I think if they could get used to their baby in a graded way – short outings within the hospital then out of the hospital, then overnight, then follow-up visits from hospital staff when the baby is at home with them – this would create a not so harsh transition.

Worker H: Even for the staff being in the NICU is a very insular experience. The nursing staff have their own particular different type of nursing;

the ward has its own culture, quite different from that of other wards. As a social worker, you come in almost like an outsider because the whole concentration is on the baby's condition. Any of our ideas that are brought in intrude on that. Also, funding for anything we ask for puts us in competition with funding for medical staff needs, and it always comes down to funding. We can do a needs assessment, we can provide all the evidence of how a home-based follow-up service would be good and how much that would cost, and we always get the same answer, 'There's no money for it!'. Each of those babies is, in a medical sense, spending a small fortune, so why would you only concentrate on the physical health and not emotional health of the mother and father and baby? Sometimes you feel as if you're like the baby, helpless and trapped in a culture. In a way it's like a mother might feel, helpless and trapped too.

Worker A: It's like you feel that whatever you say is falling on deaf ears. You feel that you're failing by not being able to give each family the help that you know they need. You feel like you're lost yourself, you don't have any control. You don't feel you've got a sense that you know where it's going for a particular mother or baby – even where they will physically be – today on that ward, tomorrow moved out; or today well, tomorrow going backwards again or worse; or today here, tomorrow going home; nothing is predictable. If I feel lost in it, what can it be doing to a mother who doesn't even belong in the system? Sometimes I wonder how much frustration I as a professional can take.

Worker B: The nursing staff burn out very frequently and get the same feelings that we have described here too. I'm wondering how many of the feelings that the mothers have are being transmitted to the ward, and the other way around as well?

Worker C: I've wondered about how much the parents pick up on staff's hostility, antipathy, ambivalence and comments about the way these parents are looking after their baby. Attitudes to how the parents want to manage their baby are always overridden by the staff's desires. When the staff are positive with some parents, it works very well and the parents cope well with the experience of the hospital, but there are times when the staff can be quite destructive and distressing. At times, the parents experience being judged in their behaviour towards their own baby, as if what they are doing isn't right and they are not all right as parents. This concerns me a lot. I have recently been involved with a family where that message was very, very strong, where I actually became quite distressed and took it home at night with me.

Worker H: I dreamt on Sunday night about this family I had been working with and I thought, 'Oh my God! I can't keep on like this!'. The next day, I took myself down to my own office, and I closed the door. I had to recreate a sense of peace within myself because I could feel I was getting more and more distressed about this particular situation, to the point at which I think I was going to become inefficient and counterproductive.

Worker B: I think it impacts on us as professionally trained workers because we are the ones on the ward who have to leave ourselves open and vulnerable to their feelings. That is our job. Some other staff may be able to protect themselves by cutting off. That is a luxury we cannot afford.

Worker A: I think you absorb the parents' sense of powerlessness and lack of control. A couple of weeks ago, we had a huge crisis in our unit, and I spent the week calming parents down and debriefing the staff. The following week I was a mess, so I had to walk out of the unit and back to my office, and get space for myself. It is as if there is no space to think.

Private Worker: It seems to me as if the ward acts out the trauma and the autism of the parents, and loses any space to think about what is going on for the parents, for the baby and for themselves in this situation. It starts to operate as if it is in its own little world, like the baby stuck in an incubator. The ward and the staff do not even feel linked to the rest of the hospital.

Worker A: It's like I live in two worlds. The ward is one world and my life's another world. And that must be what it is like for the mothers. They say, 'I don't even know what am I allowed to do in this world or even if I'm allowed to be in it. Like, how many times am I supposed or allowed to visit a day?'. It's even harder when they are actually going home and the baby is staying, and they return to be with their baby. Simple things like, 'Where is the toilet?' or 'Is there a coffee shop nearby?'. Normally, you don't even think of those things. But now I make myself remember every time. First time I see a parent, I tell them there's a parents' lounge which has a TV, where a toilet and the nearest coffee shop are, and I tell them that what my role is because they don't have any idea.

Worker B: We are all feeling powerless, and the mothers are feeling powerless; it makes us ask, 'So who's got the power on the ward?'. People think that the doctors have, but the doctors haven't got it. Is the power the power over life and death? If that is so, it doesn't seem to belong to anyone – the parents haven't got it, the staff haven't got it, no-one has it. And that's the terrible, painful understatement that runs through the whole ward, so it is not only the mother who is in an unknowing and uncertain and unsafe state, but also the whole staff.

Worker D: The staff push their lack of power and control on to the mother. They even tell her when and how she can touch her own baby. It's an incredible hurdle for these women to overcome to bond with their babies. It reinforces that feeling, I've done something to make this baby this way, otherwise why do I need such controlling?'. They often bring this up in the groups, and all the mothers sigh with relief to hear that the other mothers feel the same. There is a feeling of guilt and blame and failure in all these women.

Worker C: The same goes for the staff too! It is very frustrating for us and very frustrating for the mothers. It's worse when they go home without any support – that is the worst of all. Then they have a lot of time to think and not many supports.

Worker D: I guess one of the ways in which we as social workers get round this in our unit is that we now run what we call a Possums' Playgroup, so we invite parents to come back, after the baby's gone home, for a morning each week for seven weeks. They get to meet up with parents they've made friends with in the unit, and they get to come back to the hospital in a position of power. They trot their babies up to the unit and they say, 'Look how well my baby's doing now. I've taken my baby home and he's growing, and I've done it'.

Worker B: I am involved in follow up, and that's often an opportunity for parents to take the babies back to the ward, and most of them do. They're usually very warmly received. A lot of parents come back for other appointments with their babies and often bring their babies along to see me. It's informal, it's not planned. I don't say, 'You must come and see me *x* number of times', but I say to them, 'If you do come back to the hospital again, do come and see me; I'd love to see the baby'. Many people do for years! This indicates that the hospital has some meaning for them always.

Worker K: I think we expect parents to know more than they do. One couple were told after a few days that they could take their baby out of the humidicrib. Of course, the very first time they took the baby out and they were holding the baby, they did it wrong – the temperature dropped, and the nurse came running because the baby was blue. They were so ashamed, and I just cringed for them. It was so painful for the parents. 'We didn't know you had to keep him wrapped up; nobody said be very careful that you don't do this or that', the mother said. I think that just giving information is important because you can hang on to information, it's your security. This nebulous 'You can take the baby out whenever you like' just floats around and of course leads to panic when things don't go the way they're intended to.

Worker B: Sometimes there's miscommunication. If parents say they're coming in for a feed, they need to be there well before the feed. So they come in with this anticipation of being able to do baby's eyes and wipe the mouth and do those lovely and tender things, only to find that it's already been done because they should have been there 20 minutes earlier. The feed is at 11 but you need to be here at 10.30, but no-one told you.

Worker D: Every mother and father needs a nurturing orientation; not only are they distraught, distressed, fragile, vulnerable and all these awful things, but they also want to have a little bit of control because this is their baby. It's about a process of engaging with the mother emotionally and being able to use that engagement to give information. There are missed connections all through the ward – it's as if the missed connection between the mother and baby to do with when to be born is being endlessly repeated. Staff do it all the time – we don't consciously think that this is the first time this mother has got to do something, because we are doing it day after day.

Worker C: That's why I see my role as personalising it for the mother in an environment that can't personalise easily because it is all so medical. One of the staff said to me that they almost need to depersonalise their work to be able to do the work every day. I think that if the medical staff did personalise every mother, they would burn out so quickly and no work would get done.

Worker E: It is easy on a busy ward to lose sight of the parent as the primary care-giver. Recently, we have been talking about case conferencing, particularly with long termers. In our unit, parents are always saying, 'If we had *one* nurse to relate to it would help so much'. So we set up a brainstorming session to discuss how we could do this. The nurses all voted for case conferencing and to assign a single nurse to a mother when the baby came in. When it came time to assign a nurse to a baby, and time to have case conferencing, the nursing staff were not freed up from nursing duties to come to them. In the end no-one wanted to take on that role of being the primary carer – 'I'm busy with what I'm doing; I don't want to take on this mother's feelings'. They said that they felt threatened because they wouldn't know what to say if any parents did get upset. They felt that they had power if they were doing medical stuff with the baby, but powerless when it came to dealing with emotions of parents, and their enthusiasm waned.

Worker D: I think empowering the parents is really about the nurses and doctors and social workers feeling empowered, so they're not dumping their garbage on the parent. So if you're going to start empowering parents, you've got to start by empowering staff.

Worker C: How can you feel empowered when there's no space for you to interview parents privately? The fact is that we have a little cupboard of a social work office, and we share it with the registrars and the computer. There isn't even a space made for you. If you feel so unsupported, how supportive are you of parents? Good question! Because you might be giving over vibes without even knowing it.

Worker A: There isn't the space for us to see the parents as we would like either. You're thinly spread when you've got so much going on. You go and see someone who's been referred, but you're so conscious of, 'Oh I hope I don't get into some really deep and meaningful interaction because I've only got half an hour and then I've got to be with someone else'. Sometimes you feel like you're just doing band-aid work. Many of these families need half a day with each of them. You just can't do it. It's like trying to be a loving mother with 15 kids. There's definitely a stage with stressed mothers where they sit like statues and don't seem to be able to get anything done, and you start thinking, 'Why has it taken me an hour and a half to get this woman to walk down one floor?', and you realise that you are seeing someone who is traumatised and simply can't get things together.

Worker C: On the NICU, I always feel that there is a pressure to be doing so much more because you are conscious of how great the mothers' needs are. You know you can't do it all. There are situations of real disturbance or anger and resentment, and there isn't good support, not at any level in one's own department and certainly not in the unit one works in. I feel great support from nursing staff at times, but we come from very different spaces around certain issues – mothers who become angry and suddenly upset all the staff – and you've got to become a kind of intermediary. There's a huge range of issues that you're constantly dealing with all day. The intermediary role of the social worker is huge.

The parents are captive in a dreadful way. They have to take care of the nurses or the nurses won't take care of their baby, they think. We had one family who lived far out in the country. Their baby was a 24-weeker and he had a very very severe bleed, and that family was angry, very angry about what had happened, and there was a lot of tension between the nursing staff and the family. The nursing staff thought the family were questioning them and judging how they were looking after the baby, and they began to find constant fault with the mother, claiming that there was something not right with her, that she was too possessive, and it went on and on and on. It affected the whole unit, and when the baby was transferred up to the special care nursery, it affected that whole unit too. This baby was going to have severe disabilities, and these parents were facing an enormous situation. They didn't need to be punished on top of that. There was a kind of scapegoating of the massive tension, which doesn't necessarily belong to that family but to the whole ward, and a situation like this brings it all on, triggers it, and then everybody gets caught in it.

I felt in this case that the parents were hard to work with – and with reason I think – and there was just no support for the staff in that situation. What is going on for the staff affects the parents, and it goes the other way – the trauma that's in the minds of the parents actually affects what's going on for the staff. Everyone ends up getting paranoid. No wonder they just cut off.

Worker D: One of our staff became one of the mothers on our ward. She said that she walked in there and just realised the impact of that ward from a parent's point of view, although she's been working there every day for a year. She thought she'd be totally cool about it all, but she just freaked out. Everything the staff said to her felt like meaningless patter and meant nothing. She said, 'This is the stuff I used to say to parents, but now I knew that it was empty reassurance and that I was absolutely terrified.'

The most relevant thing is that these women aren't allowed to go mad on the ward. When we created a space for them 'to be terrified, to feel their feelings', we actually, in many cases, made difficulties for the ward that they would rather not have had. When you're that busy, that frantic, that overworked, and you're trying to control your own emotions, there's not really room for a mother's disturbance, yet their disturbance in these circumstances is normal and definitely appropriate. These mothers know that the ward can't cope with it, because they're all so well behaved on the ward and they're so compliant.

Worker F: When these mothers who have been so compliant take their babies home – and most of these NICU babies are difficult babies – all their emotions come to the fore. They are already fragile, they may have spent 24 hours with this baby, and all they are left with is a sense of being incompetent because they couldn't carry this baby full term, then they couldn't look after the baby until the baby went home, and then they take the baby home and they can't cope again. It just reinforces their sense of incompetency. A mother said to me recently that the doctor had told her to take the baby home and treat him as normal – but that was not facing the fact that the baby wasn't a normal full-term birth and she wasn't a normal full-term delivery mother. It's like saying, 'Just forget it!'.

Worker B: It is the mother who needs to hold the baby in her mind so that she can be mindful of her baby and not mindless. It is the staff who hold the mother and the baby into life, and the worker on the ward who holds the parents in her mind. Who holds the worker so that the worker can hold the mother? Who holds the institution so that the institution remains able to hold the staff? The structure that acknowledges the mother/father/ infant, the family unit, is the structure that does that. The space for thinking and feeling and holding the family, all of which is lost in trauma, is then able to have some degree of restoration and resolution.

Chapter 18
'That big glass barrier': exploring the neonatal intensive care unit

SHEILA SIM

In this chapter, I explore the paradoxical and disturbing environment that the parents in our neonatal intensive care (NICU) group encountered. Jan, mother of Lucy, born at 28 weeks' gestation, vividly described 'that big glass barrier' that lay between herself and Lucy, not simply the walls of the humidicrib, but the multitude of barriers created by the environment itself. I will consider some of these barriers: the aftermath of the birth, the sense of unreality and the status of being a visitor to their own baby. I will explore the theoretical frameworks that I find most meaningful and helpful in my work as a social worker with these NICU families, and seek an understanding of what interventions make a difference to parents whose baby is born prematurely.

The world of NICU

Listening to the interview tapes, in silence and often early in the morning, I found myself recalling the dreams that I had during my early years in that environment:

> The newborn follow-up clinic team – paediatricians, occupational therapist and myself – sit around a table, discussing a baby girl who is now severely handicapped. Tears are streaming down our cheeks in sorrow at her life.
>
> A baby, very sick and premature, is lying in a cot. I bash at him with a wooden hammer to break his neck. This seemingly violent action is to help and heal the baby. There's a loving intent ... .
>
> A baby with dark hair and huge eyes, suddenly sits up in his bassinet and says 'Let me die!'.

These dreams evoke a vivid, intense and paradoxical world: cruel death in the name of healing, babies who sit up and pronounce and weeping paediatricians. The world of NICU had a profound and often disturbing impact on me, the worker. My dreams were a reflection of the struggles I was having to make sense of this world: a world where the words 'newborn baby' and 'death' seemed to walk hand-in-hand; where women in fluffy pink dressing gowns were wheeled in from neighbouring hospitals to sit by their baby's humidicrib, leaking breast milk, tentatively sticking a hand in through the porthole; a noisy, hot, bustling and highly technological environment where monitors, intravenous lines and pagers shrieked all day long.

Now if I, the worker – at that stage a social worker of some experience – had such difficulty in making sense of the paradoxical world I found myself working in, I could not help reflecting how much more difficult it must be for the women who were the mothers of these sick and premature newborns.

In the early interviews recorded in this study, the women were mostly still in hospital; lunch arrived or 'Sister' came in with medication in a paper cup. The control group mothers' tapes were punctuated by that suctioning sound of a baby at the breast. The NICU mothers heard the clank of hospital trolleys; then all too soon they were at home, and the 'noises off' were the chiming of Rosie's cuckoo clock and the subdued chatter of Sara's family in the next room.

Birthing

Their presence at home, with none of the gurgles or cries of a baby, made it easy to disregard one critical fact: that these six women had just given birth. A premature birth is still a birth experience, compounded by all the shock and anxiety of an unexpected delivery. The NICU mothers were already hospital patients when their babies were born. Admitted because of high blood pressure, some, like Liz or Rosie, had spent weeks nurturing their pregnancies, hoping to last just one more week, and then another, so that their baby could be born as close to full term as possible.

'I got so bored I was nearly tearing my hair out' (Rosie, Interview 1). Jan was booked in for a week of 'just doing nothing' in hospital at 26 weeks. 'They took a urine sample and yes! protein city, really high.' She was rushed to the teaching hospital:

> off I went, an ambulance roaring down the street ... and they said 'very short and fast, caesarean, quick quick' ... so they had to work pretty quickly and then she was BORN.
>   The first sight of their baby is fragmented - 'all I really saw of him was a hand' (Rosie, Interview 1) – and fraught with terror. 'You had the baby and then he's gone! They hold him for a few seconds and then they took him away' (Sara, Interview 1).

Five of the six NICU mothers had already been transferred from the smaller local hospital where they had originally booked in to give birth. All six had an emergency caesarean section. They were themselves intensive care patients in their own right:

> Every time I breathed they ran in. (Jan, Interview 1)
> the first day I couldn't get out of bed. (Rosie, Interview 1)
> I didn't go the next day because I had all these tubes ... what d'you call it, the drip, I couldn't go and see him. (Sara, Interview 1)

The mothers themselves were struggling with the impact of continuing high blood pressure, analgesia, urinary catheters and the after-effects of an epidural anaesthetic. It was difficult to mobilise, and they had to make a connection with their baby the best way that they could, with photographs:

> they took two photos [of] the baby – you know, instant photos and I saw him ... with all his tubes ... this cute baby with all these tubes (Sara, Interview 1)

or with telephone calls:

> I rang up two or three times a day to see how he was. (Rosie, Interview 1)

Actually going to see their baby, even going from one floor of the hospital to another, seemed a journey of epic proportions: 'I went up to see her that night, in a wheelchair ... the little handbag of urine that you've got to take up with you, drips hanging out of everything' (Jan, Interview 1).

Unreality

Entering NICU is like entering another world: 'An almost unbearable level of diverse sensory stimuli bombard staff and patients' (Marshall and Kasman 1980). There are rituals to mark the crossing of the threshold into this highly technological environment: 'that was really interesting ... all the medical procedures and the hand-washing and the little gown' (Jan, Interview 1).

The very sight of their baby, isolated and separate in a humidicrib, reinforced the surreal qualities of that first encounter:

> ... and there she was, this little tiny lobster-red being ... does she look like a little baby monkey or a little frog with no bum? oh dear. (Jan, Interview 1)
> He's so skinny, he's got no fat on him; he just looks like a miniature human, he doesn't look like a baby. (Rosie, Interview 1)

The sight of this tiny, fragile baby, the mother's physical exhaustion and anxiety surrounding the birth, and very real fact of separation from their baby all compounded the mothers' sense of unreality:

> everyone asks us me, how does it feel? ... I say I don't know ... like I am a mother but I don't feel it at the moment. (Sara, Interview 1)
> I didn't even feel as if I'd had a baby ... like it was another miscarriage. (Rosie, Interview 1)

The numbness and detachment expressed by all the NICU mothers – their flat voice tone, jokey asides and blank silences – confirmed for me the paralysing effects of shock. The crisis of prematurity, like every other life crisis, results in disequilibrium and an insidious sense of disbelief (see, for example, Caplan 1960). This feeling of unreality surrounding their baby's birth created a barrier between the NICU mothers and their baby.

What made a difference in dispelling that sense of unreality? The mothers appreciated any tangible proof that their baby really had arrived: the Polaroid photographs, ('I use that to look at when I'm expressing', said Rosie in Interview 1) and videos shot by their proud husbands ('when I saw him breathing it was good, it was a relief', said Sara in her first interview after watching the video made by her husband Sam).

We know from the literature on other forms of pregnancy loss – stillbirth and miscarriage – that the creation of tangible mementoes and a store of memories serves an important purpose – to acknowledge the parents as mother and father of that baby – and facilitates the dissipation of the 'unreality' (see, for example, Lewis 1976). Information about the baby's condition, or about prematurity itself, also helped to ground the parents in reality: 'We're both the type of people that have to have ... the facts given to us. We wanted to know the best and the worst' (Liz, Interview 1).

The women soon realised that not all the personnel in the hospital system appreciated their need for honest fact-sharing:

> He said, 'Oh you don't have to worry, you pay us to do the worrying!'. Which made me immediately think, I don't like that, I want to know. (Liz, Interview 1)

Each nurse and doctor had an individual style of information-giving: 'Depending on who you spoke to – some would tell you, "He's fine", and they wouldn't elaborate on anything else' (Rosie, crying softly, Interview 1). The women spoke warmly of the staff who had been clear and straightforward, even when they had spelt out the risks of pre-eclampsia and prematurity for mother and baby:

> The Sister that actually met us was probably the best thing that happened to me ... I would have been lucky to know where I was by this time, I was in a world of

my own. She was so down-to-earth, so direct, so wonderful with her information ... they gave me stuff out of their library to read, and came and told me things whenever there was anything; answered our questions.(Liz, Interview 1). The more knowledge that we have, the easier the process becomes. (Jan, Interview 1)

Somebody else's baby

Even as the NICU mothers were struggling to acknowledge the reality of their baby's birth, they were simultaneously feeling their way as mother of that baby. 'Well, it still doesn't feel like my baby, it feels like I'm visiting somebody else's baby' (Rosie, Interview 1). Their abiding sense of being a visitor to their own baby, a parent by false pretences, had several contributing causes.

Needless to say, they were neither physiologically nor psychologically ready to become their baby's mother quite so soon. Liz experienced only six weeks of conscious pregnancy after her surprise diagnosis at 26 weeks: 'I had such a short pregnancy' (Interview 1). Jan wondered, 'Where's all the nice little pleasant period?' for enjoying being pregnant (Interview 1) and even after ten weeks of Lucy's stay in NICU found herself hoping for a delayed discharge (Interview 7). The abrupt curtailment of their preparation for their baby's arrival compounded the normal intrapsychic struggles of the postnatal period.

Did the dynamic of the NICU environment also impede their becoming mothers and contribute to their sense of being visitors? The very fact that their baby was being cared for by other people, neonatal nurses, acted as a barrier in itself for some women:

> I'm not seeing him in front of me all the time ... I don't know when he cries, when there's something wrong with him. (Sara, Interview 1)
> They had this pink t-shirt on him. They made him a girl! (Sara, Interview 1)
> I watched the nurses – I watch everything like a hawk! – you know, they just interact differently. (Jan, Interview 1)

Jan hovered near her baby, determinedly being wheeled down to NICU only a few hours after the birth, and jokily describing her baby's appearance as a 'little frog with no bum'. She was doing her best to enter her role as Lucy's mother. 'You get the opportunity to go down there and spend as much time as you like. I've nursed her, and changed her nappy twice, that's really nice.' Rosie, however, marooned in her district hospital for four days after Kyle's birth, already seemed alienated by her contact with Kyle's nurses:

> a lot of the time all I got on the other end of the 'phone was, 'when are you coming to see your baby' [cries], and I couldn't do anything about it, they didn't understand. (Interview 1)

The relationship between nurse and mother, at its best a supportive partnership, was often characterised by a tussle over who this baby's mother really was:

> I find it quite hard when I see him because ... I know that I can do everything that the nurses are doing for him but I get the feeling that they don't like us ... doing much for the baby. (Rosie, Interview 1)

Becoming involved in her baby's care was something that Rosie, and the other women, both longed for and shied away from:

> Yesterday I had a good day, I didn't cry at all ... the nurse that was looking after him practically threw him at us and wanted us to do all the care for him, which I liked. (Interview 1)

'I know how to bath a baby!', she said fiercely in Interview 3. And yet I could hear the ambivalence in her voice as she said rather scornfully in Interview 4, 'I leave giving the vitamins and eye drops to them', a nursing duty that she, as Kyle's mother, disdained to carry out.

This painful struggle to clarify their role as a mother of their own baby was characterised by primitive defence mechanisms such as splitting and displacement, a process expanded on in other chapters. The mothers' comments about their treatment by hospital staff, in relation to being a NICU parent, swung from genuine pleasure ('I don't have words enough for them, they are so supportive'; Liz, Interview 1) to Deedie's angry opinion of the doctors: 'a big bunch of bloody hypocritical b...s' (Interview 8). Rage and pleasure characterised the NICU mothers' affect as they spoke about their experience in NICU. The mothers of full-term babies experienced the same feelings but to a much smaller degree; a passing feeling that 'they make you feel inadequate' (G, Interview 2) was negligible in their scheme of things as, after all, they had their babies beside them. The NICU mothers had to work hard at their relationship with their baby's nurse. Jan worried: 'I feel I put my foot in it' with the NICU staff (Interview 6).

The NICU mothers were also powerless to protect their baby from uncomfortable experiences. They had been unable to prevent their baby's untimely birth; when a nurse remarked to Rosie, 'you've got him early', Rosie's voice is a study in suppressed anger and disappointment that she had failed to reach full term (Interview 3). They then had to endure seeing their baby in discomfort: 'The nurses let him cry', said Sara dully (Interview 2).

> No ... it upsets me more when I do see him ... to me he looked like he was having a lot of trouble breathing, it looked very laboured, and when I said something all I got was, Oh, he's all right. (Rosie, Interview 1)

Jan described being present while Lucy was having blood taken by a heel-prick:

> I think her little foot's about a postage-stamp in diameter ... sure enough I was
> finding it a little bit hard ... I didn't cry but still it was ... a challenge.

Her detached affect in recounting this story as a sort of joke against herself masked the despair that the NICU mothers felt as their babies endured the interventions of intensive care: those life-giving interventions that were simultaneously so invasive and destructive (as in my dreams) that no mother would undertake them. 'She said, "I wouldn't be doing this to my child if I were the mother", and I thought, "Wow"'. (Jan, Interview 1).

In tentative and halting words, the women indicated that they wanted to be involved in their baby's care: Jan stuck it out beside Lucy right through that blood test. 'Every day I used to go there ... I used to hear him cry and I used to cry with him', said Sara (Interview 1). When Rita took Harry to a children's unit to have a sleep study, she felt angry that they forgot to wake her up during the night (Interview 7). Deedie could scarcely believe that the NICU staff had given Katherine a blood transfusion without consulting her: 'Oh hallo, they're just going to brush me off' (Interview 6).

I was reminded of Ernest Freud's vivid description of a young Mexican mother in NICU who had just begun 'gingerly to touch the baby's extremities'. Her tentative contact with her baby was interrupted by the technician wheeling in 'a giant X-ray machine'. This machine had priority – in the minds of both the mother and the staff; 'how easily established medical procedures can take unquestioned precedence over psychological considerations' (Freud 1981).

The policy for visitors to NICU also took precedence over the mothers' own wishes for their baby. Jan's friends had visited Lucy (which she appreciated), but she had to have a rather solemn interview with the NICU Director because they had 'been naughty' and touched her (Interview 1). Rosie spoke bitterly about her friends not being able to see her baby: 'that really hurts'. Only her parents could visit, and 'they can see it for a short time and only one at a time'. She contrasted this reality with her picture of a birth 'on time', when she herself and her visitors could hand the baby around, admire him and spend as much time as they wanted. Instead, 'I supposedly have this baby and no-one can see it' (Interview 1). As Deedie put it, 'Does "neonatal" mean they have all rights over our baby?' (Interview 6) ... 'they don't bloody own her!' (Interview 8).

The NICU mothers' uncertain status in the hospital was emphasised by other, perhaps more subtle, messages. As patients in intensive care, they were to some extent protected, but all too soon they were transferred to the busy postnatal wards, where the crying of other women's babies emphasised their own deprived and displaced status.

Sara shared a room with two other women whose babies were in NICU. Next door, there were women with babies: 'I'd say my blood pressure was up just because of those babies; they used to cry all the night and all day' (Interview 1). The women had often not been orientated to even the most basic facilities: '[Finding] that 'phone was a big milestone, before that I was struggling up and down with my little thirty centses, in this wind tunnel next to the lifts, and [laughs] I thought there must be something better than this, I mean where am I?' (Jan, Interview 1). 'Where am I', indeed – perched on a postnatal ward but without their baby; present in NICU but with limited contact with their baby and often no control over the minutiae of their baby's treatment. It was hardly surprising that Deedie described herself as 'like a shag on a rock', a colloquialism for being isolated (Interview 1).

Even within the confines of the NICU environment, there were undoubtedly experiences that mitigated the anguish of separation from both the baby and the role of motherhood. The NICU mothers often sounded flat and detached on tape, but there was a definite softness that crept into their voices as they described being able to hold their baby. As Sara said wistfully:

> When we take him out for a cuddle I just want to sit there with him, just holding him, not putting him back … . (Interview 1)
> I touched her little hand and her little foot, very tentatively of course … Oh, it was great being able to hold her and they wrapped her up and she's so little. (Jan, Interview 1)
> The crook of me arm got sore from holding her. (Deedie, Interview 5)

Cuddling, holding and doing even little things for their baby were truly therapeutic.

The single most tangible means of demonstrating their status as their baby's mother and more than a passing visitor was, of course, their supply of breast milk. All six women expressed milk almost as a matter of course. None of them voiced any hesitation about undertaking this demanding task, which had to be carried out every four hours with an electric breast pump in between visits to the baby and their own medical care. Their labour might result in only a few millilitres of milk, but they persevered. Rosie used her first photo of Kyle 'to look at when I'm expressing, with the machine on … they say it helps bring in the milk a bit better' (Interview 1). Rita was full of praise for the lactation consultant: 'She was fabulous' (Interview 3). They all expressed anxiety that their milk supply was too low:

> I was only a dessert spoonful of milk ahead of her and anxiety city! (Jan, Interview 1)
> Yesterday and the day before I was as dry as the Sahara Desert. (Deedie, Interview 3)

In fact, all the women except Deedie, whose baby had the longest stay in NICU, persevered with expressing their milk, a measure of the NICU mothers' determination to provide at least this for their baby even if other aspects of mothering were denied them. Sara summed it up in her simple language: 'We tried him on the breast, but he didn't suck, he licked the milk ... a nice feeling, actually, when you put your baby to the breast'.

The harshness of the NICU environment was also mitigated by a simple human touch, even in the midst of the machinery:

> All this ... totally medical environment, machines, lots of graphs, but there's a touch of humanity down there with little balloons and the little pictures of houses. (Jan, Interview 1)

Liz spoke at length of Julie, the Sister who was 'the best thing that happened to me', who explained why Liz had to be admitted to hospital in easy language, 'put me a little bit at ease'. Julie, herself pregnant and at almost the same gestation as Liz, knew instinctively what to say to this stunned first-time mother. Rita appreciated the visits from the follow-up nurses after Harry was home, especially as he was an unsettled baby who gulped and choked as he fed: 'the advice from those nurses is better than books!' (Interview 5).

Many of the women expressed a sense of being held and cherished by human contact:

> really good to be surrounded by people who really care. (Jan, about her friends who have been to see Lucy, Interview 1)
> The doctors were worried about me ... they were really, really, really good. (Sara, Interview 1)

Liz considered that she reached 32 weeks' gestation '*only* because of the people here ... they were absolutely wonderful ... they'd just pop in as they were going past'. Even the cleaner greeted her on her return to her local hospital: 'You're back! What did you have?' (Interview 1).

Encountering NICU

The experience of listening to the tapes of the mothers' interviews led me, as a NICU social worker, to reflect on my own first encounters with mothers and fathers. This second part of the chapter is an exploration of the inner processes and philosophical framework that sustain me as a worker in that unique setting.

On my first morning at work, I joined the ward round. Neonatologists, registrars and nursing staff stood round each crib and reported on the baby's progress since the previous day. I did not understand a word. When they said, 'His blood gases were ...', I did not know whether that was good or bad. When they said, 'She's got haemolytic strep.', was that serious?, fatal? Later, I learnt to recognise the mix of art and science that went into the medical care of those babies. On that first day, all I could hear was a stilted technical language, crammed with acronyms and short-hand ('NETS', 'EBM' ...). I had not yet met any of the babies' parents so I would not have known what to say about them even if there had been any space for me to speak during that highly medical hand-over. As I gathered the confidence to add my input to ward rounds, or responded to a direct question, I wondered about the level at which I spoke: 'Dad's coming down from Orange' or 'Mum's living in at the parent's hostel'.

During those first days, I was not sure what to say to the babies' parents either. Since (unlike the hospital in our study) this was not a maternity hospital, the mothers had to be brought in to see their baby, often by ambulance or being driven by a nurse and wheeled up to NICU in the lift. 'I didn't see him till he was four days old' (Rosie, Interview 1). They often looked frightened and overwhelmed. I was hesitant about approaching them and interrupting this incredibly precious time with their baby. They had made a brave journey, still wincing from the pain of their caesarean section. Their escort, who had to get them back to Bankstown or Campbelltown ward before the end of this shift, would be hovering at the door and wondering aloud about the traffic. Meanwhile, the baby was asleep and the mother would be willing the baby to wake up and acknowledge her presence even with only one eye. How could I legitimately break into this tableau? How could I curtail the already brief contact between this mother and her baby?

And what could I say? The women had already been surrounded by trite reassurances, exhortations to stay positive, well-meaning words that tried to jolly them along and served to diminish and devalue the ache that they felt. 'It's been a very hard ten days', said the interviewer to Rosie in Interview 1; 'Yep ...! I don't know what else to say'. I wasn't sure that I could find the words to express the anguish of separation and powerlessness. What could I offer? I knew how to book them in to the parent's hostel, and where they could catch a bus to the city, but what else did I have that I could offer as a buffer against this agony?

Dreadful moments

I began, tentatively (just like their uncertain reaching out through the porthole to touch their baby's hand), to introduce myself, to join them in watching their baby. I am sure that some of them wondered what I was doing there. I might cautiously bring into words some of the feelings that they might have when they saw their baby so surrounded by wires, 'all these things on him, all these tubes' (Sara, Interview 1). More often we would stand by the crib in a companionable and communicative silence. I would stay for a short time and then say, 'I don't want to interrupt your time with your baby, but I want you to know that I'm available'.

I feel that I was most helpful to those mothers when I began to discard my anxieties over what I could say or do to help. Each baby's parents were thrown into a state of disequilibrium, a physical and psychological landscape so far from the 'known' that their usual coping mechanisms and resources were totally inadequate. The untimely birth of their baby made a mockery of all their careful plans, 'all these structured logical things' (Jan, Interview 1), such as planning the best month for the baby's conception. Their baby must have seemed terrifyingly fragile in the face of the unspeakable risks and possibilities that the baby faced before reaching full term:

> Everyone has them: those dreadful moments when, because something awful has happened ... we become aware of an appalling reality ... the world seems to fall away from us. (Picardie 1980)

I had no choice but to enter this 'thrown' state with these parents. They were in the midst of an existentialist crisis, a struggle with 'the ultimate concerns of human existence: death, isolation, freedom and meaninglessness' (Yalom 1985). This struggle they had previously discounted or ignored: Jan had carefully calculated the months so that her baby would be born at the 'right' time. Rosie 'wasn't meant to go through labour' – but she started contracting despite all these plans. In the face of such a paradoxical and meaningless event as this premature birth, and confronted by the utter loneliness of mother and baby, I could at first offer only to stand beside these parents at their baby's crib, to accompany them through their experience of NICU.

I could not hide safely behind my role as 'unit social worker' or categorise parents according to the severity of the crisis and the success of their coping mechanisms. It was my whole presence that I was offering in my work in NICU: the sum of my own life's experiences and obstetric history as much as my clinical skills and understanding, my capacity to bear with my clients. I was sustained not only by my professional knowledge, but also just as strongly by a personal philosophy that stemmed from reading the works of existentialist thinkers such as Heidegger, who, after all, had said 'the dreadful has already happened'.

The literature on existentialist psychotherapy offers much illumination for work with parents at a time of such acute uncertainty about the survival of their baby and their own eventual emergence as a family from this ordeal. One concept of particular relevance is the attitude described by existentialist philosophers such as Heidegger as *Gelassenheit* or 'letting-be-ness', an attitude of surrender to experiences that are threatening and unfamiliar. By allowing myself to feel overwhelmed and uncomfortable when I walked in through those plastic swing doors, I believe that I helped to evoke that same attitude of openness in the baby's parents (see Casement 1985). By resolutely not glossing over their (and my) feelings of terror and anxiety, by not dismissing them, by not providing false reassurances (that their baby would not die, that they would all emerge from this ordeal intact), I hope that both the parents and I had the courage to let ourselves 'be' in the midst of such strange experiences and surroundings. Those are:

> the moments when something new has entered into us, something unknown; our feelings grow mute in shy perplexity, everything in us withdraws, a stillness comes, and the new, which no-one knows, stands in the midst of it and is silent. (Rilke 1962)

I also wanted to bring to my first meeting with parents the lovely qualities of encounter, 'an authentic meeting between two human beings' (Laing 1967). This first encounter would have, I hoped, all the elements of any other first encounter between strangers, a sense of kindness, courtesy and welcome: introducing myself by name, finding a chair for the mother to sit on, alleviating her sense of confusion by introducing her to her new environment. My actions and presence would aim to convey an attitude of openness and respect for parents as equal and active participants in our meeting:

> The encounter is characterised by love, the active caring and concern of one person for the other. (Sinsheimer 1969)

By first acknowledging the similarities between us – being women, strangers and visitors in a medical environment – rather than the differences – my being a professional, hospital employee and 'expert' – I was seeking to convey that I would stand beside them and stay with them and their individual experience. I would not say, 'He'll be all right' as the mother stood by her baby's humidicrib. After all, we did not know that. I would not say, 'She's not coping' or 'Do those parents realise how serious this is?' or any of the other unconsciously dismissive remarks that staff can be heard to make. Instead, I would try to join with them in entering into this new and terrifying experience and to imagine the real (Buber 1951), to transcend the safety of my set role and to experience as directly as possible the mother's own felt reality, imagining and understanding it through my own experience of being in the world. 'At such a moment something can come into being which cannot be built up in any other way' (Buber 1951).

Holding

Existentialist philosophy offered an enriching perspective for me as the NICU social worker. Other, more psychodynamic constructs, in particular the concept of the holding environment, also informed my work. When the mothers who were visiting their babies became visibly distressed, the people around them – nurses, partners, family – would often put an arm round them or pat them on the shoulder. Sometimes this *was* 'an authentic meeting between two human beings', a true connection between husband and wife, or nurse and mother. More often it arose out of embarrassment and discomfort, an attempt to dampen down the terror that spilled out through the woman's tears. 'Don't cry, he'll be all right', echoed Rosie's 'All I got was, "Oh he's all right"'(Interview 1).

The mothers' tears, silences and all-pervasive anxiety were a sign that they were struggling to deal with an almost unmanageable trauma. They often met with a response that implied that their feelings were abnormal or extreme, and that they should suppress them, as seen, for example, by the comment 'You don't have to worry, you pay us to do the worrying' (Liz, Interview 1). The mothers would thus be forced to conclude that no-one could manage and survive such strength of feeling. However, 'the help being searched for is always for a *person* to be available to help with these difficult feelings' (Casement 1985), to provide the 'holding' that a mother provides for her infant. The holding environment refers to the total emotional and physical environment that the mother creates, to her capacity to hold the infant in her mind and attend intuitively to the infant's needs.

Bearing in mind

By employing a social worker, the NICU did to some extent acknowledge the enormity of the feelings that giving birth to a premature baby would elicit. The need for a holding environment, 'a person to be available', was recognised. Such holding could be (and certainly was) done by anyone;

however, it was my job to be aware of that aspect of life in the unit. This sometimes translated into creating a more facilitating physical environment: walking with a mother round to the parents' room with its comfy sofa and privacy; bringing a bunch of flowers or a home-made cake to the parents' group; providing booklets, resources, information on where to buy jumpsuits in 0000 size or help in tracking down a lost birth registration form. It meant always bearing the parents in mind, actively remembering and thinking about them, even those parents who rarely visited, rang up infrequently, were withdrawn or awkward to work with – especially those parents in fact. So I would telephone the mother directly in her maternity hospital in far-flung Coonabarabran or Deniliquin, not primarily to give her news of her baby (since the nursing staff and her husband would do that) but to establish a connection with her, to ask 'How are *you*?' in the midst of all of this unexpected event, to convey to her that I was available to her. I was someone outside the area of medical and technical care, someone who could focus my mind on her and her partner. By my bearing them in mind, they were (I hope) enabled to bear their own baby in mind, as far as that was possible. 'If you can keep that in mind how they care for you, I'm sure it helps' (Liz, Interview 8).

Every NICU has to struggle with the effects of the dynamic tension between its two opposing tasks: to treat and care for the sick or premature infant, and to facilitate the baby's eventual move home to their parents' care. Both the staff of the unit and the parents have to take part in a paradigm shift as their baby grows and matures. They have to leave behind the terror, intensity and acuity of the baby's first days or weeks, and enter into a softer, more reflective and relaxed mode. We can assume that the baby accomplishes this, albeit not without trauma. The task is for parents and staff to make their moves in tune with the baby and to 'breathe out' as the baby does. The technological culture of the institution and the deadening effects of psychological trauma often result in parents and staff alike remaining frozen in a state of disintegration and disequilibrium.

The institutional structure of a hospital to some extent reflects the consequence of the outward projection of painful feelings: safety lies in hierarchy, routine, protocols and tasks. Is it possible for the staff of a NICU, a medical environment whose focus is intervention with critically ill infants, not to take refuge in primitive defence mechanisms?:

> The nursing service bears the full, immediate and concentrated impact of stresses arising from patient care. (Menzies-Lyth 1959)

Surrounded by the raw, inchoate feelings of the parents in NICU, it is hardly surprising that staff resort to such mechanisms as splitting ('Why didn't hospital *X* transfer this baby days ago?') or denial ('We don't have any barriers to parents visiting here') just as strongly as the parents in the interview tapes do.

The NICU does let parents in, to a degree unimaginable in earlier years when mothers were limited to a daily peek at their baby through glass walls. Now, parents new to the NICU are given unit information booklets, photographs and newsletters, and they receive a card from their baby on Mother's Day, Father's Day and other holidays. They can sit for hours with their baby in a kangaroo pouch, enjoy skin-to-skin contact, and room in before their discharge. There are parents' groups, lessons in massage and swaddling techniques, follow-up home visits and after-discharge playgroups for the growing infant. Jan remarked with pleasure on the 'little balloons and houses' that softened the medical environment for her.

Other chapters in this book explore more directly the experiences of NICU staff and the crucial issue of the baby as contested terrain between staff and parents: 'They don't bloody own her!'(Deedie, Interview 8). The words of the mothers in this research reflected their felt experience of the nursing and medical staff's interactions with them. They bear witness to how far we have still to go in our work of helping families to bear the experience of prematurity. As I followed the NICU mothers and their babies from tape 1 to tape 9, I was forced to acknowledge how hard it is to create a true encounter in the fullest sense of the word, and how often those mothers had to struggle to overcome the presence of 'that big glass barrier'.

I was also heartened by the fact that as they began to be able to look back and to a certain extent reflect on their traumatic experiences, their words echoed the power of a humanising approach: 'They have become family and they have definitely become friends ... this has been such a strong thing for us. So many people have actually cared about what happened and how it was happening' (Liz, Interview 8). I am led to one overwhelming conclusion: that it is the presence of a humanising influence, the honest words, actions and existence of human beings amidst the machinery, which the mothers recalled with gratitude and which facilitated in them the capacity to bear and bear with their experiences and their baby. 'They journey together, and the therapist bears with "all that comes to be in the encounter"'(Sinsheimer 1969). Or to quote the heartfelt words of Liz (Interview 1): 'You were a person the whole time ... I can't offer any higher praise that that!'.

References

Buber M (1951) Distance and relation. Hibbert Journal XLIV(2): 105–14.
Caplan G (1960) Patterns of parental response to the crisis of premature birth. Psychiatry 23: 365–74.

Casement P (1985) On Learning from the Patient. London: Routledge.

Freud E (1981) To be in touch. Journal of Child Psychotherapy 7: 7–9.

Heidegger M (1962) Being and Time. Oxford: Blackwell.

Laing RD (1967) The Politics of Experience. Harmondsworth: Penguin Books.

Lewis E (1976) Management of stillbirth: coping with an unreality. Lancet 18 September.

Marshall R, Kasman (1980) Burnout in the neonatal intensive care unit. Paediatrics 65: 1161–5.

Menzies-Lyth I (1959) The functioning of social systems as a defence against anxiety. In Menzies-Lyth I (1988) Containing Anxiety in Institutions. London: Free Association Books.

Picardie M (1980) Dreadful moments: existentialist thoughts on doing social work. British Journal of Social Work 10: 483–90.

Rilke RM (1962) Letters to a Young Poet. New York: Norton.

Sinsheimer R (1969) The existential casework relationship. Social Casework (Feb): 67–73.

Yalom I (1985) The Theory and Practice of Group Psychotherapy. New York: Basic Books.

PART 7
UNDERSTANDING THE NATURE
OF THIS TRAUMA –
THE END OF THE JOURNEY

Chapter 19
Listening to the space between life and death

PHILIP GARNER

> As part of the overall research study involving the mothers and fathers of neonatal intensive care and full-term babies, a pilot study was undertaken to try to measure quantitatively what the mothers were thinking and feeling. As one of two raters involved in that study, I worked for more than two years listening to 108 audiotapes, identifying and measuring the intensity of emotions experienced by those mothers when talking about themselves, their babies, their partners and the medical/health care workers with whom they had contact in the first four months of their babies' lives. However, while listening to and rating those mothers, a process was taking place inside me that was largely beyond my awareness and that surfaced while examining the data in preparation for a chapter presenting the results, the working through of which changed the whole direction of the chapter. The material that follows is presented to show the powerful and profound impact that the traumatised internal world of the mothers of neonatal intensive care babies has on those around them – and how an understanding of that impact's effects on myself has provided a deepened understanding of the emotional landscape in which these mothers find themselves following the premature birth of their babies.

When I first became involved with this pilot study, I had no conception of the depth of the journey I was about to undertake, knowing only that it included the mothers of premature babies. The pilot study involved rating audiotaped interviews with six mothers of normal full-term (FT) and six of ten-week premature, low birthweight babies (NIC) who were thought likely to survive through to the end of the study. All were interviewed on nine occasions, commencing shortly after their baby's birth and finishing approximately four months later. Two raters, Sheila Sim and myself, then rated the 108 tapes on the basis of how strongly the six emotions selected for exploration were expressed in each of eleven different areas or 'Assessment Items' (Table 1), with the added instruction that we were to rate expressed emotions and were not to infer or interpret what their emotions might be. The ratings took over two years to complete.

Table 1: Emotions and assessment items rated in the pilot study

Emotions	Assessment items
1 Flatness and detachment	1 Mothers' contact with infant
2 Excitement and pleasure	2 Mothers' lack of contact with infant
3 Depression	3 Infants' health and development
4 Anxiety and fear	4 Mothers' own health
5 Rage and anger	5 Mothers' capacity to mother
6 Sadness and grief	6 Mothers' experience of staff in hospital
	7 Mothers' experience of staff
	8 Partners' support for mother*
	9 Partners' lack of support for mother*
	10 Partners' involvement with infant*
	11 Partners' non-involvement with infant*

*Not explored statistically after the pilot study, as decided by Norma Tracey and her research assistant.

Once the ratings were complete, the scores for each emotion associated with each assessment item were plotted on separate three-dimensional bar graphs to look for similarities and differences between the two groups of mothers. Of interest was the fact that, in spite of there being only a low-to-moderate degree of interrater reliability between the raters in identifying and measuring many of the links between certain emotions and assessment items, the raters, nevertheless, often came up with findings demonstrating similar 'tendencies' or 'trends' in the data over the period of time the mothers were interviewed that differed between the two groups of mothers.

As a psychotherapist having had no direct or indirect experience with neonatal intensive care units (NICUs), it was a unique experience immersing myself in the lives of 12 mothers as a rater in the first 16 weeks of their babies' lives. In order to complete the ratings, I decided from the outset that I would not attend any meetings where there was any possibility of learning, either directly or indirectly, about the pilot study's purpose or anticipated findings in order to maintain the independence and integrity of the rating process. I continued with this for three years up to the time of writing this chapter. I also believed that it was important to try to avoid any preconceptions or use of theory that would interfere with remaining open and receptive to all that the mothers were actually saying and feeling. The rating process was significantly complicated by what I was picking up in what NIC mothers were saying throughout the more than two years of the study.

When I began rating the NIC mothers, I soon found myself constantly replaying the same sections of tape, trying to stay in touch with and pick up what they were saying, only to find either that I would lose interest and repeatedly drift off somewhere in my thoughts, or that my mind would have gone blank. This happened so frequently compared with FT mothers that I came to the realisation that their emotions and experiences were having a powerful, disruptive effect on my attention. At other times, I found the implications of many of their comments both powerful and deeply moving. Having to get through and rate so many tapes meant I could not afford to dwell on my own reactions or on those of the mothers. The tape kept going, and there were more comments and emotions to rate. As time went on, there were occasions when I did not want to rate any of the tapes at all because of the degree of mental and emotional effort required to attend fully to the material, the longest being a period of 6–8 weeks when I had to force myself to continue.

It was an enormous struggle trying to make sense of the data and of the graphs, some of which demonstrated significant and meaningful differences between the two groups of mothers, while others that had appeared highly meaningful were rendered meaningless because of contradictory data obtained from the other rater. Then, as the weeks passed and I began to make sense of some of the patterns and trends in the data, I decided that it would be helpful to listen again to the tapes of two mothers from each group in order to pay particular attention to the experiences that had led to changes being detected in the data. There was plenty of time – over a month (later extended to three months) before the chapter had to be in – and I could listen to one tape a day. However, no sooner had I started listening to the very first NIC tape than I realised that I would be unable to continue. What immediately descended on me was a heavy, thick, dark, oppressive, numbing sensation that I could not escape and that I would have to work through and understand. In time, I came to see this as involving a profound sense of 'dread' and 'despair' at the thought of having to 'go through it all again', something I had actually experienced while doing the ratings but which I had to push away at the time in order to complete the task. Although I knew that the interviews had been having an impact on me during the rating process, I was surprised by the intensity of my reaction after the event. As a result, I realised that I had been the recipient of intense, raw, unprocessed, primitive anxieties and emotions throughout the two or more years of the rating process.

What follows is the result of the process of identifying and working through the often intense emotions and reactions within me as I struggled to understand the results. The factor that eventually helped to provide a framework within which to understand my reactions was the underlying belief, stemming from my work in analytical psychotherapy, that many of the thoughts, emotions and experiences that I was having represented a coming together of thoughts and emotions that had their origin in the emotions and experiences of the NIC mothers but which, at the time, they and I could not process in a thinking way. In psychoanalytical theory, the unconscious process that results in taking inside and feeling or experiencing within oneself, as if they were entirely one's own, the disavowed thoughts and feelings of another is known by the term 'projective identification' (Klein 1946, 1955, Bion 1962, 1967). Understanding those reactions, thoughts and feelings within myself would therefore provide a guide to understanding what kind of thoughts and feelings these mothers were *unable* to process within themselves, feelings that were significantly dominating their internal world beneath their flatness and detachment (Joseph 1985). There were times when I had absolutely no idea why a particular line of thought would dominate my attention. It was only later that the points came together to make sense. My delay in using this way of conceptualising my reactions stemmed from my initial uncertainty about the extent to which the process of projective identification could take place in the complete absence of any direct contact with the source of the projections and could, instead, be transmitted exclusively via a medium such as audiotape.

While looking at and trying to make sense of the results, my mind was occupied with the issue of how thoughts, emotions and experiences are conveyed from one person to another without being put into words, particularly when I had been deprived of the added benefits that visual information would have given. At this stage, I also found my thoughts dominated by recollections of work with an 18-month-old infant in a preschool for abused and neglected children in whom the staff and I were not able to make any positive changes in her capacity to relate until we tuned in to what her emotional experiences were likely to have been during the first months of her life spent in a NICU.

I came to liken the experience of listening to NIC mothers to that of following someone blindly along a particular pathway only suddenly to find they were no longer where I expected them to be, having moved off somewhere else instead. Meanwhile, there is the sense that, without necessarily thinking the thoughts that go along with it, I had gone some way along the path that they had originally been pursuing. In most cases, it was not that I actually had those thoughts consciously, the process invariably having taken place beyond my awareness. Even on those occasions when I had a conscious sense of the line of thought that these mothers would momentarily pursue, I could not afford the time to follow along these avenues of thought with my own thinking because of the need to rate some other emotion that would be brought up a moment later.

Emotions and experiences were conveyed in many different ways: through the sound of their voices, their melody and rhythm, flatness, syntax and pauses, the emphasis placed on certain words and/or syllables, and the way in which they would breath, sigh, laugh or cry. A lot of what they said was often dominated by a flatness so intense that what would be conveyed along within it, like the negative of a photograph, was the emotion or thought that was being flattened. On other occasions, the level of relief that would suddenly and momentarily burst from them once some critical milestone was reached was so intense as to indicate the depth of distress, fear or, more particularly, terror with which they were struggling.

This is all well and good, but why, when I was actually trying to write a chapter on the results of a pilot study involving mothers, was I thinking so deeply about the vital and dramatic role played by attunement with abused and neglected infants. Did it have something to do with a need for attunement with the NIC mothers and/or was it in some way concerned with babies?

The issue continued to dominate my thinking until I saw a videotape of the physical examination of a premature baby in a neonatal intensive care ward. The tape showed a premature baby who became progressively more distressed as a result of the failure of the person doing the examination to either notice or respond to the initially subtle signs of distress that the baby was making and wait until it was ready to continue, to the point at which the baby's reactions showed the same level of withdrawal and 'glassed off' detachment that I had seen in the more disturbed of infants in the preschool. This contrasted with the tape of another physical examination where the person doing the examination watched the baby and responded to the subtle cues of distress, backing off until signs from the baby indicated that it was all right to continue.

It was at this point I realised that, concealed within the verbal and non-verbal communications, and beneath the flatness and detachment of the NIC mothers (as well as beneath my preoccupation with the infant at the preschool), was the fact that they were all too aware of the vulnerability and trauma that their babies were experiencing, although this awareness was at a feeling or right-brain level, could not to be thought about consciously and was something that they were completely powerless to change. There was nothing that they could do about what was happening to their babies.

The dread against which these mothers were struggling was far more profound than they could admit – either to themselves or to others – during their interviews, and more profound than could be consciously detected and rated. Sometimes the lack of care and sensitivity shown by neonatal intensive care or other medical staff towards the mothers and/or their babies had an immediate effect in that it clearly added to the distress and trauma that they were already struggling to cope with and that was easily detected via the audiotapes.

Deep, primitive persecutory anxieties flourish in an atmosphere of suffering and vulnerability where babies are felt to be traumatised by experiences while their mothers look on helplessly, a situation similar to the reactions of police, medical and other emergency workers to disasters involving babies and young children. Data from the pilot study had shown that the intensity of excitement, flatness and anger of NIC mothers was greater when speaking of their experiences with medical/health personnel towards themselves and their babies than it was for FT mothers. I believe that the contradictory emotions expressed by these mothers was, in this case, an indication of the struggle they were going through in relation to their babies' fate. Although grateful to the staff for looking after the lives of themselves and their babies, they were clearly distressed and anxious about the emotional harm being done to their babies and because of their not being able to provide the necessary care and nurturance themselves – which they had to 'turn a blind eye and a deaf ear' to lest their persecutory anxieties were to carry them into despair.

A further understanding of these persecutory anxieties occurred after sending off the first draft of this chapter. The struggle that had enabled me to arrive at my then level of understanding had been intense, draining and difficult to put into words. Having my work out of my presence while it remained incomplete aroused an intense, unrealistic anxiety about its fate. The feeling reminded me of the profound sense of possessiveness that was briefly expressed by some NIC mothers while their babies were in neonatal intensive care as well as when their babies finally arrived home, one mother saying that she would like to lock herself and her baby away alone – away even from her husband – for a week. This led me to think about how deeply terrifying it is for these mothers when it is their 'incomplete', premature babies, and not just the chapter of a book, whom they feel forced to hand over and leave in the care of others. These mothers are clearly very much afraid and alone in the terror that their babies could literally be attacked and torn to pieces while still incomplete and not in their care, while they must struggle to survive the weeks and months until their babies are safe and at home, pushing away any thoughts and emotions that threaten to overwhelm them in the meantime.

The profound sense of possessiveness in these mothers is, I think, quite understandable and occurs in response to internal, unconscious thoughts and feelings that would be terrifying for them to express, which arise as a consequence of the perception that medical staff and technology have taken their babies from them. They want their babies but have to struggle against such thoughts as 'Whose baby is this? Does it belong to the medical and hospital staff? Or is it my baby?'. At a conscious level, some mothers seemed to express such feelings concealed within quite legitimate criticisms about how they, as the babies' mothers, were not informed of even the smallest of changes in the management of their babies by neonatal intensive care staff. Such incidents clearly exacerbated the disconnectedness they felt concerning themselves as the babies' mothers.

What my own experiences showed me was that these mothers are profoundly affected and traumatised by a host of experiences connected with what they and their babies are going through while being held suspended for so long in a space similar to that within which their babies are held – a space between life and death. They are constantly warding off powerful disruptive and destructive thoughts and feelings that threaten to penetrate and/or break out through their defences. Medical staff would, at times, become the brunt of their anger and distress, particularly on occasions when they noticed a lack of sufficient care towards themselves or their babies. This anger was expressed more on tape and not usually towards the medical/health staff directly, perhaps because they feared that its expression could have disastrous consequences for their babies. Happiness was always muted and short lived because of this constant threat of loss and death hanging over themselves and their babies.

In thinking about all of my reactions while doing the ratings, I came to the realisation that I, like the NIC mothers, had erected a barrier, the purpose of which was to keep disturbing interferences outside while protecting an internal space within which I could work. To have heard about the study would have been disturbing to the rating process that lay in front of me. In forming the barrier, the effect was a type of numbing to the outside that helped to keep the irrelevant and potentially disturbing outside while I continued to focus my mind and energies on staying in touch with and rating the mothers.

Using this awareness, I wondered whether the numbing response of the NIC mothers was, in part, one aspect of a barrier that they were *actively* seeking to create, not only to ward off and dull any unthinkable and 'unprocessable' primitive anxieties and dread, but also to attempt to create and maintain the fantasy of an alive, womb-like space and umbilical cord-like connection with which to hold onto their babies in the hope that their babies would survive, all of this taking place at an unconscious level. In a sense, these mothers could be said to be in a state of primitive identi-fication with the baby within the humidicrib-like/womb-like space as a way of maintaining a sense of connectedness with which to hold onto their babies.

Once there is knowing, dread disappears, something I experienced within myself when, as a result of realising my active desire and role in creating the barrier, the weight of the dread that had been hanging over me up until that time rapidly dissipated. A mother cannot truly begin to know her baby until she knows that her baby will live and until, after that, her baby comes home. Until that time, the mother's experience of her baby is at a feeling or right-brain level. She is functioning at the level of her emotions. There can be little left-brain/thought processing while her baby's life is held in that unknown space between life and death. Once her baby is known to be safe and alive, she can allow herself to begin to know her baby and become a mother in the sense described by Winnicott (1960) when he says, 'There can be no mother without a baby'.

Having myself gone through such intense experiences, I wondered what sense could be made of the data emerging from the pilot study using the benefit of insights gained from understanding those reactions. For a start, differences in the data obtained from the two raters appeared to reflect different degrees of attunement to the emotions and/or comments made by the mothers during the rating process at different times. For example, the level of agreement between raters for the highest overall level of depression detected for each mother at each interview was greater than that seen with any other emotion. Despite this, differences were still found when it came to the detection of depression within the different assess-ment items studied.

Figure 19.1 clearly shows how NIC mothers expressed more intense levels of flatness and detachment than FT mothers. This difference was found in all areas under study: when talking about their babies, about themselves, or about the treatment of themselves and their babies by the various health professionals involved. Whereas the flatness of most FT mothers tended to lessen as time went on, that of NIC mothers tended to remain higher throughout the four months of the study. However, what the pilot study did not show was that the flatness differed in quality between the two groups. While that of FT mothers was less intense, more

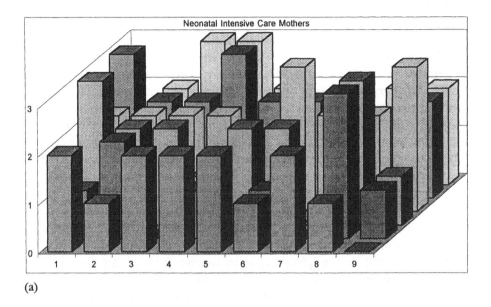

(a)

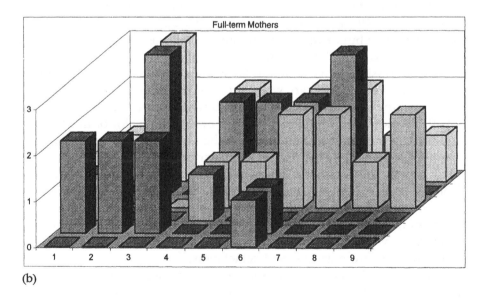

(b)

Figure 19.1: Highest level of flatness experienced by (a) neonatal intensive care and (b) full-term mothers.

short lived and linked to experiences they often went on to discuss, the flatness of NIC mothers was far more intense and pervasive, involving either a dulling or a numbing of affect or, more frequently, a switching off when they spoke that was not usually followed up by any further exploration later on. They were clearly 'absent' in mind.

Figure 19.2 indicates that the intensity of excitement in all mothers tended to increase as time went on, being more intense in FT mothers when they spoke of contact with their babies and of their capacity to mother. Although the 'excitement' of NIC mothers also tended to increase with time when talking of their capacity to mother, it was not as high as for FT mothers and was not consistent within the NIC mothers' group.

As with flatness, there was a significant difference in the meaning of 'excitement' between the two groups of mothers, which, again, the ratings did not show. For NIC mothers, 'excitement' tended to involve expressions of relief that their babies had achieved some small but nevertheless critical milestone in their physical progress, pointing to a 'hint' or a 'suggestion' that they might be able to survive. This would occur when their babies were taken off oxygen, when their babies' weight increased, or when they, as mothers, were able to provide even the slightest demonstration of maternal care. It also happened when they became aware that their babies had been moved from the more critical, more central, 'at risk' section of the NIC unit (a space that did not seem to have been explicitly labelled as such but of which the mothers would clearly have been all too aware) to a less central, less 'at-risk' section of the unit.

The expression of excitement/relief by these mothers was clearly more constrained and momentary when they spoke about their baby's health and development, whereas FT mothers were more openly happy and joyful. FT mothers were clearly buoyed up by the health of their babies and the corresponding development in their capacities as mothers as they came to know and adapt to the particular moods and requirements of their babies, despite occasions when they spoke of painful, depressed feelings. A discernible change occurred in NIC mothers when their babies arrived home and they could begin to get to know them as their true mothers rather than as merely their birth mothers, at which point their excitement would last longer. Nevertheless, their excitement/relief was never fully free from flatness and detachment.

Figure 19.3 shows FT mothers to have experienced more intense levels of depression than NIC mothers, particularly when talking of their own health and welfare. Unlike FT mothers, the depression of NIC mothers tended to lessen as time went on. NIC mothers also expressed more depression when they spoke about their lack of contact with their babies. For these mothers, it was better to minimise contact with their babies so

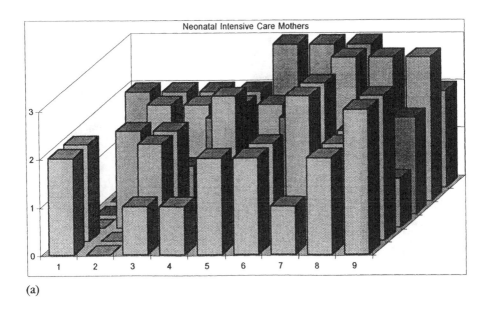

(a)

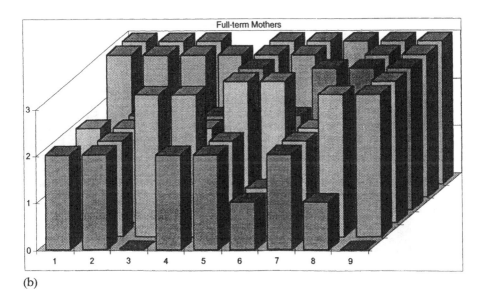

(b)

Figure 19.2: Highest level of excitement experienced by (a) neonatal intensive care and (b) full-term mothers.

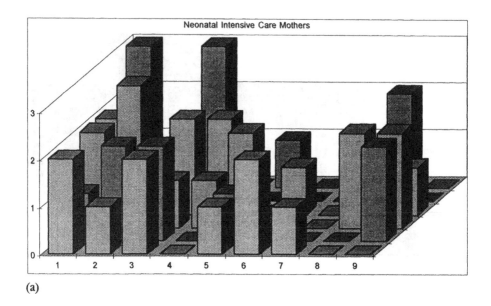

(a)

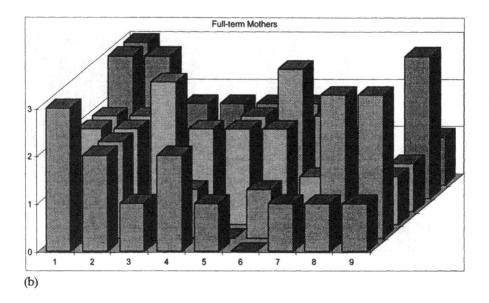

(b)

Figure 19.3: Highest level of depression experienced by (a) neonatal intensive care and (b) full-term mothers.

that feelings of separation and loss were not as unbearable, which gave these mothers the appearance of being detached and uninterested in their babies. The numbing/dissociative response – similar to my own feeling of oppression and dread when I did not want to 'visit' the tapes – was clearly serving the purpose for which it was intended, that is, protecting them at a time when they were intensely preoccupied internally and acutely vulnerable. The depression had become lost as a result of the detachment.

Figure 19.4 outlines how the intensity of anxiety/fear expressed by all mothers tended to be high, particularly in the NIC group. Their anxiety/fear tended to diminish as time progressed, albeit more gradually among NIC mothers. FT mothers expressed significantly more fear when talking of a lack of contact with their babies. As with all other emotions, anxiety/fear was found to differ in quality between the two groups. Whereas FT mothers tended to express their fears more openly, NIC mothers were far more deadened in its expression, often to the point of detachment. This was particularly the case when talking of the health and development of their babies as well as their capacity to mother. What the ratings did not pick up was the profound intensity of terror and dread that lay beyond the conscious awareness of these mothers.

Sadness and anger were the emotions least expressed and detected throughout the period of the study, the differences between the two groups of mothers being slight as well as inconsistent between the raters except in the case of medical/health personnel, where NIC mothers expressed more intense levels of anger.

What the above factors demonstrate is that certain emotions and experiences of NIC mothers could not be detected and rated, the extent of their impact being largely beyond the conscious awareness of both the mothers and myself except that they had an impact on my unconscious. There would clearly be an atmosphere of a struggle for life hanging over neonatal intensive care wards that is beyond words. After having personally experienced the cumulative effect of listening to the distress of these mothers, even though my exposure was limited to the medium of audio-taped recordings, I wondered about similar unconscious effects of NIC mothers on doctors, nurses, social workers and others who come into daily contact with them. From the experience of doing the ratings, I know that having 'a job to do' (such as keeping strictly to some form of procedure or timetable) can be a way for medical and hospital staff (as well as therapists or a rater) to protect themselves from emotions that are felt to be too much to bear and that threaten to put anxiety and despair in the place of hope.

Being aware of and acknowledging what NIC mothers and their babies (as well as oneself) are experiencing carries with it the potential to reduce

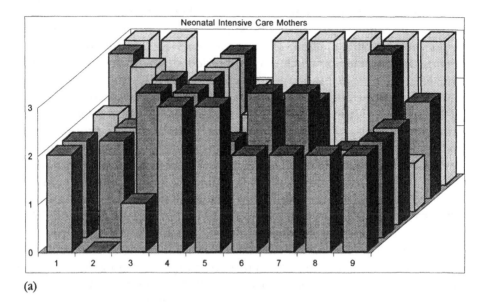

(a)

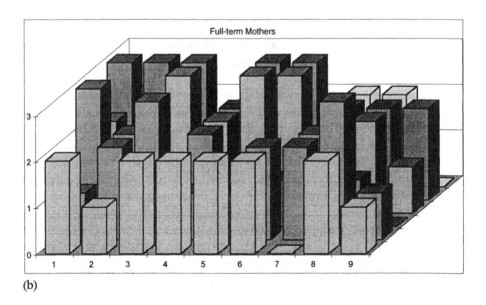

(b)

Figure 19.4: Highest level of fear experienced by (a) neonatal intensive care and (b) full-term mothers.

the level of trauma and detachment with which these mothers and their babies (and oneself) are faced. This helps to prevent mothers who want to remain in NICUs with their babies and ask questions being seen as 'getting in the way' or as 'asking too many questions', which one experienced neonatal intensive care worker once told me was an attitude among some staff. Just as the emotions of mothers can be conveyed to others, so too can even the merest hint of negative emotions and attitudes of staff be conveyed to the mothers. What is essential is that the flatness and detachment of these mothers gives way to bonding and good enough attunement as soon as possible after the baby returns to their care.

What may be helpful to those working with such mothers is a way of conceptualising the process of projective identification that takes place between the mothers and the carers that is beyond words, an understanding of which can lead to a greater depth of comprehension of what is going on in their internal worlds. In thinking about the effects of the NIC mothers on myself, I saw a metaphorical equivalent to projective identification in the Big Bang theory of the universe. Using data gained from a variety of observations and experiments of seemingly separate phenomena occurring throughout the universe, scientists were led to develop a unified theory to explain the origins of much of what was being observed. In this theory, an enormous explosion is thought to have resulted in a spreading outwards of many particles from its source, eventually leading to the formation of numerous 'gaseous' clouds, many millions of light years in diameter and containing particles, atoms and molecules. Out of these clouds, and under the influence of enormous gravitational forces, came the development of many separate galaxies containing solar systems, planets and moons.

The value of this metaphor is that, through an examination of separate phenomena, scientists were led back to an understanding of what happened at the source of those phenomena in much the same way as an examination of the thoughts and feelings that arose within me led me to a deepened understanding of what was happening at the source of the catastrophe in the internal worlds of these mothers. Both during and after listening to the audiotapes, a process similar to the formation of galaxies took place within me, in which many separate 'particles' in the form of separate, unconsidered emotions and thoughts beyond what was being consciously conveyed by these mothers came together around areas of sensitivity within myself to create disturbances of thought and emotion within my own internal world. Through examining those effects, I was eventually led back to an understanding of the traumatic emotional landscape within which these mothers found themselves in the aftermath of the premature birth of their babies.

Data from the pilot study show that NIC mothers are unable to experience the full intensity and range of emotions, including excitement, anxiety and depression while in the midst of the trauma within which they find themselves. Once expressed, any intense emotion must immediately be cut short and/or deadened. It is impossible and unrealistic for them to relax their grip on their defensive barriers until they know that their babies are safe and that they will survive. To the outside world, the mothers can appear detached to the point of disinterest, although this is done to conceal from themselves, and from others, the true depth of their disturbed inner worlds. For example, from the ratings it was found that three NIC mothers had expressed excitement when talking about a *lack* of contact with their babies. Using the understanding gained from the impact of the NIC mothers on myself, it seems that the excitement expressed by some of these mothers was actually an expression of their wish to be relieved of the burden of an intensification of pain provoked by *not* seeing their babies, noting that they had *also* expressed an intensification of depression when talking about their lack of contact with their babies.

These processes of flattening, detachment and/or dissociation are similar to those experienced by other trauma victims whose attention is preserved almost exclusively in the interests of surviving the period of the trauma as well as in shutting out physical as well as emotional pain. This being so, it is highly likely that NIC mothers would go on to experience a release of these intense levels of emotion after their babies come home were it not for the fact that the conscious experience of such thoughts and emotions would be terrifying alongside simultaneously learning to know their babies. Their extended exposure to trauma would then serve further to exacerbate the sense of disconnection that they were already experiencing at the very time when their babies were in absolute need of their attunement and care if they were to grow and develop normal, emotional, cognitive and relationship skills in later life.

These mothers do not require analytic treatment in the midst of this most difficult of situations. Verbal interpretation is not necessary and could, in fact, be highly inappropriate and destructive at such a time. What they instead need is something similar to what was received by the infants in the preschool mentioned previously and was experienced by the mothers in this study as reported to the interviewer. They need someone capable of being attentive and attuned, someone who has the potential to be in touch with and know the depth of the dread that they are experiencing beneath their flatness and detachment.

While reading the final draft of this chapter before sending it to the editor, I again read the paragraph in which I discussed the 'space between life and death', by which I had meant an emotional space within the mothers resulting from a taking inside of the outside physical space within the neonatal intensive care ward. Thinking again of the excited relief that suddenly and momentarily burst from one of the mothers when describing how her baby had been moved to a less critical part of the NICU, I pondered anew the emotions of mothers on entering such units to find babies lost beneath mechanical, life-sustaining medical apparatus in a space that is, quite literally, one between life and death, where other babies have been placed to live and grow, where some have died, and where one finds one's own baby has now been placed, the measure of how near or how far one's baby is from that undefined space being a measure of the extent to which he/she needs to be in the minds of the medical and nursing staff because of his/her more precarious hold on health and on life. Just how terrifying, but unspeakable and unthinkable, that literal space must be.

For true empathy and attunement to occur, workers must be prepared to rediscover that space again for the very first time with every new mother – whatever that space may be.

Acknowledgement

I wish to express my thanks to my fellow rater, Sheila Sim, Research Assistant Angela Todd, Dr Celia Pickworth and my wife Vicki, for their invaluable thoughts, care and support. This chapter is dedicated to Dr Alan Bull.

References

Klein M (1946) Notes on some schizoid mechanisms. In Envy and Gratitude and Other Works (1975). New York: Dell Publishing.

Klein M (1955) On identification. In Envy and Gratitude and Other Works. New York: Dell Publishing.

Bion WR (1962) Learning from Experience. London: Heinemann.

Bion WR (1967) Second Thoughts. London: Heinemann.

Joseph B (1985) Projective identification: some clinical aspects. In Feldman M, Spillius EB (Eds) Psychic Equilibrium and Psychic Change (1989). London: Routledge.

Winnicott DW (1960) The theory of the parent–infant relationship. In The Maturational Processes and the Facilitating Environment. London: Hogarth Press.

Chapter 20
The trauma of prematurity: the impact on the parents

NORMA TRACEY

This chapter aims to gather together some of the ideas explored in this book that might give us a way of thinking about the trauma that these mothers and fathers suffer. Although any full-term pregnancy and birth is fraught with psychic difficulties as parents move from the chaos to the order of new parenthood, this chaos turns to trauma through prematurity. Kierkegard (1941) wrote of the 'heartbreak at the centre of existence'. I am proposing that the trauma suffered by the parents of premature infants hurls them into the heartbreak at the very core of their own and their infant's exsistence.

We know that the growth of a woman to motherhood and a man to fatherhood adds more than just another dimension to their lives. We have known since as early as Bibring (1959), Bibring et al (1961), Pines (1972, 1978), Raphael-Leff (1982, 1991, 1993), Brazleton (1980, 1982) and, more recently, Brazleton and Cramer (1991) and Stern (1995) that a far deeper and more intrinsic change is taking place as the woman, in a psychic sense, gives birth to herself as mother and the man gives birth to himself as father. It is not only the psychic unit of 'mother–baby' that comes into being as a symbiotic entity at this time, but also the psychic unit of 'mother–father–baby'. Little (1960), Mahler et al (1975) and Tustin (1981) highlight the dangers of a premature psychic separating out from these symbiotic units. The disturbance created by the prematurity and by the infant being cared for by others seriously intrudes on the sensitive process of movement from fusion to differentiation, which needs to be in minute and tolerable doses over a long period of time.

This situation is quite different from that of the immediate rupturing caused by prematurity, which is often so massive that it can only be coped with by the mother's initially denying the emotional affect of what she has suffered. We were able as a group to discern relevant features from which we could attempt to formulate a theory and which fitted all too well the massive literature on trauma. I would like to show this pattern and then move into the actual thinking processes of the mother and father and the disruption of these through the trauma of prematurity.

In the initial interview, each parent's narration lacked affect. It was as if it had no meaning for them personally, as if the story they told was another person's rather than their own. Their particular attention to minute external detail was in marked contrast to the lack of internal meaning of the events for them. Deedie's narration is a typical first interview.

Parents did not, however, return to a normal emotional state. As they recovered from the shock and as their infant thrived, they displayed an initial overt raging or inwardly paranoid and primitive response to the surrender of this 'autistic-like' defence. While the general pattern of loss of affect was the same for each of the six mothers and six fathers in the study group, there was a marked individual difference in their expression of the experience as they 'came to life' emotionally. The basic template of each parent's personality at its most primitive level was exposed and expressed. These emotions were at their worst as the infant began to recover and was given more into the mother's care on the ward. It seemed that only then was it safe to allow the expression of the emotions the parents had not dared know before.

The central theme of all these emotions was their terror of death, sometimes for the mother, always for the baby. Interestingly, these fears seemed greater in intensity and more freely enacted and expressed as the infant was discharged from hospital. The terror of the possible loss of their baby became more powerful as the parents assumed personal responsibility. Only then did the task of mothering and fathering seem more relevant than the trauma suffered.

The preoccupation with their infants was much more intense and longer lasting. There were also marked differences in the parents' feelings and attitudes towards parenting and towards their infant at this early stage after they came home from hospital, compared with the parents of the full-term infants.

The 'shock' of an early birth

These parents have had the 'shock' of an early birth, often by caesarean section. Even when a mother and father know that their infant will be premature, the decision of 'when' and 'how' this will happen always seems to shock them. All the mothers and fathers felt cheated of a full-term pregnancy and of a birth. The caesarean birth sometimes causes a mother to feel as if she has not 'had' her baby – not only that she has been cheated of the birth, but also that there has not been a birth.

After the birth, the mother's infant is taken away from her and placed in a humidicrib with tubes, intravenous lines, strange machines and space-age-like equipment. Her infant, being cared for by others rather than by her, feels inaccessible to her. She has 'failed' as a physical carrier of an infant to full term and may feel ashamed or punished as machinery and medical staff take over. Her baby feeds not with milk suckled from her breast but with milk expressed from her breast by a machine. All this separates the mother even more from her baby and reminds her constantly of how ill her baby is. Events are out of her and her partner's control, and the vulnerable family unit can feel fractured, fearing that they have failed in their primary task of being, by their own capacity, able to protect their baby. The mother and her partner are ambivalent. Their dependence on the hospital is extraordinary, their gratitude to the staff for saving their infant balanced by their rage at having the infant removed from them.

Instead of the reward of holding their baby and feeling ownership, the parents can initially only 'sit and look'. There is a total lack of privacy. The stillness, the private culture that a mother–infant or mother–father–infant create between each other in those early days is not possible. A third party has entered the intimate circle of the mother–infant dyad – the staff, with whom a mother must negotiate to hold, bath or feed her baby. Every inter-action that a mother has with her infant is a negotiated moment that binds them together. The continuous thousands of negotiated moments that form the threads of interrelatedness between a mother and her infant are limited by her lack of contact and often by the illness of her infant. Through all of this, defining herself as a mother is a constant challenge. When she takes the infant home, there is another kind of shock: reality telling her she did have a baby.

So, what happens in the inner world of the father? A father with an infant in neonatal intensive care lives in fear of his infant's death. He has little sensory contact with his infant. His baby is in a machine instead of in the protection of his partner's womb. He has to communicate with the staff about his infant. He may also need to sustain his position in the workplace and hold and support a seriously distressed partner. Rarely is the father's role in the drama seen as anything more than an adjunct to that of his partner. The father of a premature infant has no space for his own feelings and needs, everything being focused on his wife and baby. The research presented in this book gives the father a central position and, by its interest in him, the space of a stage on which to play out the events from without and the drama from within.

We will now move in closer and analyse what happens to these parents in trauma.

Emotional events are stripped of their meaning by this trauma

Tustin (1972, 1978, 1981, 1983) developed the concept of autism, initially as a developmental stage and later as a pathological one. Tracey (1991, 1993, Tracey et al 1995, 1996) took this concept and demonstrated that, in trauma, the same lack of affect, loss of emotional meaning and deadened centre occurred for those mothers who had been traumatised by the birth of a premature, sick or dying infant. This autistic or deadened psychic space is where 'emotional meaning' and 'thinking about' the baby would be, but the experience is so painful that it is unthinkable. Thus, an otherwise normally emotionally loaded space becomes deadened and autistic-like. This is particularly serious at such an early time when, as a beginning to the bonding process, the mother's links with her infant require her to be minutely in touch and in a state of constant preoccupation.

When emotional meaning is lost, there is interference with the processes of attachment and bonding between the mother and her infant and the father and his infant, and a disruption of the close protective pattern of the three. In the first interview of each research subject, their flat affect, as if they were drained of emotion, caused us to look at these processes. It was as if their feelings were disconnected from the events and they could not give emotional meaning to the birth of their baby.

The 'I' in the narrator seemed to be absent during the trauma. How much had the rupturing of the normal birth processes also ruptured the ongoing emotional meaning of 'us' in the mother–baby and mother–father–baby unit? Had the historical continuity of 'self' been lost? In this autistic-like, non-relating centre, the external baby could not be related to, but the parents' relatedness to their internal infant also seemed to be lost. In the beginning, we saw that the infant was like a 'thing' to them, and only when they could nurse 'it' did it dawn on them that it was a baby, their baby. The mothers would often say, 'It's like I haven't had a baby' or 'It's hard to believe that little thing lying there in the midst of all that machinery has anything to do with me'. One mother said, 'Holding her for the first time in my arms, I thought, she's a baby, not just a wired up "thing" – a baby, my baby!'.

With all the parents interviewed, some of the elements of behaviour during recovery could be described as psychotic and paranoid. Utmost was a sense of terror, as if death were too close and the protection from it too precarious. It is important to know that the responses at this stage were highly individual and seemed to be an exaggeration of each person's usual way of responding and experiencing emotional processes. For example, one mother would not leave her infant for a second and even took her into the toilet with her; another raged at the staff and felt that they were trying to cut her out and keep her baby from her; a third covered all the windows with sheets for fear of germs entering the infant's room, also developing an obsession with lead in the paint and the soil around the house; another refused to let anyone look at her baby and would not take her baby girl out for weeks.

Parents are psychically wounded by this trauma. The trauma can be likened to a psychic wound caused by a violent intrusion, an excess of psychic pain flooding their inner self. They could not 'hold' it; it was too much to cope with. Freud (1916–17), speaking of trauma, said, 'We apply it to an experience which within a short period of time presents the mind with an increase of stimulus too powerful to be dealt with or worked off in the normal manner'. There is a psychic hole or space in trauma. 'Trauma' in medicine means 'wound'. In Greek, 'wound' means 'pierce'. Freud's comments in a draft (1895) seem to be a metaphor of what is happening: 'It is like a wound, an internal haemorrhage, a hole in the psychic sphere' .

Laplanche and Pontalis (1981) found three implicit ideas in psychic trauma: 'The idea of violent shock, the idea of a wound, and the idea of consequences affecting the organisation'. Pontalis (1981) adds, 'An excess of excitation hinders any binding activity at the level of primary process'. Janet's (1889) concept was that the traumatised person actually disassociates from the experience. Bion (1967) wrote of a violent explosion, accompanied by an immense psychotic fear or panic, that was expressed by a sudden total silence to get away from the devastation. Bowlby (1973) described a state of protest, which, if unmet, brings despair and psychic detachment. This detachment correlates with the autistic deadened space.

Parents' internal objects are severely affected by this trauma

The parents' sense of shock was obvious, but the effect on their inner world was less obvious. For all parents, good internal objects remain as protectors against bad and damaging internal objects. We propose that, with the shock of prematurity, the normal tension between protective and persecutory objects is halted and frozen, and there is a terror that the bad objects have triumphed or will triumph.

Matte-Blanco (1959) defined differences between the laws governing our unconscious mind and those of our conscious mind. The unconscious mind neither discriminates between the present and the past nor has a concept of time. It does not discriminate between persons, and it does not discriminate between what is fantasy and what is real. The relevance of understanding this is important because the more conscious processes of judgement and logical thinking are diminished or suspended during trauma. This leaves these parents open to all sorts of fantasies and fears. They cannot discriminate between past and present, past traumas return to haunt them, and they are unable to judge what is real and what they are imagining. The parents in this study imagined that the hospital was trying to steal their infants or that there were external forces that could take and damage their baby. One father spent two hours of his interviews speaking only of the poor security on the ward and how he feared that someone could come in and steal his baby without the staff even knowing. Perhaps he felt that his baby had already been stolen from the mother's womb, from the family unit.

The new mother and father seem to move between internal objects that love and protect, and internal objects that persecute and destroy. The capacity to 'hold' a previous good experience in the face of a present bad one is lost. Past experiences that gave positive meaning to their lives seem lost to them because of present shocking negative ones. Persecutory internal objects seem to take over from protective ones, and the murderous or destructive elements appear temporarily to triumph over the loving, life-giving ones. There is guilt from not only what has been done, but also what has been fantasised as having been done. Instead of a neutral space where good and bad and love and hate can meet, there is an overwhelming sense of bad feeling and an irrational sense of being bad, of deserving this punishment.

Most of the mothers interviewed seemed to seek proof of where they went wrong. They described feelings of depression at the loss of their internal good mother, as if they were cursed rather than blessed. They doubted whether they had the capacity to shield themselves or their infants from harm. Later, their depression changed to rage – 'Why me? I don't deserve this. It's unfair'. This rage similarly expressed itself towards those close to the parents for not shielding them from the painful experience, and towards those who had 'caused it' or were witnesses to it, these often being seen as the staff of the neonatal intensive care unit (NICU). With the loss of the psychic centre of self, the archaic splitting of good and bad internal objects returns. This presented itself in the parents' expressing anger towards different members of their family or of staff, and gratitude towards others, defining people around them as either good or bad. During the trauma, it was the 'absence' of those who should care, such as close family members, or perhaps a doctor who had not made the time to talk to them, that caused the anger and hurt. In the post-traumatic stage when feeling was returning, it was the 'intrusiveness' of close family members, perhaps by the expression of the most minute remark unwittingly made, that became the object of the parent's anger and hurt. The support of 'good' people in their family, particularly their partner, assumed great relevance, as did caring staff.

The vulnerability of this time cannot be overemphasised. The traumatised mothers and fathers interviewed all recalled past traumas, be it of a mother's death, a father's abuse in childhood, a parent's death by suicide, the loss of a sibling or a previous miscarriage. There was often what we came to term a 'litany of losses'. More than this, it sometimes seemed as if the past and the present traumas had become confused and were one and the same.

The parents' capacity to think is affected by this trauma

Bion writes that when an experience is good enough, it can be 'thought about' and that the emotional meaning in it can be stored by being symbolised and abstracted. Once stored, these satisfying experiences can be called upon in difficult times. The memory 'holds' us.

However, the timing and the amount of frustration before relief are relevant. With prematurity, the interruption of the pregnancy process through ill-health, the frustration of not being in control, the timing and the intrusion on the normal process is so disturbing that thought is lost. When an experience is so terrible that it cannot be thought about, it remains in its raw and unprocessed state with all the original dread and fear. This is not a new thought: Janet in 1887 first linked trauma with disassociation. When an event in a person's life was too bizarre, terrifying or overstimulating to fit into a pre-existing schema, Janet believed that it was split off from consciousness into a separate system of 'fixed ideas'. These would not be affected by future experiences. This disassociation, in contrast to repression, involved foreclosure rather than events being thought about and the experience stored.

In the earliest stages of thinking about experiences, good hallucinations are needed to balance bad ones. If the experience has been good enough, this will happen and create in the mind a neutral territory where the experience can be thought about (de Monchaux 1963). When the experience is more bad than good, the more powerful negative hallucinatory images attack the positive ones and fragment them, stripping them of all meaning. There is a dead, autistic-like space with no meaning where the 'alive' thoughts that are linked to positive emotion should be (Tustin 1972, 1981, 1986, Tracey 1991). This will be seen clearly in the interviews reported throughout the book. When the emotions do surface, they do so as the dreaded experience itself, raw and unprocessed. We saw in these mothers and fathers an awful dichotomy between a factual narration stripped of all 'meaning' so that they even made the baby into a 'thing', and the opposite, which was a situation so loaded with feeling that they were in a kind of negative hell of fear and paranoia.

Recent work by Van der Kolk (1987, 1996) confirms that 'disassociation always seems to be a response to traumatic events'. He says that it is not uncommon for such people to be on the verge of a psychotic breakdown.

Van der Kolk describes extreme splitting as having no continuous sense of self, having little sense of cause and affect, as if good and bad actions are not being performed by the same person, and feeling shame, blame and a degree of self-hatred. We observed that, for many of the mothers interviewed, closeness and distancing from their infant seemed to lack synchrony. One mother could not separate from her baby even to go to the bathroom yet the next day was planning to go to work two days a week. Another mother was doing everything possible to breastfeed but suddenly weaned her infant to the bottle overnight. Tustin (1986) sees rage at the root of all these responses: rage at what has been done to them, rage at what they cannot defend against.

This does not mean that the parents remain in this state. They seem to recover as their infant recovers, although we are not able to say what the lasting effects of the trauma will be in their relationship with their infant, as this book covers only the first 12 weeks of the infant's life. For the parents interviewed, one of the most important sources of recovery, apart from their infant's health, was their own health, followed by how much trauma they had suffered in their past life. The single most important factor in their recovery was the amount of support they received during the crisis.

Through the occurrence of the 'unexpected', there is a shattering of the parents' expectations for their infant and a loss of belief that things could go right for them. Affleck et al (1991) found that 70 per cent of the mothers of premature infants who participated in their study had no warning of a premature or hazardous delivery. The pregnancies had proceeded uneventfully, but the mothers' expectations were abruptly shattered by a premature birth. Janoff-Bulman (1989) wrote:

> The psychological disequilibrium and emotional upheaval experienced is largely a reflection of this intense, serious challenge to their basic assumptions ... All of a sudden they are confronted with a world that is malevolent and meaningless, and a view of themselves as having been singled out for misfortune.

Janoff-Bulman and Frieze (1983) and Thompson and Janigian (1988) wrote of the tendency to see ourselves as having control over events; to view ourselves as relatively invulnerable; to regard the things that happen to us as being orderly, predictable and meaningful; and to see ourselves as worthy and others as benevolent or at least benign. The centrality of these assumptions in our lives is revealed most starkly when we face a personal catastrophe that challenges this validity. Half of the mothers who participated in Affleck et al's study said that when they were pregnant, they had imagined no possibility of their baby needing hospitalisation in a neonatal intensive care ward. In addition to the shattering of expectations of invulnerability and control, the crisis of neonatal intensive care caused some parents to question the meaning of life and the fairness of these events.

Tennen et al (1986) report a relatively high incidence of self-blame in the parents of these infants. This has also been reported in studies of parents of acutely ill or handicapped newborn babies by Affleck et al (1982, 1985) and by Affleck et al (1985). The purpose of their studies was to examine the relationship between the severity of victimisation and self-blame, and perceived control over recurrence and adaptation. In the studies, mothers whose infants who had been treated in NICU attributed a significant proportion of their child's serious medical condition at least in part to their own behaviour. For those involved in a tragic event, there is a need to believe that the event could have been averted and thus could not happen to them again. They desperately seek a cause over which they have control. If they caused it, they can also cause it not to happen. Other people also blame the victims of uncontrollable events for the same reason. This often means that the mother is isolated, judged harshly or avoided at the very time when she needs most support.

Internal holding and the capacity to project is damaged by the trauma of prematurity. The concept of internal holding is linked to projective identification, an early mechanism of ego defence, which Klein wrote about in 1946. Unable to hold an image of good and bad in the one person, the infant splits and projects so that 'good' may go to one person and 'bad' to another. This defends his ego from intolerable anxiety by splitting off and projecting unbearable feelings and impulses, either good or bad, onto his mother. His mother 'holds' these, thus relieving him of unbearable feelings that he cannot deal with himself. At a later stage, he could experience them both as belonging to the same person and in so doing could also experience his ambivalence of both loving and hating his mother. Winnicott and Klein both called this the depressive position, Winnicott going on to define the capacity to feel both love and hate as the beginning of guilt and reparation.

Bion (1967) defined it as an ongoing process, a never-ending dynamic moving from integration to disintegration, from chaos to order throughout life. He further defined projective identification not as a defence but more as a mode of communication by which the infant lets his mother know what he is feeling. She becomes the container of his emotions, tolerating and understanding them. She 'processes' them for the infant, giving them back in a form that is tolerable and can therefore be 'used' by the baby. This containing, sometimes called attunement or empathy, is the most fundamental emotional intercourse between two people. In normal processes, it brings opposites together in a neutralised way that is tolerable rather than fused or split. In that neutral area, thinking can take place.

What happens as a result of trauma is that this ongoing process is frozen. For the traumatised mother of the premature infant, there is a breakdown in this container. She may well experience the good internal mother as turning into a destructive one and robbing her of her infant or wanting to kill it (Bion 1962). When there is no attunement or empathy and no container, this 'results in the introjection of an object that is hostile to understanding' (Harris and Bick 1987). This is then experienced as a nameless dread. For many of the parents of premature infants, the trauma they suffer causes their internal container to break down. This is the centre of our thinking. When 'holding' is lost, there is disintegration, a split and a loss of affect on one side, and an overflow of affect that is primitive and uncontained on the other – the neutral thinking space is lost. Projective identification does not work, the psychic pain becomes unbearable, and there is fear of fragmentation and death. There is unthinkable fear, so there is no thinking.

Memory and storage of memories are distorted by trauma. To be stored, an experience needs to be thought about and thus processed. Because the traumatised person cannot hold the pain of the experience, he/she cannot think about it. If it cannot be processed, it remains repressed and is stored in its original raw state. The experience has no links with other experiences: it is cut off and emotionally denied. This means that it does not have a place in the person's 'self' or in their internal history. The internal narrator of that history is absent from the trauma.

Many of the parents' narrations in this book seem to fit this model, with a 'cut-off' quality in the initial narrating, as if telling someone else's story. When events begin to settle and the infant is on the road to recovery, what is remembered is not a 'memory of' but an abreaction of the emotions linked with the event. This makes sense of the depth and power of the primitive emotions expressed in the interviews when the initial numbness has gone and the infant is beginning to recover. Tustin (1986) says:

> The bereft person is frozen with shock, is numb and dumb. I have come to see that this state has been preceded by flaming and blinding rage about this disappointment. This has been unbearable because it has not been sufficiently received and understood. Thus it seems to implode back.

Bion (1967) says that the traumatised person experiences 'pain but not the suffering. They are in the pain, overwhelmed by it, the pain is not in them'.

For each subject in this research, we were aware of such traumatisation. The aloneness experienced by these parents is overwhelming. Far from celebrating, these parents, no matter how many supports they have, are in mourning for the full-term birth, the healthy baby and indeed their own parenting. They are, in a terrible sense, alone, and even the sharing with the other mothers on the ward is tainted by whose baby is doing well and whose is not, who will retain motherhood and who will lose it. Every minute of improvement gives rise to an 'emotional high', and any hint of reversal throws the parents into despair.

Tuned into a possible threat of impending disaster, they live in an agonised state of hypervigilance or cut out completely. There is a terrible problem of ambivalence: the parents need the staff but resent their power over and knowledge of the baby. The normal dependence–independence process of the new mother is severely distorted as a result of this. One of the mothers 'disappeared' for two weeks, refusing to face taking her infant home. She later explained this, saying that the responsibility for such a small infant was awesome. For the professional, knowing the depth and strength of the wound shows all too clearly how important it is to give the mother full support as the trauma is taking place. When the womb of the mother can no longer safely contain her baby, something similar occurs for her psychically. When internal holding is lost, external holding must be there for the trauma to be alleviated. Holding for the parents and the staff who care for them is vital.

References

Affleck G, Allen D, McGrade BJ, McQueeney M (1982) Maternal caretaking perceptions and reported mood disturbance at hospital discharge of a high risk infant and nine months later. Mental Retardation 20: 220–5.

Affleck G, McGrade B, Allen D, McQueeney M (1985) Mothers' beliefs about behavioural causes of their developmentally disabled infant's condition: what do they signify? Journal of Pediatric Psychology 10: 293–303.

Affleck G, Roll J, Tennen H (1991) Infants in Crisis. New York: Springer-Verlag.

Bibring GL (1959) Some considerations of the psychological processes in pregnancy. The Psychoanalytical Study of the Child, Volume 14. New York: International Universities Press.

Bibring GL, Dwyer TF, Huntington DS, Valenstein AF (1961) A study of the psychological processes in pregnancy and of the earliest mother–child relationship. I: Some propositions and comments. II: Methodological considerations. In Eissler RS, Freud A, Hartmasnn H et al (Eds) The Psychoanalytic Study of the Child, Volume 16. New York: International Universities Press.

Bion WR (1962) Learning from Experience. London: Heinemann.

Bion WR (1963) Elements of Psychoanalysis. London: Heinemann.

Bion WR (1965) Transformations. London: Heinemann.

Bion WR(1967) Second Thoughts. London: Heinemann.

Bion WR (1970) Attention and Interpretation. London: Tavistock Publications.

Bowlby J (1969) Attachment and Loss, Volume 1. New York: Basic Books.

Bowlby J (1973) Attachment and Loss, Volume 2. Separation, Anxiety and Anger. London: Hogarth Press.

Brazleton TB (1980) New Knowledge About the Infant from Current Research: Implications for Psychoanalysis. Paper presented at the American Psychoanalytic Association Meeting, California.

Brazelton TB (1982) Joint Regulation of Neonate Parent Behaviour. Social Interchange in Infancy. Baltimore: Medical University Park Press.

Brazleton TB, Cramer BG (1991) The Earliest Relationship. London: Karnac Books.

Freud S (1895) Extracts from the Fliess papers. Draft a. The Aetiology of Neurosis. SE 1: The Standard Edition of the Complete Psychological Works of Sigmund Freud. London: Hogarth Press/Institute of Psychoanalysis.

Freud S (1909) Some General Remarks on Hysterical Attacks, C.P., 11, 100. SE IX: The Standard Edition of the Complete Psychological Works of Sigmund Freud. London: Hogarth Press/Institute of Psychoanalysis.

Freud S (1916–17) Introductory Lectures on Psychoanalysis. Vienna GS.,7. GW.,XI. London 1929. Revised edition New York 1966:S.E. XV–XVI.

Harris M, Bick E (1987) Collected Papers of Martha Harris and Esther Bick. Section II: Papers on Child Development and the Family 2. Perthshire: Clunie Press for The Roland Harris Trust.

Janet P (1889) L'automatisme psychologique. Translated by Hull RFC (1960)as On the Nature of the Psyche. London: Routledge & Kegan Paul.

Janoff-Bulman R (1989) The benefits of illusions, the threat of disillusionment and the limitations of inaccuracy. Journal of Social and Clinical Psychology 8: 158–75.

Janoff-Bulman R, Frieze I (1983) A theoretical perspective for understanding reactions to victimization. Journal of Social Issues 39: 1–17.

Kierkergaard, S. (1941) Fear, Trembling and Sickness Unto Death (translation Walter Lowrie). Princeton NJ: Princeton University Press.

Klein M (1946) Notes on Some Schizoid Mechanisms. Envy and Gratitude and Other Works. London: Hogarth Press/Institute of Psychoanalysis. (Original publication 1938.)

Laplanche J, Pontalis JB (1973) The Language of Psychoanalysis. London: Karnac Books/Institute of Psychoanalysis.

Little M (1960) On basic unity. International Journal of Psychoanalysis 41: 377–84.

Mahler MS, Pine F, Bergman A (1975) The Psychological Birth of the Human Infant. London: Hutchinson.

Matte-Blanco (1959) Expression in symbolic logic of the characteristics of the system unconscious. International Journal of Psychoanalysis 40: 1–5.

Monchaux C de (1963) Realisation. The psychoanalytic study of thinking. III: Thinking and negative hallucination. International Journal of Psychoanalysis: 311–14.

Pines D (1972) Pregnancy and motherhood. Interaction between fantasy and reality. British Journal of Medical Psychology 45: 333–43.

Pines D (1978) On becoming a parent. Journal of Child Psychotherapy 4(4): 257–73.

Pines D (1982) The relevance of early psychic development to pregnancy and abortion. International Journal of Psychoanalysis 63: 311–18.

Pontalis JB (1981) Frontiers in Psychoanalysis: Between the Dream and Psychic Pain (translated by Cullen C, Cullen P). London: Hogarth Press/Institute of Psychoanalysis.

Raphael-Leff J (1982) Psychotherapeutic needs of mothers to be. Journal of Child Psychotherapy 8: 3–13.

Raphael-Leff J (1991) Psychological Processes of Childbearing. London: Chapman & Hall.

Raphael-Leff J (1993) Pregnancy. The Inside Story. London: Sheldon Press.

Stern DN (1977) The First Relationship: Infant and Mother. Cambridge, MA: Harvard University Press.

Stern DN (1995) The Motherhood Constellation: A Unified View of Parent–Infant Psychotherapy. New York: Basic Books.

Tennen H, Affleck G, Gershman K (1986) Self blame among parents with infants with perinatal complications the role of self protected motives. Journal of Personality and Social Psychology 50: 690–6.

Thompson S, Janigian A (1988) Life schemes: a framework for understanding the search for meaning. Journal of Social and Clinical Psychology 7: 260–80.

Tracey N (1991) The psychic space in trauma. Journal of Child Psychotherapy 17(2): 29–45.

Tracey N (1993) Mothers and Fathers Speak. Sydney: Apollo Books.

Tracey N, Blake P, Warren B, Hardy H, Enfield S, Schein P (1995) A mother's narrative of a premature birth. Journal of Child Psychotherapy 21(1): 43–64.

Tracey N, Blake P, Warren B, Hardy H, Enfield S, Schein P (1996) Will I be to my son as my father was to me? Journal of Child Psychotherapy 22(21): 168–95.

Tustin F (1972) Autism and Childhood Psychosis. London: Hogarth Press.

Tustin F. (1978) Psychotic elements in the neurotic disorders of childhood. Journal of Child Psychotherapy 4:5–18.

Tustin F (1981) Autistic states in children. Journal of Child Psychotherapy 7: 193.

Tustin F (1983) Psychological birth and psychological catastrophe. In Grotstein J (Ed.) Do I Dare Disturb the Universe? London: Marsefield Reprints. (First published in 1981 by Caesura Press.)

Tustin F (1986) Autistic Barriers in Neurotic Patients. London: Karnac Books.

Tustin F (1995) Autism and Childhood Psychosis. London: Karnac Books.

Van der Kolk B (1987) Psychological Trauma. Washington, DC: American Psychiatric Press.

Van der Kolk B, with McFarlane AC (Eds)(1996) Traumatic Stress: Human Adaptations to Overwhelming Experience. New York: Guilford Press.

Concluding remarks

NORMA TRACEY, BRYANNE BARNETT, BEULAH WARREN,
LORRAINE ROSE AND SHEILA SIM

Trauma is associated with any birth. From the intensity of the narratives in this book, it is clear that prematurity creates greater trauma for mother, father and baby. The reality of the question of the infant's, and sometimes the mother's, survival is terrifyingly present day after day. For the parents, the core of the trauma is 'terror of death'.

Evident in every chapter is the parents' need for someone to be available to absorb the shock and hold the emotional overload. Staff on the ward may offer this support, or they may enlist a close family member to undertake this task. In some cases, the community itself needs to be mobilised to fulfil this role. We want to emphasise here that, without this support, the trauma remains unresolved – with serious consequences for the mother, father and infant.

In the case of prematurity, there has been a rupture of the continuity from pregnancy to birth. Staff need to facilitate the reunion between the mother and baby as soon as possible after birth. All the parents in the research suffered deprivation because of a lack of contact, both emotional and physical, with their infant. The constant refrain was, 'It is as if I haven't had a baby. I don't know what it means to be a mother'. We do not see the staff role as being merely the provision of medical and technological care: the establishment of a partnership between staff and parents around the care of their baby is critical. This means that the ward has to create an atmosphere in which the family feel welcome and comfortable.

The staff are deeply affected by the vulnerability and hypersensitivity of both parents and babies. The latter chapters show how critical support for the staff is. Their well-being and the professional support they receive are an intrinsic part of the resolution of the trauma for the family.

Index

Printed and bound by CPI Group (UK) Ltd, Croydon, CR0 4YY

Printed and bound by CPI Group (UK) Ltd, Croydon, CR0 4YY

27/10/2024

14580141-0004